Respiratory Disorders
SOURCEBOOK

Second Edition

Health Reference Series

Second Edition

Respiratory Disorders SOURCEBOOK

Basic Consumer Health Information about Infectious, Inflammatory, and Chronic Conditions Affecting the Lungs and Respiratory System, Including Pneumonia, Bronchitis, Influenza, Tuberculosis, Sarcoidosis, Asthma, Cystic Fibrosis, Chronic Obstructive Pulmonary Disease, Lung Abscesses, Pulmonary Embolism, Occupational Lung Diseases, and Other Bacterial, Viral, and Fungal Infections

Along with Facts about the Structure and Function of the Lungs and Airways, Methods of Diagnosing Respiratory Disorders, and Treatment and Rehabilitation Options, a Glossary of Related Terms, and a Directory of Resources for Additional Help and Information

Edited by
Sandra J. Judd

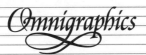

P.O. Box 31-1640, Detroit, MI 48231

Bibliographic Note

Because this page cannot legibly accommodate all the copyright notices, the Bibliographic Note portion of the Preface constitutes an extension of the copyright notice.

Edited by Sandra J. Judd

Health Reference Series

Karen Bellenir, *Managing Editor*
David A. Cooke, M.D., *Medical Consultant*
Elizabeth Collins, *Research and Permissions Coordinator*
Cherry Stockdale, *Permissions Assistant*
EdIndex, Services for Publishers, *Indexers*

* * *

Omnigraphics, Inc.

Matthew P. Barbour, *Senior Vice President*
Kevin M. Hayes, *Operations Manager*

* * *

Peter E. Ruffner, *Publisher*

Copyright © 2008 Omnigraphics, Inc.

ISBN 978-0-7808-1007-5

Library of Congress Cataloging-in-Publication Data

Respiratory disorders sourcebook : basic consumer health information about infectious, inflammatory, and chronic conditions affecting the lungs and respiratory system, including pneumonia, bronchitis, influenza, tuberculosis, sarcoidosis, asthma, cystic fibrosis, chronic obstructive pulmonary disease, lung abscesses, pulmonary embolism, occupational lung diseases, and other bacterial, viral, and fungal infections; along with facts about the structure and function of the lungs and airways, methods of diagnosing respiratory disorders, and treatment and rehabilitation options, a glossary of related terms, and a directory of resources for additional help and information / edited by Sandra J. Judd. -- 2nd ed.
   p. cm. -- (Health reference series)
  Includes bibliographical references and index.
  Summary: "Provides basic consumer health information about symptoms, diagnosis, and treatment of diseases and disorders of the respiratory system. Includes index, glossary of related terms, and other resources"--Provided by publisher.
  ISBN 978-0-7808-1007-5 (hardcover : alk. paper) 1. Respiratory organs--Diseases. I. Judd, Sandra J.
  RC731.R468 2008
  616.2--dc22
                                                    2008028424

Table of Contents

Visit www.healthreferenceseries.com to view *A Contents Guide to the Health Reference Series*, a listing of more than 14,000 topics and the volumes in which they are covered.

Part II: Symptoms, Diagnosis, and Treatment of Respiratory Disorders

Part III: Infectious and Inflammatory Diseases of the Respiratory System

Part IV: Other Medical Conditions Affecting the Lungs

ix

Part V: Additional Help and Information

Preface

About This Book

Breathing is an activity many people take for granted. An average person takes almost 25,000 breaths a day and processes more than 10,000 liters of air. When the respiratory system functions properly, this work is done automatically. When things go awry, however, a wide range of conditions can develop that lead to outcomes varying in severity from transient to chronic and from mild to fatal. Furthermore, respiratory disorders are widespread, affecting people at all stages of life. Consider, for example, the following U.S. statistics:

- More than 3.6 million children and 22 million adults suffer from chronic respiratory diseases.

- Asthma leads to 14 million missed school days, 2 million emergency room visits, and 5,000 deaths per year.

- Lung cancer is the leading cause of cancer-related deaths for both men and women. According to the American Lung Association, more than 200,000 new cases of lung cancer are expected to occur in 2008.

- Approximately 30,000 Americans have cystic fibrosis, and an additional thousand cases are diagnosed annually.

- Chronic obstructive pulmonary disease is the nation's fourth-leading cause of death, and its numbers are on the rise.

- Occupational lung disease is the number one cause of work-related illness.

Respiratory Disorders Sourcebook, Second Edition provides up-to-date information about infectious, inflammatory, occupational, and other types of respiratory disorders, including influenza, tuberculosis, pneumonia, asthma, chronic obstructive pulmonary disease, cystic fibrosis, and lung cancer. It describes common symptoms, diagnostic techniques, and the most current pharmacological and surgical treatment options. The book also explains known causes of lung disease, including genetic, environmental, and lifestyle factors, and it discusses lung disorders that may be caused by bioterrorism or chemical agents. Tips for managing chronic respiratory diseases and suggestions for ways to promote lung health are presented, and the book concludes with a glossary of related terms and a list of additional resources.

How to Use This Book

This book is divided into parts and chapters. Parts focus on broad areas of interest. Chapters are devoted to single topics within a part.

Part I: Introduction to Respiratory Disorders provides basic information about how the lungs work and how they are affected by aging. It describes common lung irritants, such as air pollution and cigarette smoke, and explains how to minimize their effects. Tips for preserving lung health, including suggestions on how to quit smoking, are also included.

Part II: Symptoms, Diagnosis, and Treatment of Respiratory Disorders describes the most common symptoms of lung diseases, including coughing, breathing difficulties, and skin discoloration. Diagnostic tests and procedures, commonly prescribed medications, and the use of inhalers, nebulizers, and home oxygen therapy are explained. Pulmonary rehabilitation, airway clearance techniques, and surgical treatment options are also discussed.

Part III: Infectious and Inflammatory Diseases of the Respiratory System provides a description of the most common bacterial, viral, and fungal infections, including the common cold, influenza, and tuberculosis, as well as emerging infectious diseases, such as avian flu and severe acute respiratory syndrome. Common symptoms, diagnostic techniques, and treatment options are also detailed for other chronic and inflammatory lung diseases, such as asthma, cystic fibrosis, chronic obstructive pulmonary disease, bronchitis, and pneumonia. In addition, facts about respiratory diseases associated with specific occupations are provided.

Part IV: Other Medical Conditions Affecting the Lungs describes physical ailments that impact respiratory function. These include lung cancer, acute respiratory distress syndrome, pulmonary hypertension, sleep apnea, and traumatic injuries. Concerns related to breathing disorders in infants and young children are addressed, and the part concludes with a discussion about respiratory disorders that may be caused by bioterrorism or chemical agents.

Part V: Additional Resources for Help and Information includes a glossary of terms related to respiratory disorders and their treatment and a directory of organizations able to provide additional help and support.

Bibliographic Note

This volume contains documents and excerpts from publications issued by the following U.S. government agencies: Agency for Toxic Substances and Disease Registry; Centers for Disease Control and Prevention (CDC); Consumer Product Safety Commission (CPSC); Environmental Protection Agency (EPA); NIH Warren Grant Magnuson Clinical Center; Mine Safety and Health Administration; National Cancer Institute (NCI); National Heart, Lung, and Blood Institute (NHLBI); National Human Genome Research Institute (NHGRI); National Institute for Occupational Safety and Health (NIOSH); National Institute of Allergy and Infectious Diseases (NIAID); National Institute of Diabetes and Digestive and Kidney Diseases (NIDDK); National Women's Health Information Center (NWHIC); Occupational Safety and Health Administration (OSHA); and the Office of the Surgeon General.

In addition, this volume contains copyrighted documents from the following organizations and individuals: A.D.A.M., Inc.; American Academy of Otolaryngology–Head and Neck Surgery; American Association for Respiratory Care; American College of Chest Physicians; American Lung Association; American Lung Association of San Diego and Imperial Counties; American Medical Association; American Thoracic Society; Ascend Media; Asthma and Allergy Foundation of America; British Lung Foundation; California Department of Public Health; Canadian Centre for Occupational Health and Safety; Cedars-Sinai Medical Center; Children's Hospital of Philadelphia; Cincinnati Children's Hospital Medical Center; CNY Thoracic Surgery; David Cooke, M.D.; Cystic Fibrosis Foundation; Todd Demmy, M.D.; Immunization Action Coalition;

Infectious Disease Epidemiology, Prevention and Control Division, Minnesota Department of Health; MyDR.com.au; National Jewish Medical and Research Center; Nemours Foundation; New Zealand Dermatological Society; NSW Health (New South Wales, Australia); PCD Foundation; St. Jude Medical; Texas Department of State Health Services; University of Southern California, Department of Cardiothoracic Surgery; University of Maryland, Greenbaum Cancer Center; Virginia Department of Health; Virtual Medical Centre; and the Wisconsin Department of Health and Family Services.

Full citation information is provided on the first page of each chapter. Every effort has been made to secure all necessary rights to reprint the copyrighted material. If any omissions have been made, please contact Omnigraphics to make corrections for future editions.

Acknowledgements

Thanks go to the many organizations, agencies, and individuals who have contributed materials for this *Sourcebook* and to medical consultant Dr. David Cooke and document engineer Bruce Bellenir. Special thanks go to managing editor Karen Bellenir and permissions coordinator Liz Collins for their help and support.

About the Health Reference Series

The *Health Reference Series* is designed to provide basic medical information for patients, families, caregivers, and the general public. Each volume takes a particular topic and provides comprehensive coverage. This is especially important for people who may be dealing with a newly diagnosed disease or a chronic disorder in themselves or in a family member. People looking for preventive guidance, information about disease warning signs, medical statistics, and risk factors for health problems will also find answers to their questions in the *Health Reference Series*. The *Series*, however, is not intended to serve as a tool for diagnosing illness, in prescribing treatments, or as a substitute for the physician/patient relationship. All people concerned about medical symptoms or the possibility of disease are encouraged to seek professional care from an appropriate healthcare provider.

A Note about Spelling and Style

Health Reference Series editors use *Stedman's Medical Dictionary* as an authority for questions related to the spelling of medical terms and the *Chicago Manual of Style* for questions related to grammatical structures, punctuation, and other editorial concerns. Consistent adherence is not always possible, however, because the individual volumes within the *Series* include many documents from a wide variety of different producers and copyright holders, and the editor's primary goal is to present material from each source as accurately as is possible following the terms specified by each document's producer. This sometimes means that information in different chapters or sections may follow other guidelines and alternate spelling authorities. For example, occasionally a copyright holder may require that eponymous terms be shown in possessive forms (Crohn's disease *vs.* Crohn disease) or that British spelling norms be retained (leukaemia *vs.* leukemia).

Locating Information within the Health Reference Series

The *Health Reference Series* contains a wealth of information about a wide variety of medical topics. Ensuring easy access to all the fact sheets, research reports, in-depth discussions, and other material contained within the individual books of the series remains one of our highest priorities. As the *Series* continues to grow in size and scope, however, locating the precise information needed by a reader may become more challenging.

A Contents Guide to the Health Reference Series was developed to direct readers to the specific volumes that address their concerns. It presents an extensive list of diseases, treatments, and other topics of general interest compiled from the Tables of Contents and major index headings. To access *A Contents Guide to the Health Reference Series*, visit www.healthreferenceseries.com.

Medical Consultant

Medical consultation services are provided to the *Health Reference Series* editors by David A. Cooke, M.D. Dr. Cooke is a graduate of Brandeis University, and he received his M.D. degree from the University of Michigan. He completed residency training at the University of Wisconsin Hospital and Clinics. He is board-certified in Internal Medicine. Dr. Cooke currently works as part of the University of Michigan Health System and practices in Ann Arbor, MI. In his free time, he enjoys writing, science fiction, and spending time with his family.

Our Advisory Board

We would like to thank the following board members for providing guidance to the development of this series:

Dr. Lynda Baker,
Associate Professor of Library and Information Science,
Wayne State University, Detroit, MI

Nancy Bulgarelli,
William Beaumont Hospital Library, Royal Oak, MI

Karen Imarisio,
Bloomfield Township Public Library, Bloomfield Township, MI

Karen Morgan,
Mardigian Library, University of Michigan-Dearborn,
Dearborn, MI

Rosemary Orlando,
St. Clair Shores Public Library, St. Clair Shores, MI

Health Reference Series *Update Policy*

The inaugural book in the *Health Reference Series* was the first edition of *Cancer Sourcebook* published in 1989. Since then, the *Series* has been enthusiastically received by librarians and in the medical community. In order to maintain the standard of providing high-quality health information for the layperson the editorial staff at Omnigraphics felt it was necessary to implement a policy of updating volumes when warranted.

Medical researchers have been making tremendous strides, and it is the purpose of the *Health Reference Series* to stay current with the most recent advances. Each decision to update a volume is made on an individual basis. Some of the considerations include how much new information is available and the feedback we receive from people who use the books. If there is a topic you would like to see added to the update list, or an area of medical concern you feel has not been adequately addressed, please write to:

Editor
Health Reference Series
Omnigraphics, Inc.
P.O. Box 31-1640
Detroit, MI 48231
E-mail: editorial@omnigraphics.com

Part One

Introduction to Respiratory Disorders

Chapter 1

How the Respiratory System Works

The Respiratory System

Our lungs are the main organs of the respiratory system. The lungs are located inside the upper part of our chest on either side of the heart, and they are protected by the ribcage. The breastbone (sternum) is at the center front of the chest, and the spine is at the center of the back of the chest.

The inside of the chest cavity and the outside of the lungs are covered by the pleura, a slippery membrane that allows the lungs to move smoothly as they fill up with and empty out air when we inhale and exhale. Normally, there is a small amount of lubricating fluid between the two layers of the pleura. This helps the lungs glide inside the chest as they change size and shape during breathing.

With each breath, our lungs are filled with air that comes into our body through the nose or mouth. It flows down the throat (pharynx) and through the voice box (larynx). A small flap of tissue (epiglottis) covers the entrance to the larynx, and it automatically closes when we swallow to prevent food or liquids from getting into our airways.

Our largest airway is the windpipe (trachea), which is between three-and-a-half and six inches long and a little over half an inch in

Reprinted from "The Respiratory System," "How We Breathe," "How the Lungs Protect Themselves," "The Respiratory System," and "The Gas Exchange," all © Cedars-Sinai Medical Center. All rights reserved. Reprinted with permission. The text of these documents is available online at http://www.csmc.edu; accessed September 24, 2007.

diameter. It brings air to the chest, where it branches into two smaller airways: the left and right bronchi, which lead to the left and right lungs.

The bronchi themselves divide many times into smaller and smaller airways (bronchioles). Because the pattern of these increasingly smaller passages looks like an upside-down tree, this part of the system is sometimes called the bronchial tree. The airways are held open by flexible, fibrous connective tissue called cartilage. Circular airway muscles can make the airways wider or narrower. The smallest bronchiole is only half a millimeter across.

At the end of each bronchiole are clusters of air sacs called alveoli. Each air sac is surrounded by a dense network of tiny blood vessels (capillaries). The extremely thin barrier between the air and the blood allows the blood to pick up oxygen and release carbon dioxide into the alveoli.

How We Breathe

The body's ability to breathe involves the nose, mouth, chest muscles, and diaphragm. Breathing is usually automatic and controlled by the respiratory center at the base of the brain. We breathe during sleep and usually even during unconsciousness. Small sensors in the brain and aorta and carotid arteries monitor the blood. If there is too little oxygen in the blood these sensors trigger faster or deeper breathing. (In quiet breathing, the average adult inhales and exhales about fifteen times a minute.)

The work of breathing is done by the diaphragm and the muscles between the ribs, in the neck, and in the abdomen. The diaphragm, a bell-shaped sheet of muscle that separates the lungs from the abdomen, is the most important muscle used for breathing. The diaphragm is attached to the base of the breastbone, the lower parts of the ribcage, and the spine.

Inhaling

A breath starts when the ribs and the chest wall expand and the diaphragm tightens and flattens, which causes the lungs to fill with air. All the muscles used in breathing contract only if the nerves connecting them to the brain are healthy. In some neck and back injuries, the spinal cord can be severed, in which case, a person will die unless he or she has a machine to help with breathing.

As the air enters our mouth and nose, the mucus membranes lining the mouth and nose make the air moist and warm, and they trap

4

any particles. The air then passes down the throat into the trachea (or windpipe), the bronchi, the bronchioles, and then the alveoli.

When the air rushes into the lungs, it fills the alveoli like balloons. Each alveolus is surrounded by tiny blood vessels. The oxygen that moves across the walls of the air sacs is picked up by the blood and carried to the rest of the body. The carbon dioxide and waste gases that the blood carried to the lungs pass into the air sacs and are exhaled.

Exhaling

Once the blood has picked up fresh oxygen and released carbon dioxide into the alveoli, the diaphragm and chest muscles relax. This relaxation pushes the air out of the alveoli, through the bronchioles and the bronchi, up through the windpipe, and out through the nose or mouth.

When we are at rest, the process of breathing out requires no effort from the respiratory muscles. During vigorous exercise, however, many muscles assist in exhalation. The abdominal muscles are the most important of these. Abdominal muscles contract, raise abdominal pressure, and push a relaxed diaphragm against the lungs, causing air to be expelled.

How the Lungs Protect Themselves

Because the lungs are continuously pulling in air (as well as germs, particles, and dirt), a system to protect the lungs is needed.

The mucus membranes that line the nose, mouth, throat, and airways of the lungs are the first line of defense. The mucus traps dirt and foreign matter that we may breathe in. Tiny hairs (cilia) beat back and forth more than one thousand times a minute in the airways to move the mucus and dirt up to where it can be coughed out of the body or swallowed.

Because of the requirements of gas exchange, alveoli are not protected by mucus and cilia. Mucus is too thick and would impair movement of oxygen and carbon dioxide.

Macrophages (special cells in the airways that consume toxins) are the next line of defense. Mobile cells on the alveolar surface (called phagocytes) seek out deposited particles, bind to them, ingest them, kill any that are living, and digest them. Phagocytes in the lungs are called alveolar macrophages.

When the lung is exposed to serious threats, white blood cells in the circulation can help. For example, when the person inhales a great

5

deal of dust or is fighting a respiratory infection, more macrophages are produced and white blood cells are recruited.

The Gas Exchange

The purpose of breathing is to provide a way for the body to receive fresh oxygen in exchange for the carbon dioxide and other waste gases that the cells of the body have produced. During this exchange of gases, between six and ten liters of fresh air per minute is brought into the lungs.

Inhaled air fills the alveoli, which are only one cell thick and are surrounded by capillaries that are also one cell thick. Oxygen passes through the air-blood barrier quickly and into the blood in the capillaries. About 0.3 of a liter of oxygen are transferred from the alveoli to the blood each minute. In much the same way, the carbon dioxide passes from the blood into the alveoli and is then exhaled. About 0.3 of a liter of carbon dioxide flows across the walls of the capillaries and the alveoli to be exhaled each minute.

Blood loaded with fresh oxygen flows out of the lungs through the pulmonary veins and into the left side of the heart, which pumps the blood to the rest of the body. Oxygen-depleted, carbon dioxide–rich blood returns to the right side of the heart through two large veins, the superior vena cava and the inferior vena cava. Then the blood is pumped through the pulmonary artery to the lungs, where it picks up oxygen and releases carbon dioxide.

During exercise, we can breathe in as much as one hundred liters of air per minute. The rate at which oxygen enters the body is one way to measure how much energy the body is using.

Chapter 2

Effects of Aging on the Lungs

The lungs have two primary functions: to acquire oxygen from the air, which is required for life, and to remove carbon dioxide from the body, which is a byproduct of many of the chemical reactions that sustain life.

During breathing, air enters and exits the lungs. It flows in through increasingly small airways, finally filling tiny sacs called alveoli. Blood circulates around the alveoli through capillaries. Where the capillaries and alveoli meet, oxygen crosses into the bloodstream. At the same time, carbon dioxide crosses from the bloodstream into the alveoli to be exhaled.

The lungs are continuously being exposed to particles in the air, including smoke, pollen, dust, and microorganisms. Therefore, another major function of the lungs is to protect from any diseases that may be caused by inhaled particles.

Aging Changes

An average person continues to slowly make new alveoli until about age twenty. After this age, the lungs begin to lose some of their tissue. The number of alveoli decreases, and there is a corresponding decrease in lung capillaries. The lungs also become less elastic due to various factors including the loss of a tissue protein called elastin.

Reprinted from "Aging Changes in the Lungs," © 2007 A.D.A.M., Inc. Reprinted with permission. Updated November 13, 2006.

Changes in the bones and muscles result in a slightly increased front-to-back chest diameter. Loss of bone mass in the ribs and vertebrae, and mineral deposits in the rib cartilage, change the spine curvature. There may be front-to-back curvature (kyphosis or lordosis) or side-to-side curvature (scoliosis).

The maximal force one can generate on inspiration (breathing in) or expiration (breathing out) decreases with age, as the diaphragm and muscles between the ribs (intercostals) become weaker. The chest is less able to stretch to breathe, and the pattern of breathing may change slightly to compensate for decreased ability to expand the chest.

Effect of Changes

Maximum lung function decreases with age. The amount of oxygen diffusing from the air sacs into the blood decreases, the rate of airflow through the airways slowly declines after age thirty, and the maximal force one is able to achieve on inspiration and expiration decreases. Usual breathing should remain adequate, and even a very old person should, under most circumstances, be able to breathe without effort.

However, when there is a need for increased breathing, the lungs may not be able to keep up with the demand. As aging continues, there may be a decreased capacity for exercise, and high altitude may cause problems.

An important change for many older people is that the airways close more readily. The airways tend to collapse when an older person breathes shallowly or when in bed for a prolonged time. Breathing shallowly because of pain, illness, or surgery causes an increased risk for pneumonia or other lung problems. As a result, it is important for older people to be out of bed as much as possible, even when ill or after surgery.

Normally, breathing is controlled by your brain. It receives information from various parts of the body telling it how much oxygen and carbon dioxide are in the blood. Low oxygen levels or high carbon dioxide levels trigger an increased rate and depth of breathing. It is normal for even healthy older people to have a reduced response to both decreased oxygen and increased carbon dioxide levels.

The voice box (larynx) also changes with aging. This causes the pitch, loudness, and quality of the voice to change. The voice may become quieter and slightly hoarse. The pitch may be decreased (becoming lower) in women and increased (becoming higher) in men. The voice may sound "weaker," but most people remain quite capable of effective communication. Some people may be emotionally sensitive to the voice's perceived loss of appeal or effectiveness.

Common Problems

Elderly people are at increased risk for lung infections. The body has many ways to protect against lung infections. With aging, these defenses may weaken.

The cough reflex may not trigger as readily, and the cough may be less forceful. The hairlike projections that line the airway (cilia) are less able to move mucus up and out of the airway. In addition, the nose and breathing passages secrete less of a substance called immunoglobulin A (IgA), an antibody that protects against viruses. Thus, the elderly are more susceptible to pneumonia and other types of lung infections.

Common lung problems in the elderly include chronically low oxygen levels (reducing tolerance to illness), decreased exercise tolerance, abnormal breathing patterns including sleep apnea (episodes of no breathing during sleep), increased risk of lung infections such as pneumonia or bronchitis, and diseases caused by tobacco damage such as emphysema or lung cancer.

Prevention

Avoidance of smoking is the most important way to minimize the effect of aging on the lungs. Exercise and good overall fitness improve breathing capacity. Exercise tolerance can be affected by changes in the heart, blood vessels, muscles, and skeleton, as well as lung changes. However, studies have shown that exercise and training can improve the reserve capacity of the lungs.

Secondly, more than any other group the elderly need to be aware of the need to be up and about and should consciously try to increase deep breathing during illness or after surgery.

Continued use of the voice helps maintain overall vocal performance.

Chapter 3

Lung Disease Statistics

Chapter Contents

Section 3.1

How Common Is Lung Disease?

"Lung Disease: A Statistical Overview" is excerpted from the *2006 NHLBI Fact Book*, Chapter 4: Disease Statistics, National Heart Lung and Blood Institute, 2006. "Chronic Obstructive Pulmonary Disease (COPD)," "Asthma," and "Bronchitis" (February 22, 2007); "Pneumonia" (October 6, 2006); and "Smoking" (January 24, 2007) are excerpted from FASTATS, National Center for Health Statistics, Centers for Disease Control and Prevention.

Lung Disease: A Statistical Overview

- Lung diseases, excluding lung cancer, caused an estimated 231,000 deaths in 2004.

- Chronic obstructive pulmonary disease (COPD) caused 120,000 deaths in 2004 and is the fourth-leading cause of death.

- Between 1999 and 2004, death rates for COPD and asthma decreased in both black and white men and women, with one exception: the COPD death rate increased slightly in white women.

- Between 1980 and 2004, infant death rates for various lung diseases declined markedly.

- Of the ten leading causes of infant mortality, four are lung diseases or have a lung disease component. Between 1994 and 2004, changes in mortality for the causes were as follows:

  - Congenital anomalies (-15 percent)

  - Disorders of short gestation (-5 percent)

  - Sudden infant death syndrome (-50 percent)

  - Respiratory distress syndrome (-42 percent)

- One in five deaths in children under one year of age is due to a lung disease.

- The COPD death rate for women in the United States is increasing significantly compared with the rates in several other countries.

- Between 1985 and 2003, death rates for COPD increased for women in all racial/ethnic groups except Asian. For men, they increased in American Indians, decreased in whites and Asians, and were essentially flat in blacks and Hispanics.

- Sleep disorders are increasingly being recognized as an important health problem. The number of physician office visits for sleep apnea, restless legs syndrome, and narcolepsy increased from 1,046,927 in 1990 to 6,549,402 in 2004.

- Asthma is a common chronic condition, particularly in children.

- The economic cost of lung diseases is expected to be $154 billion in 2007—$95 billion in direct health expenditures and $59 billion in indirect cost of morbidity and mortality.

Chronic Obstructive Pulmonary Disease (COPD)

Morbidity

- Number of noninstitutionalized adults with diagnosed chronic bronchitis in the past year: 8.9 million

- Percentage of noninstitutionalized adults with diagnosed chronic bronchitis in the past year: 4.1

- Number of noninstitutionalized adults who have ever been diagnosed with emphysema: 3.8 million

- Percentage of noninstitutionalized adults who have ever been diagnosed with emphysema: 1.7

- Number of noninstitutionalized adults who have ever been diagnosed with asthma: 23.3 million

- Percentage of noninstitutionalized adults who have ever been diagnosed with asthma: 11

Source: Summary Health Statistics for U.S. Adults: National Health Interview Survey, 2005, tables 3, 4, Appendix III, table V

Home Health Care

- Number of current patients with COPD as primary diagnosis: 71,900

- Percentage of current patients with COPD as primary diagnosis: 5.3

Source: 2000 National Home and Hospice Care Survey, table 12

Hospice Care

- Number of current patients with COPD as primary diagnosis: 4,500
- Percentage of current patients with COPD as primary diagnosis: 4.3

Source: 2000 National Home and Hospice Care Survey, table 12

Mortality

- Number of deaths: 123,884
- Deaths per 100,000 population: 42.2
- Cause of death rank: 4

Source: Preliminary Data for 2004, table 7

Asthma

Morbidity

- Number of noninstitutionalized adults who currently have asthma: 15.7 million
- Percentage of noninstitutionalized adults who currently have asthma: 7.2

Source: Summary Health Statistics for U.S. Adults: National Health Interview Survey, 2005, tables 3 and 4, Appendix III, table V

- Number of children who currently have asthma: 6.5 million
- Percentage of children who currently have asthma: 8.9

Source: Summary Health Statistics for U.S. Children: National Health Interview Survey, 2005, table 1, Appendix III, table IV

Health Care Use

- Number of visits to office-based physicians: 13.6 million

Source: National Ambulatory Medical Care Survey: 2004 Summary, table 13

- Number of hospital outpatient department visits: 1 million

Source: National Hospital Ambulatory Medical Care Survey: 2004 Outpatient Department Summary, table 12

- Number of hospital emergency department visits: 1.8 million

(Source: National Hospital Ambulatory Medical Care Survey: 2004 Emergency Department Summary, table 10)

Mortality

- Number of deaths: 3,780
- Deaths per 100,000: 1.3

Source: Deaths: Preliminary Data for 2004, table 2

Bronchitis

- Number of noninstitutionalized adults with diagnosed chronic bronchitis in the past year: 8.9 million
- Percentage of noninstitutionalized adults with diagnosed chronic bronchitis: 4.1

Source: Summary Health Statistics for U.S. Adults: National Health Interview Survey, 2005, tables 3, 4, Appendix III, table V

Pneumonia

Hospital Inpatient Care

- Number of discharges: 1.3 million
- Average length of stay: 5.5 days

Source: 2004 National Hospital Discharge Survey, tables 2,4

Home Health Care

- Number of current patients with pneumonia as primary diagnosis: 20,300 (2000)
- Percentage of current patients with pneumonia as primary diagnosis: 1.5 (2000)

Source: The National Home and Hospice Care Survey, table 12

Nursing Home Care

- Number of residents with pneumonia: 22,500
- Percentage of residents with pneumonia at time of survey: 1.4

- Average length of stay for discharges with pneumonia as primary diagnosis: 124 days

Source: National Nursing Home Survey: 1999 Summary, tables 26, 58

Mortality

- Number of deaths: 60,207
- Deaths per 100,000 population: 20.5

Source: Preliminary Data for 2004, tables 2

- Percentage of hospital inpatient deaths from pneumonia: 5.4

Source: National Hospital Discharge Survey: 2004 Annual Summary With Detailed Diagnosis and Procedure Data, table 25

Smoking

- Percentage of adults eighteen years of age and over who currently smoke cigarettes (2004): 21

Source: Health, United States, 2006, table 63

- Percentage of high school students who smoked cigarettes in the past thirty days (2005): 23

Source: Health, United States, 2006, data table for figure 10)

Section 3.2

Lung Disease in Diverse Communities: At-Risk Populations

Excerpted from "State of Lung Disease in Diverse Communities: 2007," © 2007 American Lung Association. Reprinted with permission. For more information about the American Lung Association or to support the work it does, call 1-800-LUNG-USA (1-800-586-4872) or log on to http://www.lungusa.org.

Both indoor and outdoor air pollution are linked to breathing problems and communities of color are especially vulnerable: Studies have linked air pollution to heart disease, cancer, asthma, and other respiratory illnesses, even death. Children, the elderly, and those with chronic lung and heart disease are most vulnerable to the adverse effects of air pollution. Communities of color are more likely to reside near industrial sources of air pollution.[1] This report shows that certain communities of color have higher prevalence and death rates from some of the most common respiratory illnesses, such as asthma, and most often reside in high-pollution areas.

Puerto Ricans have the highest asthma prevalence: Asthma is found in all populations, but some racial and ethnic groups experience it at higher rates, particularly the inner-city African American and Puerto Rican communities. Presently, Puerto Ricans living in the United States have the highest asthma prevalence of any population.[2]

African Americans are less likely to develop or die from chronic obstructive pulmonary disease (COPD), yet they have more emergency room visits and similar disease severity when compared to whites who have smoked cigarettes over a longer period of time and are heavier smokers: COPD is the fourth leading cause of death in the United States.[3] Smoking is the main cause of the disease, but other risk factors including air pollution, occupational exposures, and secondhand smoke can worsen the condition. White Americans in the United States are more likely to develop the disease than other racial or ethnic groups.

17

Native Americans have the second highest incidence rate of cystic fibrosis; whites have the highest: Cystic fibrosis is a life-long hereditary disease that is most common among white babies, but Native Americans have the second highest incidence.

African Americans represent half of all human immunodeficiency virus (HIV) diagnoses. HIV and acquired immunodeficiency syndrome (AIDS) is the leading cause of death among African American women aged twenty-five to thirty-four: Since the beginning of the HIV epidemic, individuals of color have constituted 61 percent of AIDS cases. Hispanics with HIV are more likely than whites and African Americans to have their condition turn into AIDS within twelve months of diagnosis. Because the lung is the major target of infection in HIV/AIDS patients, some persons infected with HIV are in danger of contracting various forms of lung disease, such as pneumonia or tuberculosis, especially extensively drug-resistant tuberculosis (XDR TB), strains resistant to usual and second-line drugs in the treatment of tuberculosis.[4]

Influenza/pneumonia is the fourth leading cause of death among Asian Americans/Pacific islanders over the age of sixty-five: Within the Asian/Pacific islander population, influenza and pneumonia ranks as the sixth leading cause of death overall. Surveys show that African Americans over age sixty-five are less likely to receive an influenza or pneumonia vaccine than their white counterparts. Approximately 72.5 percent of all influenza and pneumonia deaths in African Americans occur in this age group.[5]

Lung cancer kills more African Americans and American Indians/Alaska natives than any other cancer: In 2007, an estimated 213,380 new cases of lung cancer and an estimated 160,390 deaths from lung cancer will occur in the United States.[6] American Indians/Alaska natives had higher mortality rates (33.1 per 100,000) for lung cancer than Asian Americans (27.2 per 100,000) and Hispanics (23.9 per 100,000). Asian Americans are more likely than any other racial or ethnic group to develop and die from lung cancer, although they have lower overall exposure to tobacco smoke.[7]

African American children are more than three times more likely than children of other races to develop sleep disordered breathing: Sleep apnea or sleep disordered breathing occurs in all age groups and both sexes, but is most common in males and those over the age of forty. It is also more common among people who are moderately overweight to obese. Strong evidence suggests that obesity may increase the risk of obstructed breathing during sleep. Lack of awareness by the public and healthcare professionals has resulted in the vast majority of people with the illness remaining undiagnosed and, therefore, untreated.[8]

Hispanics are more likely to be employed in high-risk occupations than any other racial or ethnic group: Traditionally, certain racial and ethnic groups have been overexposed to occupational respiratory hazards because they are more likely to be employed in industries associated with lung disease. Occupational asthma is the most prevalent occupational lung disease in the United States, with approximately 15 to 23 percent of new onset asthma cases in the United States attributed to occupational exposure.[9]

American Indians/Alaska natives have high rates of respiratory syncytial virus (RSV): One study found that age-adjusted RSV hospitalization rates among Navajo and White Mountain Apache children less than one year old to be three times higher than rates reported for other children of the same age group in the United States.[10]

African Americans have the highest prevalence rates of sarcoidosis in the United States: In 2003, the mortality rate from sarcoidosis was thirteen times higher among African Americans than whites.[11] The cause of the disease is still a mystery, but researchers have several theories, including genetic predisposition to increased susceptibility and progression of the disorder.[12]

American Indians/Alaska natives have sudden infant death syndrome (SIDS) rates over two times higher than the overall U.S. population: SIDS is the third leading cause of death among infants under one year of age. Infants of American Indian and Alaska native mothers have the highest SIDS rates of all racial and ethnic groups. American Indian infants were 2.5 times more likely than white babies to die of SIDS. The cause of the disease remains unknown, but research has found that maternal smoking during pregnancy could double the risk of an infant developing the disease[13]

Smoking prevalence is highest among American Indians, but Chinese American males and lesbian, gay, bisexual, and transgender (LGBT) communities also have high rates: About

19

8.6 million people in the United States have at least one serious illness caused by smoking. Exposure to tobacco smoke is projected to cause to some 438,000 deaths each year.[14] Data indicate smoking prevalence is highest among American Indians. In addition, recent studies indicate there is widespread occurrence of smoking in LGBT (lesbian, gay, bisexual, and transgender) communities, which puts them at an increased risk for lung cancer, COPD, and coronary heart disease.[15]

Tuberculosis (TB) case rates are dramatically higher among Asians/Pacific islanders than other racial groups: The highest TB case rates in the U.S. population occur in persons of Asian and Native Hawaiian/other Pacific islander descent (25.8 and 13.8 per 100,000, respectively). Asian Americans also have the highest percentage of new TB cases among foreign-born persons living in the United States. African Americans account for the highest percentage of TB cases in the U.S.-born population. African Americans accounted for 28 percent of new TB cases in 2005, while Asian Americans accounted for 23 percent.[16]

References

1. Perlin SA, Sexton K, Wong DW. An examination of race and poverty for populations living near industrial sources of air pollution. *J Expo Anal Environ Epidemiol.* January–February 1999; 9(1):29–48; Perlin SA, Wong DW, Sexton K. Residential proximity to industrial sources of air pollution: Interrelationships among race, poverty and age. *Journal of the Air Waste Management Association* March 2001; 51(3):406–21.

2. Homa DM, Mannino DM, Lara M. Asthma mortality in U.S. Hispanics of Mexican, Puerto Rican and Cuban heritage, 1990–1995. *American Journal of Respiratory and Critical Care Medicine* 2000; 161:504–9.

3. Centers for Disease Control and Prevention. Deaths: Leading causes for 2003. *National Vital Health Statistics.* Available at: http://www.cdc.gov/nchs/data/hestat/leadingdeaths03_tables .pdf#3. Accessed March 19, 2007.

4. Centers for Disease Control and Prevention. Cases of HIV infection and AIDS in the United States, 2005. *HIV AIDS Surveillance Report.* Vol. 17. Revised June 2007.

5. Centers for Disease Control and Prevention. Deaths: Leading causes for 2003. National Vital Health Statistics. Available at: http://www.cdc.gov/nchs/data/hestat/leadingdeaths03_tables .pdf#3. Accessed March 19, 2007.

6. American Cancer Society. Cancer facts and figures, 2007. Available at: http://www.cancer.org/downloads/SST/CAFF2007 PWSecured.pdf. Accessed May 31, 2007.

7. Ibid.

8. U.S. Department of Health and Human Services. National Institutes of Health. National Heart, Lung and Blood Institute. Sleep apnea. What is sleep apnea. February 2006. Available at: http://www.nhlbi.nih.gov/health/dci/Diseases/Sleep Apnea/SleepApnea_WhatIs.html. Accessed May 2, 2007.

9. Healthy People. Available at: http://www.healthypeople.gov/. Accessed May 16, 2007.

10. Bockova J, O'Brien KL, Oski J, et al. Respiratory syncytial virus infection in Navajo and White Mountain Apache children. *Pediatrics* August 2002; 110(2).

11. Centers for Disease Control and Prevention. CDC Wonder. Underlying cause of death. Sarcoidosis. Available at: http://wonder .cdc.gov/controller/datarequest/D17;jsessionid=763 D9B069 BEAD1DCA4E87341CED98BB8. Accessed March 8, 2007.

12. Rybicki B, Iannuzzi MC, Frederick MM, et al. Familial aggregation of sarcoidosis. *American Journal of Respiratory and Critical Care. Medicine* 2001; 164:2085–91.

13. Yu E, Chen E, Kim K, Abdulrahim S. Smoking among Chinese Americans: Behavior, knowledge and beliefs. *American Journal of Public Health* 2002; 92(6):1007–12.

14. Centers for Disease Control and Prevention. Annual smoking-attributable mortality, years of potential life lost and productivity losses-U.S., 1997–2001. *Morbidity and Mortality Weekly Report*. July 2005; 54:35.

15. Gay and Lesbian Medical Association (GLMA). Healthy People 2010: Companion Document for lesbian, gay, bisexual and transgender health. Available at http://www.lgbthealth.net/downloads/ np2010doc.pdf. Accessed July 16, 2007.

16. Centers for Disease Control and Prevention. Reported tuberculosis in the U.S., 2005. Available at: http://www.cdc.gov/nchstp/tb/surv/surv2005/PDF/TBSurvFULLReport.pdf. Accessed March 26, 2007.

Chapter 4

Air Pollution and Respiratory Disease

Chapter Contents

Section 4.1

Indoor Air Pollutants:
Steps to Reduce Exposure

Excerpted from "The Inside Story: A Guide to Indoor Air Quality,"
U.S. Environmental Protection Agency, August 27, 2007.

The pollutants listed in this section have been shown to cause the health effects mentioned. However, it is not necessarily true that the effects noted occur at the pollutant concentration levels typically found in the home. In many cases, our understanding of the pollutants and their health effects is too limited to determine the levels at which the listed effects could occur.

Radon (Rn)

Sources: Earth and rock beneath home; well water; building materials.

Health effects: No immediate symptoms. Estimated to contribute to between seven thousand and thirty thousand lung cancer deaths each year. Smokers are at higher risk of developing radon-induced lung cancer.

Levels in homes: Based on a national residential radon survey completed in 1991, the average indoor radon level is 1.3 picocuries per liter (pCi/L). The average outdoor level is about 0.4 pCi/L.

Steps to Reduce Exposure

- Test your home for radon—it's easy and inexpensive.
- Fix your home if your radon level is 4 picocuries per liter (pCi/L) or higher.
- Radon levels less than 4 pCi/L still pose a risk, and in many cases may be reduced.
- If you want more information on radon, contact your state radon office.

Environmental Tobacco Smoke (ETS)

Source: Cigarette, pipe, and cigar smoking.

Health effects: Eye, nose, and throat irritation; headaches; lung cancer; may contribute to heart disease. Specifically for children, increased risk of lower respiratory tract infections, such as bronchitis and pneumonia, and ear infections; buildup of fluid in the middle ear; increased severity and frequency of asthma episodes; decreased lung function.

Levels in homes: Particle levels in homes without smokers or other strong particle sources are the same as, or lower than, those outdoors. Homes with one or more smokers may have particle levels several times higher than outdoor levels.

Steps to Reduce Exposure

- Do not smoke in your home or permit others to do so.
- Do not smoke if children are present, particularly infants and toddlers.
- If smoking indoors cannot be avoided, increase ventilation in the area where smoking takes place. Open windows or use exhaust fans.

Biologicals

Sources: Wet or moist walls, ceilings, carpets, and furniture; poorly maintained humidifiers, dehumidifiers, and air conditioners; bedding; household pets.

Health effects: Eye, nose, and throat irritation; shortness of breath; dizziness; lethargy; fever; digestive problems. Can cause asthma; humidifier fever; influenza and other infectious diseases.

Levels in homes: Indoor levels of pollen and fungi are lower than outdoor levels (except where indoor sources of fungi are present). Indoor levels of dust mites are higher than outdoor levels.

Steps to Reduce Exposure

- Install and use fans vented to outdoors in kitchens and bathrooms.
- Vent clothes dryers to outdoors.

- Clean cool mist and ultrasonic humidifiers in accordance with manufacturer's instructions and refill with clean water daily.

- Empty water trays in air conditioners, dehumidifiers, and refrigerators frequently.

- Clean and dry or remove water-damaged carpets.

- Use basements as living areas only if they are leak-proof and have adequate ventilation. Use dehumidifiers, if necessary, to maintain humidity between 30 and 50 percent.

Carbon Monoxide (CO)

Sources: Unvented kerosene and gas space heaters; leaking chimneys and furnaces; back-drafting from furnaces, gas water heaters, woodstoves, and fireplaces; gas stoves; automobile exhaust from attached garages; environmental tobacco smoke.

Health effects: At low concentrations, fatigue in healthy people and chest pain in people with heart disease. At higher concentrations, impaired vision and coordination; headaches; dizziness; confusion; nausea. Can cause flu-like symptoms that clear up after leaving home. Fatal at very high concentrations.

Levels in homes: Average levels in homes without gas stoves vary from 0.5 to 5 parts per million (ppm). Levels near properly adjusted gas stoves are often 5 to 15 ppm and those near poorly adjusted stoves may be 30 ppm or higher.

Steps to Reduce Exposure

- Keep gas appliances properly adjusted.

- Consider purchasing a vented space heater when replacing an unvented one.

- Use proper fuel in kerosene space heaters.

- Install and use an exhaust fan vented to outdoors over gas stoves.

- Open flues when fireplaces are in use.

- Choose properly sized woodstoves that are certified to meet Environmental Protection Agency (EPA) emission standards. Make certain that doors on all woodstoves fit tightly.

- Have a trained professional inspect, clean, and tune up central heating system (furnaces, flues, and chimneys) annually. Repair any leaks promptly.

- Do not idle the car inside garage.

Nitrogen Dioxide (NO₂)

Sources: Kerosene heaters, unvented gas stoves and heaters. Environmental tobacco smoke.

Health effects: Eye, nose, and throat irritation. May cause impaired lung function and increased respiratory infections in young children.

Levels in homes: Average level in homes without combustion appliances is about half that of outdoors. In homes with gas stoves, kerosene heaters, or unvented gas space heaters, indoor levels often exceed outdoor levels.

Steps to reduce exposure: See steps under carbon monoxide.

Organic Gases

Sources: Household products including: paints, paint strippers, and other solvents; wood preservatives; aerosol sprays; cleansers and disinfectants; moth repellents and air fresheners; stored fuels and automotive products; hobby supplies; dry-cleaned clothing.

Health effects: Eye, nose, and throat irritation; headaches, loss of coordination, nausea; damage to liver, kidney, and central nervous system. Some organics can cause cancer in animals; some are suspected or known to cause cancer in humans.

Levels in homes: Studies have found that levels of several organics average two to five times higher indoors than outdoors. During and for several hours immediately after certain activities, such as paint stripping, levels may be one thousand times background outdoor levels.

Steps to Reduce Exposure

- Use household products according to manufacturer's directions.

- Make sure you provide plenty of fresh air when using these products.

- Throw away unused or little-used containers safely; buy in quantities that you will use soon.

- Keep out of reach of children and pets.

- Never mix household care products unless directed on the label.

Respirable Particles

Sources: Fireplaces, woodstoves, and kerosene heaters; environmental tobacco smoke.

Health effects: Eye, nose, and throat irritation; respiratory infections and bronchitis; lung cancer. (Effects attributable to environmental tobacco smoke are listed elsewhere.)

Levels in homes: Particle levels in homes without smoking or other strong particle sources are the same as, or lower than, outdoor levels.

Steps to Reduce Exposure

- Vent all furnaces to outdoors; keep doors to rest of house open when using unvented space heaters.

- Choose properly sized woodstoves, certified to meet EPA emission standards; make certain that doors on all woodstoves fit tightly.

- Have a trained professional inspect, clean, and tune up central heating system (furnace, flues, and chimneys) annually. Repair any leaks promptly.

- Change filters on central heating and cooling systems and air cleaners according to manufacturer's directions.

Formaldehyde

Sources: Pressed wood products (hardwood plywood wall paneling, particleboard, fiberboard) and furniture made with these pressed wood products. Urea-formaldehyde foam insulation (UFFI). Combustion sources and environmental tobacco smoke. Durable press drapes, other textiles, and glues.

Health effects: Eye, nose, and throat irritation; wheezing and coughing; fatigue; skin rash; severe allergic reactions. May cause cancer. May also cause other effects listed under "organic gases."

Levels in homes: Average concentrations in older homes without UFFI are generally well below 0.1 ppm. In homes with significant amounts of new pressed wood products, levels can be greater than 0.3 ppm.

Steps to Reduce Exposure

- Use "exterior-grade" pressed wood products (lower-emitting because they contain phenol resins, not urea resins).
- Use air conditioning and dehumidifiers to maintain moderate temperature and reduce humidity levels.
- Increase ventilation, particularly after bringing new sources of formaldehyde into the home.

Pesticides

Sources: Products used to kill household pests (insecticides, termiticides, and disinfectants). Also, products used on lawns and gardens that drift or are tracked inside the house.

Health effects: Irritation to eye, nose, and throat; damage to central nervous system and kidney; increased risk of cancer.

Levels in homes: Preliminary research shows widespread presence of pesticide residues in homes.

Steps to Reduce Exposure

- Use strictly according to manufacturer's directions.
- Mix or dilute outdoors.
- Apply only in recommended quantities.
- Increase ventilation when using indoors. Take plants or pets outdoors when applying pesticides to them.
- Use nonchemical methods of pest control where possible.
- If you use a pest control company, select it carefully.
- Do not store unneeded pesticides inside home; dispose of unwanted containers safely.

- Store clothes with moth repellents in separately ventilated areas, if possible.

- Keep indoor spaces clean, dry, and well ventilated to avoid pest and odor problems.

Asbestos

Sources: Deteriorating, damaged, or disturbed insulation, fireproofing, acoustical materials, and floor tiles.

Health effects: No immediate symptoms, but long-term risk of chest and abdominal cancers and lung diseases. Smokers are at higher risk of developing asbestos-induced lung cancer.

Levels in homes: Elevated levels can occur in homes where asbestos-containing materials are damaged or disturbed.

Steps to Reduce Exposure

- It is best to leave undamaged asbestos material alone if it is not likely to be disturbed.

- Use trained and qualified contractors for control measures that may disturb asbestos and for cleanup.

- Follow proper procedures in replacing woodstove door gaskets that may contain asbestos.

Lead (Pb)

Sources: Lead-based paint, contaminated soil, dust, and drinking water.

Health effects: Lead affects practically all systems within the body. Lead at high levels (lead levels at or above 80 micrograms per deciliter [80 ug/dl] of blood) can cause convulsions, coma, and even death. Lower levels of lead can cause adverse health effects on the central nervous system, kidney, and blood cells. Blood lead levels as low as 10 ug/dl can impair mental and physical development.

Steps to Reduce Exposure

- Keep areas where children play as dust-free and clean as possible.

- Leave lead-based paint undisturbed if it is in good condition; do not sand or burn off paint that may contain lead.

- Do not remove lead paint yourself.

- Do not bring lead dust into the home.

- If your work or hobby involves lead, change clothes and use doormats before entering your home.

- Eat a balanced diet, rich in calcium and iron.

Section 4.2

Biological Pollutants in the Home

Excerpted from Consumer Product Safety Commission.
The text of this document is available online at http://www.cpsc.gov/
cpscpub/pubs/425.html; accessed September 18, 2007.

Outdoor air pollution in cities is a major health problem. Much effort and money continues to be spent cleaning up pollution in the outdoor air. But air pollution can be a problem where you least expect it, in the place you may have thought was safest—your home. Many ordinary activities such as cooking, heating, cooling, cleaning, and redecorating can cause the release and spread of indoor pollutants at home. Studies have shown that the air in our homes can be even more polluted than outdoor air.

Many Americans spend up to 90 percent of their time indoors, often at home. Therefore, breathing clean indoor air can have an important impact on health. People who are inside a great deal may be at greater risk of developing health problems, or having problems made worse by indoor air pollutants. These people include infants, young children, the elderly, and those with chronic illnesses.

What Are Biological Pollutants?

Biological pollutants are or were living organisms. They promote poor indoor air quality and may be a major cause of days lost from work

31

or school, and of doctor and hospital visits. Some can even damage surfaces inside and outside your house. Biological pollutants can travel through the air and are often invisible.

Some common indoor biological pollutants are as follows:

- Animal dander (minute scales from hair, feathers, or skin)
- Dust mite and cockroach parts
- Infectious agents (bacteria or viruses)
- Pollen

Some of these substances are in every home. It is impossible to get rid of them all. Even a spotless home may permit the growth of biological pollutants. Two conditions are essential to support biological growth: nutrients and moisture. These conditions can be found in many locations, such as bathrooms, damp or flooded basements, wet appliances (such as humidifiers or air conditioners), and even some carpets and furniture.

Modern materials and construction techniques may reduce the amount of outside air brought into buildings, which may result in high moisture levels inside. Using humidifiers, unvented heaters, and air conditioners in our homes has increased the chances of moisture forming on interior surfaces. This encourages the growth of certain biological pollutants.

The Scope of the Problem

Most information about sources and health effects of biological pollutants is based on studies of large office buildings and two surveys of homes in the northern United States and Canada. These surveys show that 30 to 50 percent of all structures have damp conditions that may encourage the growth and buildup of biological pollutants. This percentage is likely to be higher in warm, moist climates.

Some diseases or illnesses have been linked with biological pollutants in the indoor environment. However, many of them also have causes unrelated to the indoor environment. Therefore, we do not know how many health problems relate only to poor indoor air.

Health Effects of Biological Pollutants

All of us are exposed to biological pollutants. However, the effects on our health depend upon the type and amount of biological pollution and the individual person. Some people do not experience health reactions from certain biological pollutants, while others may experience one or more of the following reactions:

- Allergic
- Infectious
- Toxic

Except for the spread of infections indoors, allergic reactions may be the most common health problem with indoor air quality in homes. They are often connected with animal dander (mostly from cats and dogs), with house dust mites (microscopic animals living in household dust), and with pollen. Allergic reactions can range from mildly uncomfortable to life threatening, as in a severe asthma attack. Some common signs and symptoms are as follows:

- Watery eyes
- Runny nose and sneezing
- Nasal congestion
- Itching
- Coughing
- Wheezing and difficulty breathing
- Headache
- Fatigue

Health experts are especially concerned about people with asthma These people have very sensitive airways that can react to various irritants, making breathing difficult. The number of people who have asthma has greatly increased in recent years. The number of people with asthma has gone up by 59 percent since 1970, to a total of 9.6 million people. Asthma in children under fifteen years of age has increased 41 percent in the same period, to a total of 2.6 million children. The number of deaths from asthma is up by 68 percent since 1979, to a total of almost 4,400 deaths per year.

Talking to Your Doctor

Are you concerned about the effects on your health that may be related to biological pollutants in your home? Before you discuss your concerns with your doctor, you should know the answers to the following questions. This information can help the doctor determine whether your health problems may be related to biological pollution:

- Does anyone in the family have frequent headaches, fevers, itchy watery eyes, a stuffy nose, dry throat, or a cough? Does anyone complain of feeling tired or dizzy all the time? Is anyone wheezing or having difficulties breathing on a regular basis?

- Did these symptoms appear after you moved to a new or different home?

- Do the symptoms disappear when you go to school or the office or go away on a trip, and return when you come back?

- Have you recently remodeled your home or done any energy conservation work, such as installing insulation, storm windows, or weather stripping? Did your symptoms occur during or after these activities?

- Does your home feel humid? Can you see moisture on the windows or on other surfaces, such as walls and ceilings?

- What is the usual temperature in your home? Is it very hot or cold?

- Have you recently had water damage?

- Is your basement wet or damp?

- Is there any obvious mold or mildew?

- Does any part of your home have a musty or moldy odor?

- Is the air stale?

- Do you have pets?

- Do your houseplants show signs of mold?

- Do you have air conditioners or humidifiers that have not been properly cleaned?

- Does your home have cockroaches or rodents?

Infectious diseases caused by bacteria and viruses, such as flu, measles, chicken pox, and tuberculosis, may be spread indoors. Most infectious diseases pass from person to person through physical contact. Crowded conditions with poor air circulation can promote this spread. Some bacteria and viruses thrive in buildings and circulate through indoor ventilation systems. For example, the bacterium causing Legionnaires disease, a serious and sometimes lethal infection, and Pontiac fever, a flu-like illness, have circulated in some large buildings.

Toxic reactions are the least studied and understood health problem caused by some biological air pollutants in the home. Toxins can damage a variety of organs and tissues in the body, including the liver, the central nervous system, the digestive tract, and the immune system.

Coping with the Problem

Checking Your Home

There is no simple and cheap way to sample the air in your home to determine the level of all biological pollutants. Experts suggest that sampling for biological pollutants is not a useful problem-solving tool. Even if you had your home tested, it is almost impossible to know which biological pollutants cause various symptoms or health problems. The amount of most biological substances required to cause disease is unknown and varies from one person to the next.

Does this make the problem sound hopeless? On the contrary, you can take several simple, practical actions to help remove sources of biological pollutants, to help get rid of pollutants, and to prevent their return.

Self-Inspection: A Walk through Your Home

Begin by touring your household. Follow your nose, and use your eyes. Two major factors help create conditions for biological pollutants to grow: nutrients and constant moisture with poor air circulation.

Dust and construction materials, such as wood, wallboard, and insulation, contain nutrients that allow biological pollutants to grow. Firewood also is a source of moisture, fungi, and bugs.

Appliances such as humidifiers, kerosene and gas heaters, and gas stoves add moisture to the air.

A musty odor, moisture on hard surfaces, or even water stains, may be caused by any of the following:

- Air-conditioning units
- Basements, attics, and crawlspaces
- Bathrooms
- Carpets
- Heating and air-conditioning ducts
- Humidifiers and dehumidifiers
- Refrigerator drip pans

35

What You Can Do about Biological Pollutants

Before you give away the family pet or move, there are less drastic steps that can be taken to reduce potential problems. Properly cleaning and maintaining your home can help reduce the problem and may avoid interrupting your normal routine. People who have health problems such as asthma, or are allergic, may need to do this and more. Discuss this with your doctor.

Moisture Control

Water in your home can come from many sources. Water can enter your home by leaking or by seeping through basement floors. Showers or even cooking can add moisture to the air in your home. The amount of moisture that the air in your home can hold depends on the temperature of the air. As the temperature goes down, the air is able to hold less moisture. This is why, in cold weather, moisture condenses on cold surfaces (for example, drops of water form on the inside of a window). This moisture can encourage biological pollutants to grow.

There are many ways to control moisture in your home:

- Fix leaks and seepage. If water is entering the house from the outside, your options range from simple landscaping to extensive excavation and waterproofing. (The ground should slope away from the house.) Water in the basement can result from the lack of gutters or a water flow toward the house. Water leaks in pipes or around tubs and sinks can provide a place for biological pollutants to grow.

- Put a plastic cover over dirt crawlspaces to prevent moisture from coming in from the ground. Be sure crawlspaces are well ventilated.

- Use exhaust fans in bathrooms and kitchens to remove moisture to the outside (not into the attic). Vent your clothes dryer to the outside.

- Turn off certain appliances (such as humidifiers or kerosene heaters) if you notice moisture on windows and other surfaces.

- Use dehumidifiers and air conditioners, especially in hot, humid climates, to reduce moisture in the air, but be sure that the appliances themselves don't become sources of biological pollutants.

- Raise the temperature of cold surfaces where moisture condenses. Use insulation or storm windows. (A storm window installed on the inside works better than one installed on the outside.) Open doors between rooms (especially doors to closets, which may be colder than the rooms) to increase circulation. Circulation carries heat to the cold surfaces Use fans and move furniture from wall corners to promote air and heat circulation. Be sure that your house has a source of fresh air and can expel excessive moisture.

- Pay special attention to carpet on concrete floors. Carpet can absorb moisture and serve as a place for biological pollutants to grow. Use area rugs, which can be taken up and washed often. In certain climates, if carpet is to be installed over a concrete floor, it maybe necessary to use a vapor barrier (plastic sheeting) over the concrete and cover that with sub-flooring (insulation covered with plywood) to prevent a moisture problem.

- Moisture problems and their solutions differ from one climate to another. The northeast is cold and wet, the southwest is hot and dry, the south is hot and wet, and the western mountain states are cold and dry. All of these regions can have moisture problems. For example, evaporative coolers used in the southwest can encourage the growth of biological pollutants. In other hot regions, the use of air conditioners that cool the air too quickly may prevent the air conditioners from running long enough to remove excess moisture from the air. The types of construction and weatherization for the different climates can lead to different problems and solutions.

Maintain and Clean All Appliances That Come in Contact with Water

Have major appliances, such as furnaces, heat pumps, and central air conditioners, inspected and cleaned regularly by a professional, especially before seasonal use. Change filters on heating and cooling systems according to manufacturer's directions. (In general, change filters monthly during use.) When first turning on the heating or air conditioning at the start of the season, consider leaving your home until it airs out.

Have window or wall air-conditioning units cleaned and serviced regularly by a professional, especially before the cooling season. Air conditioners can help reduce the entry of allergy-causing pollen. But they may also become a source of biological pollutants if not properly maintained. Clean the coils and rinse the drain pans according to manufacturer's instructions, so water cannot collect in pools.

Have furnace-attached humidifiers cleaned and serviced regularly by a professional, especially before the heating season.

Follow manufacturer's instructions when using any type of humidifier. Experts differ on the benefits of using humidifiers. If you do use a portable humidifier (approximately one- to two-gallon tanks), be sure to empty its tank every day and refill with distilled or demineralized water, or even fresh tap water if the other types of water are unavailable. For larger portable humidifiers, change the water as recommended by the manufacturer. Unplug the appliance before cleaning. Every third day, clean all surfaces coming in contact with water with a 3 percent solution of hydrogen peroxide, using a brush to loosen deposits. Some manufacturers recommend using diluted household bleach for cleaning and maintenance, generally in a solution of one-half cup bleach to one gallon water. When using any household chemical, rinse well to remove all traces of chemical before refilling humidifier.

Empty dehumidifiers daily and clean often. If possible, have the appliance drip directly into a drain. Follow manufacturer's instructions for cleaning and maintenance. Always disconnect the appliance before cleaning.

Clean refrigerator drip pans regularly according to manufacturer's instructions. If refrigerator and freezer doors don't seal properly, moisture may build up and mold can grow. Remove any mold on door gaskets and replace faulty gaskets.

Clean Surfaces

Clean moist surfaces, such as showers and kitchen counters.

Remove mold from walls, ceilings, floors, and paneling. Do not simply cover mold with paint, stain, varnish, or a moisture-proof sealer, as it may resurface.

Replace moldy shower curtains, or remove them and scrub well with a household cleaner and rinse before rehanging them.

Dust Control

Controlling dust is very important for people who are allergic to animal dander and mites. You cannot see mites, but you can either remove their favorite breeding grounds or keep these areas dry and clean. Dust mites can thrive in sofas, stuffed chairs, carpets, and bedding. Open shelves, fabric wallpaper, knickknacks, and Venetian blinds are also sources of dust mites. Dust mites live deep in the carpet and are not removed by vacuuming. Many doctors suggest that their mite-allergic patients use washable area rugs rather than wall-to-wall carpet.

Always wash bedding in hot water (at least 130° F) to kill dust mites. Cold water won't do the job. Launder bedding at least every seven to ten days.

Use synthetic or foam rubber mattress pads and pillows, and plastic mattress covers if you are allergic. Do not use fuzzy wool blankets, feather or wool-stuffed comforters, and feather pillows.

Clean rooms and closets well and dust and vacuum often to remove surface dust. Vacuuming and other cleaning may not remove all animal dander, dust mite material, and other biological pollutants. Some particles are so small they can pass through vacuum bags and remain in the air. If you are allergic to dust, wear a mask when vacuuming or dusting. People who are highly allergy-prone should not perform these tasks. They may even need to leave the house when someone else is cleaning.

Before You Move

Protect yourself by inspecting your potential new home. If you identify problems, have the landlord or seller correct them before you move in, or even consider moving elsewhere.

Have professionals check the heating and cooling system, including humidifiers and vents. Have duct lining and insulation checked for growth.

Check for exhaust fans in bathrooms and kitchens. If there are no vents, do the kitchen and bathrooms have at least one window apiece? Does the cook top have a hood vented outside? Does the clothes dryer vent outside? Are all vents to the outside of the building, not in attics or crawlspaces?

Look for obvious mold growth throughout the house, including attics, basements, and crawlspaces and around the foundation. See if there are many plants close to the house, particularly if they are damp and rotting. They are a potential source of biological pollutants. Downspouts from roof gutters should route water away from the building.

Look for stains on the walls, floor, or carpet (including any carpet over concrete floors) as evidence of previous flooding or moisture problems. Is there moisture on windows and surfaces? Are there signs of leaks or seepage in the basement?

Look for rotted building materials, which may suggest moisture or water damage.

If you or anyone else in the family has a pet allergy, ask if any pets have lived in the home.

Examine the design of the building. Remember that in cold climates, overhanging areas, rooms over unheated garages, and closets on outside walls may be prone to problems with biological pollutants. Look for signs of cockroaches.

Warning

Carefully read instructions for use and any cautionary labeling on cleaning products before beginning cleaning procedures:

- Do not mix any chemical products. Especially, never mix cleaners containing bleach with any product (such as ammonia) that does not have instructions for such mixing. When chemicals are combined, a dangerous gas can sometimes be formed.

- Household chemicals may cause burning or irritation to skin and eyes.

- Household chemicals may be harmful if swallowed or inhaled.

- Avoid contact with skin, eyes, mucous membranes, and clothing.

- Avoid breathing vapor. Open all windows and doors and use an exhaust fan that sends the air outside.

- Keep household chemicals out of reach of children.

- Rinse treated surface areas well to remove all traces of chemicals.

Correcting Water Damage

What if damage is already done? Follow these guidelines for correcting water damage:

- Throw out mattresses, wicker furniture, straw baskets, and the like that have been water damaged or contain mold. These cannot be recovered.

- Discard any water-damaged furnishings such as carpets, drapes, stuffed toys, upholstered furniture, and ceiling tiles, unless they can be recovered by steam cleaning or hot water washing and thorough drying.

- Remove and replace wet insulation to prevent conditions where biological pollutants can grow.

Section 4.3

Outdoor Air Pollution and Your Health

Air quality is a major pubic health concern. Unfortunately, millions
of Americans live in areas where the pollution in the outdoor air all
too often puts their health and even their lives at risk. Studies have
tied air pollution to heart disease, cancer, asthma, and other respiratory illnesses, and even death.

The Clean Air Act provides the principal framework for air quality in the United States, including national air quality standards that safeguard the public against the following six damaging pollutants:[1]

- Ozone (O_3) is a highly reactive form of oxygen that results from sunlight mixing with volatile organic compounds (including hydrocarbons) and nitrogen oxides released in fuel combustion. New research shows that breathing ozone over a short period, even at levels currently considered safe, increases the risk of premature death.[2, 3, 4, 5] Exposure to ozone can cause shortness of breath and coughing, trigger asthma attacks, and reduce lung function, often leading to hospital admissions and emergency room visits. Ozone is the main component of smog.[6]

- Particulate matter air pollution (PM) is a complex mixture of substances, including carbon-based particles, dust, and acid aerosols. Exposure to particle pollution is associated with increased risk of premature death, heart attacks, and lung cancer, and can trigger asthma attacks, wheezing, coughing, and lung irritation in people with sensitive airways.[7]

- Nitrogen dioxide (NO_2) forms when fossil fuels are burned at high temperatures. It can irritate the lungs and lower one's resistance to lung infections such as influenza. Exposure to concentrations

41

that are higher than normal may increase the rate of acute respiratory illness in children. Nitrogen oxides are also a key ingredient in the formation of ozone and some particle pollution.[8]

- Sulfur dioxide (SO_2) forms during the burning of fuel containing sulfur (mainly coal and oil), and during metal smelting and other industrial processes. Major health concerns associated with exposure to high concentrations of SO_2 include difficulty breathing, lung illness, changes in pulmonary defenses, and aggravation of existing heart disease. Sulfur dioxide is a key ingredient in the formation of some particle pollution as well.[9]

- Carbon monoxide (CO) is colorless and odorless, but at high levels it can be deadly. CO forms when carbon in fuel does not burn completely. It can cause harmful health effects by reducing oxygen delivery to the body's organs and tissues. At low levels of exposure, CO can be poisonous, creating headaches, nausea, and sleepiness. At higher levels, which can develop indoors, CO can be life threatening. CO exposure may also cause injury to the eyes, reduced work capacity, difficulty doing manual and complex tasks, and poor learning ability.[10]

- Lead is a highly toxic metal found naturally in the environment as well as in manufactured products. Due to the phase out of leaded gasoline between 1975 and 1986, outdoor lead levels have decreased by more than 90 percent. While the primary impact is not on the lungs, the respiratory system is the major route of entry into the body for lead particles. Lead harms the brain and nervous system and damages the kidneys, liver, and other organs. High levels of exposure to lead can cause seizures, behavioral disorders, and death. Even at low doses, lead exposure is associated with damage to the nervous systems of fetuses and children six years and under. They are most at risk because their bodies are growing quickly.[11,12]

In addition to these six major pollutants, there are other hazardous or toxic air pollutants that may not be as widespread but can be found in high concentrations, especially in industrial areas or near roadways and coal-fired power plants. These include pollutants known to cause cancer, such as benzene, and others that damage the nervous system or brain, such as mercury.

Much outdoor air pollution stems from burning fossil fuels, whether from generating electricity, operating industrial processes, or driving the family car. Over the past twenty years, the national air quality and emission levels for all six principal pollutants have improved. Despite this progress, about 141 million tons of air pollution were released into the air in the United States in 2005. Approximately 122 million people lived in counties that did not meet U.S. Environmental Protection Agency standards for at least one of the pollutants.[13]

References

1. U.S. Environmental Protection Agency. The Plain English Guide to the Clean Air Act. 2001. Available at http://www.epa.gov/air/caa/peg/. Accessed July 16, 2007.

2. Bell ML, Dominici F, Samet JM. A meta-analysis of time-series studies of ozone and mortality with comparison to the national morbidity, mortality and air pollution study. *Epidemiology.* 2005; 16:436–45.

3. Levy JI, Chermerynski SM, Sarnat JA. Ozone exposure and mortality: An empiric Bayes metaregression analysis. *Epidemiology.* 2005;16:458–68.

4. Ito K, De Leon SF, Lippmann M. Associations between ozone and daily mortality: Analysis and meta-analysis. *Epidemiology.* 2005; 16:446–57.

5. Goodman SN. The methodologic ozone effect. *Epidemiology.* 2005; 16:430–35.

6. U.S. Environmental Protection Agency. Air quality criteria for ozone and oxidative air pollutants. March 2006.

7. U.S. Environmental Protection Agency. Air quality criteria for particulate matter. October 2004.

8. U.S. Environmental Protection Agency. Air quality trends report, 2003.

9. Ibid.

10. Ibid.

11. U.S. Environmental Protection Agency. Six Common Air Pollutants. Available at: http://www.epa.gov/air/urbanair/lead/hlth.html. Accessed July 16, 2007.

12. U.S. Environmental Protection Agency. Lead in paint, dust and soil. Fact sheet. Available at: http://www.epa.gov/lead. Accessed July 13, 2007.

13. U.S. Environmental Protection Agency. Air trends: Basic information fact sheet. Available at: http://www.epa.gov/air/airtrends/sixpoll.html. Accessed May 5, 2007.

Section 4.4

Minimizing the Effects of Outdoor Air Pollution

"Minimizing the Effects of Outdoor Air Pollution,"
© 2005 American Association for Respiratory Care. Reprinted with permission. For additional information, visit www.yourlunghealth.org.

Everyone is adversely affected by poor air quality; however, individuals who suffer from pulmonary problems are much more sensitive to irritants in the atmosphere. For them, pollutants can cause more severe symptoms, such as chest tightness or cough, along with burning of the eyes and throat.

Here are some tips for helping you avoid exposure to, and complications from, poor outdoor air quality.

Avoid Exposure to Noxious Fumes

The Environmental Protection Agency (EPA) includes 188 substances on its list of toxic air pollutants, including components found in gasoline, chemicals emitted by dry cleaning facilities, solvents and paint strippers used by numerous industries, and substances like asbestos, dioxin, lead compounds, and mercury. We can't avoid all of these pollutants all of the time, but there are simple things we can do to minimize our exposure:

- If you are working on your car in the garage, make sure your garage door is completely open and don't let exhaust fumes from the garage enter your house.

- Minimize your exposure to strong chemicals by replacing the lids on solvent containers securely and disposing of saturated rags in a sealed container. Don't mix any chemical solutions.

- When painting, use a brush rather than a sprayer.

- Be careful not to overfill or spill gasoline when filling up your car or lawn and garden equipment. Make sure your equipment is properly maintained.

- Be aware of ozone levels in your community and try to stay inside when levels are high.

Check Local Pollution Reports

Be aware of ozone levels in your community and try to stay inside when levels are high. The EPA issues a daily air quality index (AQI) for most of the United States indicating the concentration of five major air pollutants: ground-level ozone, particle pollution, carbon monoxide, sulfur dioxide, and nitrogen dioxide. The AQI categories, which are color-coded to make them easy to understand, are shown in Table 4.1.

Table 4.1. Air Quality Index

Air Quality Index Levels of Health Concern	Numerical Value	Meaning
Good	0–50	Air quality is considered satisfactory, and air pollution poses little or no risk.
Moderate	51–100	Air quality is acceptable; however, for some pollutants there may be a moderate health concern for a very small number of people who are unusually sensitive to air pollution.
Unhealthy for Sensitive Groups	101–150	Members of sensitive groups may experience health effects. The general public is not likely to be affected.
Unhealthy	151–200	Everyone my begin to experience health effects; members of sensitive groups may experience more serious health effects.
Very Unhealthy	201–300	Health alert: Everyone may experience more serious health effects.
Hazardous	>300	Health warnings of emergency conditions. The entire population is more likely to be affected.

Those with lung disease may experience increased symptoms when the AQI is Moderate, but more often at Unhealthy for Sensitive Groups level, and these symptoms should alert you to take measures to protect your lungs:

- Stay indoors as much as possible.

- Limit outside activities to the early morning hours or after sunset. Ozone levels, in particular, tend to go down with the sun.

- Refrain from exercising outdoors when levels are high. Exercising causes you to breathe faster, which means you take in even more pollutants than you would during normal activities.

- Stay away from high-traffic areas, and avoid exercising near these areas at all times.

Follow Your Care Plan

No matter how careful you are while you're outside, atmospheric pollutants and irritants may cause respiratory problems. If you have asthma or another respiratory condition, ask your doctor or respiratory therapist to provide you with a care plan to follow in case of increasing symptoms. Follow the plan carefully, and if you are still having problems, contact your doctor or therapist for further advice.

Chapter 5

Smoking and Respiratory Disease

Chapter Contents

Section 5.1

Health Effects of Cigarette Smoking

Reprinted from the Centers for Disease Control and Prevention,
December 2006.

Smoking harms nearly every organ of the body; causing many diseases and reducing the health of smokers in general.[1] The adverse health effects from cigarette smoking account for an estimated 438,000 deaths, or nearly one of every five deaths, each year in the United States.[2,3] More deaths are caused each year by tobacco use than by all deaths from human immunodeficiency virus (HIV), illegal drug use, alcohol use, motor vehicle injuries, suicides, and murders combined.[2,4]

Cancer

Cancer is the second-leading cause of death and was among the first diseases casually linked to smoking.[1]

Smoking causes about 90 percent of lung cancer deaths in women and almost 80 percent of lung cancer deaths in men. The risk of dying from lung cancer is more than twenty-three times higher among men who smoke cigarettes, and about thirteen times higher among women who smoke cigarettes compared with never smokers.[1]

Smoking causes cancers of the bladder, oral cavity, pharynx, larynx (voice box), esophagus, cervix, kidney, lung, pancreas, and stomach, and causes acute myeloid leukemia.[1]

Rates of cancers related to cigarette smoking vary widely among members of racial/ethnic groups, but are generally highest in African American men.[5]

Cardiovascular Disease (Heart and Circulatory System)

Smoking causes coronary heart disease, the leading cause of death in the United States.[1] Cigarette smokers are two to four times more likely to develop coronary heart disease than nonsmokers.[6]

Cigarette smoking approximately doubles a person's risk for stroke.[7,8]

Cigarette smoking causes reduced circulation by narrowing the blood vessels (arteries). Smokers are more than ten times as likely as nonsmokers to develop peripheral vascular disease.[9]

Smoking causes abdominal aortic aneurysm.[1]

Respiratory Disease and Other Effects

Cigarette smoking is associated with a tenfold increase in the risk of dying from chronic obstructive lung disease.[7] About 90 percent of all deaths from chronic obstructive lung diseases are attributable to cigarette smoking.[1]

Cigarette smoking has many adverse reproductive and early childhood effects, including an increased risk for infertility, preterm delivery, stillbirth, low birth weight, and sudden infant death syndrome (SIDS).[1]

Postmenopausal women who smoke have lower bone density than women who never smoked. Women who smoke have an increased risk for hip fracture than never smokers.[10]

References

1. U.S. Department of Health and Human Services. The Health Consequences of Smoking: A Report of the Surgeon General. U.S. Department of Health and Human Services, Centers for Disease Control and Prevention, National Center for Chronic Disease Prevention and Health Promotion, Office on Smoking and Health, 2004 [cited 2006 Dec 5]. Available from: http://www.cdc.gov/tobacco/data_statistics/sgr/sgr_2004/index.htm.

2. Centers for Disease Control and Prevention. Annual Smoking-Attributable Mortality, Years of Potential Life Lost, and Productivity Losses—United States, 1997–2001. *Morbidity and Mortality Weekly Report* [serial online]. 2002; 51(14):300–303 [cited 2006 Dec 5]. Available from: http://www.cdc.gov/mmwr/preview/mmwrhtml/mm5114a2.htm.

3. Centers for Disease Control and Prevention. Health United States, 2003, With Chartbook on Trends in the Health of Americans. Hyattsville, MD: CDC, National Center for Health Statistics; 2003 [cited 2006 Dec 5]. Available from: http://www.cdc.gov/nchs/data/hus/tables/2003/03hus031.pdf.

4. McGinnis J, Foege WH. Actual Causes of Death in the United States. *Journal of the American Medical Association* 1993; 270:2207–12.

5. Novotny TE, Giovino GA. Tobacco Use. In: Brownson RC, Remington PL, Davis JR (eds). *Chronic Disease Epidemiology and Control*. Washington, DC: American Public Health Association; 1998; 117–48 [cited 2006 Dec 5].

6. U.S. Department of Health and Human Services. *Reducing the Health Consequences of Smoking—25 Years of Progress: A Report of the Surgeon General*. Atlanta, GA: U.S. Department of Health and Human Services, CDC; 1989. DHHS Pub. No. (CDC) 89–8411 [cited 2006 Dec 5]. Available from: http://profiles.nlm .nih.gov/NN/B/B/X/S/.

7. U.S. Department of Health and Human Services. *Tobacco Use Among U.S. Racial/Ethnic Minority Groups—African Americans, American Indians and Alaska Natives, Asian Americans and Pacific Islanders, and Hispanics: A Report of the Surgeon General*. Atlanta, GA: U.S. Department of Health and Human Services, CDC; 1998 [cited 2006 Dec 5]. Available from: http:// www.cdc.gov/tobacco/data_statistics/sgr/sgr_1998/index.htm.

8. Ockene IS, Miller NH. Cigarette Smoking, Cardiovascular Disease, and Stroke: A Statement for Healthcare Professionals From the American Heart Association. *Journal of American Health Association*. 1997; 96(9):3243–47 [cited 2006 Dec 5].

9. Fielding JE, Husten CG, Eriksen MP. Tobacco: Health Effects and Control. In: Maxcy KF, Rosenau MJ, Last JM, Wallace RB, Doebbling BN (eds.). *Public Health and Preventive Medicine*. New York: McGraw-Hill; 1998; 817–45 [cited 2006 Dec 5].

10. U.S. Department of Health and Human Services. *Women and Smoking: A Report of the Surgeon General*. Rockville, MD: U.S. Department of Health and Human Services, CDC; 2001 [cited 2006 Dec 5]. Available from: http://www.cdc.gov/tobacco/data _statistics/sgr/sgr_2001/index.htm.

Section 5.2

Secondhand Smoke

"Facts about Secondhand Smoke" is reprinted from "Secondhand Smoke," Centers for Disease Control and Prevention, September 2006. "How to Protect Yourself and Your Loved Ones from Secondhand Smoke" is reprinted from the U.S. Department of Health and Human Services, January 4, 2007.

Facts about Secondhand Smoke

Definition of Secondhand Smoke

Secondhand smoke, also known as environmental tobacco smoke, is a complex mixture of gases and particles that includes smoke from the burning cigarette, cigar, or pipe tip (side stream smoke) and exhaled mainstream smoke.[1]

Secondhand smoke contains at least 250 chemicals known to be toxic, including more than 50 that can cause cancer.[1]

Health Effects of Secondhand Smoke Exposure

Secondhand smoke exposure causes heart disease and lung cancer in nonsmoking adults.[2]

Nonsmokers who are exposed to secondhand smoke at home or work increase their heart disease risk by 25 to 30 percent and their lung cancer risk by 20 to 30 percent.[2]

Breathing secondhand smoke has immediate harmful effects on the cardiovascular system that can increase the risk of heart attack. People who already have heart disease are at especially high risk.[2]

Secondhand smoke exposure causes respiratory symptoms in children and slows their lung growth.[2]

Secondhand smoke causes sudden infant death syndrome (SIDS), acute respiratory infections, ear problems, and more frequent and severe asthma attacks in children.[2]

There is no risk-free level of secondhand smoke exposure. Even brief exposure can be dangerous.[2]

51

Current Estimates of Secondhand Smoke Exposure

Exposure to nicotine and secondhand smoke is measured by testing the saliva, urine, or blood for the presence of a chemical called cotinine. Cotinine is a byproduct of nicotine metabolization, and tobacco is the only source of this marker.[2]

From 1988–91 to 2001–02, the proportion of nonsmokers with detectable levels cotinine was halved (from 88 percent to 43 percent).[3]

Over that same time period, cotinine levels in those who were exposed to secondhand smoke fell by 70 percent.[3]

More than 126 million nonsmoking Americans continue to be exposed to secondhand smoke in homes, vehicles, workplaces, and public places.[2]

Most exposure to tobacco smoke occurs in homes and workplaces.[2]

Almost 60 percent of U.S. children aged three to eleven years—or almost twenty-two million children—are exposed to secondhand smoke.[2]

About 25 percent of children aged three to eleven years live with at least one smoker, compared to only about 7 percent of nonsmoking adults.[2]

The California Environmental Protection Agency estimates that secondhand smoke exposure causes approximately 3,400 lung cancer deaths and 22,700 to 69,600 heart disease deaths annually among adult nonsmokers in the United States.[4]

Each year in the United States, secondhand smoke exposure is responsible for 150,000 to 300,000 new cases of bronchitis and pneumonia in children aged less than eighteen months. This results in 7,500 to 15,000 hospitalizations annually.[5]

References

1. National Toxicology Program. 11th Report on Carcinogens, 2005. Research Triangle Park, NC: U.S. Department of Health and Human Sciences, National Institute of Environmental Health Sciences, 2000 [cited 2006 Sep 27]. Available from: http://ntp.niehs.nih.gov/ntp/roc/eleventh/profiles/s176toba.pdf.

2. U.S. Department of Health and Human Services. The Health Consequences of Involuntary Exposure to Tobacco Smoke: A Report of the Surgeon General. Atlanta, Georgia: U.S. Department of Health and Human Services, Centers for Disease Control and Prevention, Coordinating Center for Health Promotion, National Center for Chronic Disease Prevention and Health

Promotion, Office on Smoking and Health, 2006 [cited 2006 Sep 27]. Available from: http://www.surgeongeneral.gov/library/secondhandsmoke/report/.

3. Pirkle JL, Bernert JT, Caudill SP, Sosnoff CS, Pechacek TF. Trends in the Exposure of Nonsmokers in the U.S. Population to Secondhand Smoke: 1988–2002. *Environmental Health Perspectives*. 2006; 114(6):853–58 [cited 2006 Sep 27].

4. California Environmental Protection Agency. Proposed Identification of Environmental Tobacco Smoke as a Toxic Air Contaminant. Final report, September 29, 2005, approved by Scientific Review Panel on June 24, 2005 [cited 2006 Sep 27]. Available from: http://www.arb.ca.gov/toxics/ets/ets.htm.

5. United States Environmental Protection Agency. *Respiratory Health Effects of Passive Smoking: Lung Cancer and Other Disorders*. Office of Research and Development, EPA/600/6-90/006F, Washington, D.C., December 1992 [cited 2006 Sep 27]. Available from: http://oaspub.epa.gov/eims/eimscomm.getfile?p_download _id=36793. Also published as: National Institutes of Health. National Cancer Institute. *Respiratory Health Effects of Passive Smoking: Lung Cancer and Other Disorders: The Report of the U.S. Environmental Protection Agency*. Smoking and Tobacco Control Monograph Number 4. NIH Publication No. 93-3605, Washington, D.C., August 1993.

How to Protect Yourself and Your Loved Ones from Secondhand Smoke

The Surgeon General has concluded that there is no risk-free level of exposure to secondhand smoke. Breathing even a little secondhand smoke can be harmful.

The Surgeon General has concluded that the only way to fully protect yourself and your loved ones from the dangers of secondhand smoke is through 100 percent smoke-free environments.

Opening a window, sitting in a separate area, or using ventilation, air conditioning, or a fan cannot eliminate secondhand smoke exposure.

You can protect yourself and your loved ones by doing the following things:

*   Making your home and car smoke-free

- Asking people not to smoke around you and your children

- Making sure that your children's daycare center or school is smoke-free

- Choosing restaurants and other businesses that are smoke-free. Thanking businesses for being smoke-free. Letting owners of businesses that are not smoke-free know that secondhand smoke is harmful to your family's health.

- Teaching children to stay away from secondhand smoke

- Avoiding secondhand smoke exposure especially if you or your children have respiratory conditions, if you have heart disease, or if you are pregnant

- Talking to your doctor or healthcare provider more about the dangers of secondhand smoke

If you are a smoker, the single best way to protect your family from secondhand smoke is to quit smoking. In the meantime, you can protect your family by making your home and vehicles smoke-free and smoking only outside. A smoke-free home rule can also help you quit smoking.

Section 5.3

Smoking: Benefits of Quitting

The following material "Benefits of Quitting Smoking" has been reproduced with the permission of the NSW Department of Health from its
publication "Tobacco and Health Fact Sheet." © December 2006 NSW
Department of Health.

The best thing a smoker can do for their health is to quit smoking.
There are health benefits of quitting for all smokers, regardless of age,
sex, or length of time that they have been smoking. People who have
already developed smoking-related health problems, like heart disease, can still benefit from quitting.

For example, compared to continuing smokers, people who quit
smoking after having a heart attack reduce their chances of having
another heart attack by 50 percent.[1]

There are many benefits to quitting, some even occur within hours
of stopping smoking. The changes that occur once you have quit show
how your body can make an amazing recovery from smoking.[1]

Benefits for All Ages

Are you under thirty-five? If you quit before age thirty-five, then
your life expectancy is similar to someone who has never smoked.

Are you under fifty? If you quit before age fifty, then your risk of
dying in the next fifteen years is reduced by half when compared to
people who continue to smoke.

For people of all ages: Best of all, quitting at any age doesn't just
increase life expectancy—it also improves quality of life!

By quitting smoking you will reduce your chance of having:

- Cancer of the lungs, throat, mouth, lips, gums, kidneys, and
  bladder;
- Heart disease and hardening of the arteries;
- A stroke;
- Emphysema and other lung diseases;
- Gangrene and other circulation problems.

Benefits of Quitting

Appearance, Vision, and Aging

As an ex-smoker, you are also less likely to have:

- Macular degeneration;
- Cataracts;
- Brittle bones (that break easily);
- Wrinkles and look older faster;
- Yellow teeth and bad breath.

Reproductive Health

By quitting you will reduce your chances of:

- Impotence;
- Having difficulty getting pregnant;
- Having premature births, babies with low birth weights, and miscarriage.

Children's Health

If you have children, your quitting can lower their risk of:

- Sudden Infant Death Syndrome (SIDS)—(cot death);
- Being smokers themselves;
- Ear infections;
- Allergies;
- Asthma;
- Bronchitis and other lung problems.

What Are the Other Benefits of Quitting?

Although reducing your chances of premature death and illness is important, they aren't the only benefits of quitting smoking:

- Think of the money you will save by not having to buy tobacco, around $3,500 a year for a pack a day smoker!
- Your costs for cleaning clothes, carpets, and furniture may go down.

Table 5.1. Benefits of Quitting Smoking

Time since quitting	Beneficial health changes that take place[2]
Within 20 minutes	Your body begins a series of changes that continue for years. Your heart rate reduces.
12 hours	The carbon monoxide level in your blood reduces dramatically.
2–12 weeks	Your heart attack risk begins to reduce. Circulation improves. Exercise is easier. Lung function improves.
1–9 months	Coughing and shortness of breath decrease.
1 year	Your risk of coronary heart disease is halved compared to a continuing smoker.
5 years	Your risk of cancer of the mouth, throat, and esophagus decreases and your risk of stroke is dramatically reduced.
10 years	Your risk of lung cancer falls to about half that of a smoker and your risk of cancers of the bladder, kidney, and pancreas also decreases.
15 years	Your risk of coronary heart disease and risk of death fall to about the same as someone who has never smoked.

- Your sense of taste and smell will be enhanced. You will enjoy your food more.

- You will have more energy to do the things you love.

- Exercising will be easier.

- You'll feel proud of your ability to overcome something so challenging. Many smokers remember the exact day they quit because it is a source of great pride.

- Cigarettes will no longer control your life.

- You will be setting a great example for children and other smokers.

References

1. U.S. Department Of Health and Human Services 1990, *Surgeon General Report: The Health Benefits of Smoking Cessation*, Center for Health Promotion and Education Centers for Disease Control, Office on Smoking and Health, Rockville, Maryland 20857.

2. U.S. Department of Health and Human Services 2004, *The Health Consequences of Smoking: A Report of the Surgeon General*, U.S. Department of Health and Human Services, Centers for Disease Control and Prevention, National Center for Chronic Disease Prevention and Health Promotion, Office on Smoking and Health, 2004.

Section 5.4

How to Quit Smoking

Excerpted from "Independence from Smoking: A Breath of Fresh Air!
How to Quit," National Women's Health Information Center, March 2007.

Make the Decision to Quit and Feel Great

If you have made the decision to quit smoking, congratulations! Not only will you improve your own health, you will also protect the health of your loved ones by no longer exposing them to secondhand smoke.

We know how hard it can be to quit smoking. Did you know that many people try to quit two or three times before they give up smoking for good? Nicotine is a very addictive drug—as addictive as heroin and cocaine. The good news is that millions of people have given up smoking for good. It's hard work to quit, but you can do it. Freeing yourself of an expensive habit that is dangerous to your health and the health of others will make you feel great.

Many people who smoke worry that they will gain weight if they quit. In fact, nearly 80 percent of people who quit smoking do gain weight, but the average weight gain is just five pounds. Keep in mind, however, that 56 percent of people who continue to smoke will gain weight too. The bottom line: The health benefits of quitting far exceed any risks from the weight gain that may follow quitting.

How to Quit

Research has shown that these five steps will help you to quit for good:

- **Pick a date to stop smoking:** Before that day, get rid of all cigarettes, ashtrays, and lighters everywhere you smoke. Do not allow anyone to smoke in your home. Write down why you want to quit and keep this list as a reminder.

- **Get support from your family, friends, and coworkers:** Studies have shown you will be more likely to quit if you have help. Let the people important to you know the date you will be quitting and ask them for their support. Ask them not to smoke around you or leave cigarettes out.

- **Find substitutes for smoking and vary your routine:** When you get the urge to smoke, do something to take your mind off smoking. Talk to a friend, go for a walk, or go to the movies. Reduce stress with exercise, meditation, hot baths, or reading. Try sugar-free gum or candy to help handle your cravings. Drink lots of water and juice. You might want to try changing your daily routine as well. Try drinking tea instead of coffee, eating your breakfast in a different place, or taking a different route to work.

- **Talk to your doctor or nurse about medicines to help you quit:** Some people have withdrawal symptoms when they quit smoking. These symptoms can include depression, trouble sleeping, feeling irritable or restless, and trouble thinking clearly. There are medicines to help relieve these symptoms. Most medicines help you quit smoking by giving you small, steady doses of nicotine, the drug in cigarettes that causes addiction. Talk to your doctor or nurse to see if one of these medicines may be right for you:

  - *Nicotine patch:* Worn on the skin and supplies a steady amount of nicotine to the body through the skin

  - *Nicotine gum or lozenge:* Releases nicotine into the bloodstream through the lining in your mouth

  - *Nicotine nasal spray:* Inhaled through your nose and passes into your bloodstream

  - *Nicotine inhaler:* Inhaled through the mouth and absorbed in the mouth and throat

  - *Bupropion:* An antidepressant medicine that reduces nicotine withdrawal symptoms and the urge to smoke

  - *Varenicline (Chantix®):* A medicine that reduces nicotine withdrawal symptoms and the pleasurable effects of smoking

- **Be prepared for relapse:** Most people relapse, or start smoking again, within the first three months after quitting. Don't get discouraged if you relapse. Remember, many people try to quit several times before quitting for good. Think of what helped and didn't help the last time you tried to quit. Figuring these out before you try to quit again will increase your chances for success. Certain situations can increase your chances of smoking. These include drinking alcohol, being around other smokers, gaining weight, stress, or becoming depressed. Talk to your doctor or nurse for ways to cope with these situations.

Chapter 6

Disease Prevention and Lung Health

Chapter Contents

Section 6.1

Exercise and Lung Health

"Exercise and the Lungs," © 2007 British Lung Foundation
(www.lunguk.org). Reprinted with permission.

The amount of air you need to breathe in depends on how active you are.

When you are sitting down you only take in about fifteen breaths a minute, giving you around twelve liters of air (a liter is one and three-quarter pints). From this your lungs will extract just one-fifth of a liter of oxygen.

During exercise your breathing and heart rate increase. Exercising flat out, a top-class athlete can expect to increase his or her breathing rate to around forty to sixty breaths a minute. This means they take in an incredible 100 to 150 liters of air, extracting around five liters of oxygen every single minute.

Even those of us with more modest goals need to double our lung intake when we exercise. Our lungs must be able to respond to our body's increased demands for oxygen.

What Happens When You Exercise?

As you start to move about, the muscles in your body send messages to your brain that they need more oxygen. Your brain then sends signals to the muscles that control breathing—your diaphragm and the muscles between your ribs—so that they shorten and relax more often. This causes you to take more breaths.

More oxygen will be absorbed from your lungs and carried to the muscles you are using to exercise—mainly your arms and legs.

Why Do Muscles Need More Oxygen?

For you to become more active your muscles will need to produce more energy. They do this by breaking down glucose from your food, but to do this they need oxygen. If there is too little oxygen they will try to produce energy in a different way. But this can lead to a build-up of a chemical called lactic acid, which causes cramps—something that many athletes are all too familiar with.

Athletes train so that their lungs and muscles become more efficient and it takes longer for lactic acid to build up. This means that their muscles can work harder. In fact, everyone can benefit from exercise to strengthen their lungs and muscles.

What Happens When Your Lungs Don't Work Properly?

People with long-term lung problems such as COPD (chronic obstructive pulmonary disease), may find their lungs unable to provide enough oxygen for their muscles to perform even simple activities. When walking short distances their lungs may struggle to keep up, which causes breathlessness.

Physical Training

Through exercise you can train your body so that more oxygen is delivered to your muscles.

Unfortunately, many people with long-term lung problems are afraid to exercise. This is partly because they are worried that being breathless may be harming them. This isn't true. By gradually building up the exercise you take, you can help to improve your breathing and feel better.

People with severe lung problems benefit a lot from even small amounts of exercise, so it really is worth keeping as active as possible.

Begin slowly by doing arm and leg movements while you are sitting down. Then set yourself targets for walking about: from room to room, going to the front door, the bottom of the garden, down the road, and so on. It's surprising how quickly you'll be able to do more.

Breathing Control

The "breathing control" techniques featured here are not suitable for everyone. Please check with your health professional whether you should use them.

Breathing control concentrates on using the lower chest with relaxation of the upper chest and shoulders. This encourages you to use the diaphragm more efficiently. Concentrate on allowing your abdomen (tummy) to move out as you breathe in, rather than allowing it to be sucked inwards. Practice breathing control with one hand on your abdomen.

Breathing control will help slow down your breathing rate and will reduce any anxiety if you do become breathless.

Discuss with your doctor or chest specialist the possibility of being referred to a physical therapist to help teach you breathing control and breathing exercises.

Can Extra Oxygen Help You Exercise?

Some people with chronic lung disease can exercise more if they receive extra oxygen.

However, not everyone can benefit, so it is very important to be assessed by your health professional before receiving treatment.

Section 6.2

Influenza Vaccine

Reprinted from "Key Facts about Seasonal Flu Vaccine,"
Centers for Disease Control and Prevention, September 19, 2007.

The single best way to protect against the flu is to get vaccinated each year.

There are two types of vaccines:

- **The "flu shot":** An inactivated vaccine (containing killed virus) that is given with a needle, usually in the arm. The flu shot is approved for use in people older than six months, including healthy people and people with chronic medical conditions.

- **The nasal-spray flu vaccine:** A vaccine made with live, weakened flu viruses that do not cause the flu (sometimes called LAIV for "live attenuated influenza vaccine"). LAIV (FluMist®) is approved for use in healthy people two to forty-nine years of age who are not pregnant.

Each vaccine contains three influenza viruses—one A (H3N2) virus, one A (H1N1) virus, and one B virus. The viruses in the vaccine change each year based on international surveillance and scientists' estimations about which types and strains of viruses will circulate in a given year.

About two weeks after vaccination, antibodies that provide protection against influenza virus infection develop in the body.

When to Get Vaccinated

October or November is the best time to get vaccinated, but you can still get vaccinated in December and later. Flu season can begin as early as October and last as late as May.

Who Should Get Vaccinated

In general, anyone who wants to reduce their chances of getting the flu can get vaccinated. However, it is recommended by the Advisory Committee on Immunization Practices (ACIP) that certain people should get vaccinated each year. They are either people who are at high risk of having serious flu complications or people who live with or care for those at high risk for serious complications. During flu seasons when vaccine supplies are limited or delayed, ACIP makes recommendations regarding priority groups for vaccination.

People who should get vaccinated each year are as follows:

- People at high risk for complications from the flu, including:
  - Children aged six months until their fifth birthday;
  - Pregnant women;
  - People fifty years of age and older;
  - People of any age with certain chronic medical conditions;
  - People who live in nursing homes and other long term care facilities.
- People who live with or care for those at high risk for complications from flu, including:
  - Household contacts of persons at high risk for complications from the flu (see above);
  - Household contacts and out of home caregivers of children less than six months of age (these children are too young to be vaccinated);
  - Healthcare workers.

Use of the Nasal Spray Flu Vaccine

It should be noted that vaccination with the nasal-spray flu vaccine is always an option for healthy persons aged two to forty-nine years who are not pregnant. On September 19, 2007, the U.S. Food and Drug Administration approved use of the nasal influenza vaccine LAIV (FluMist®) for healthy children ages two to four years old (24–59 months old) without a history of recurrent wheezing, as well as for healthy persons ages five to forty-nine years who are not pregnant. Previously, approval was for healthy persons ages five to forty-nine years who are not pregnant.

Who Should Not Be Vaccinated

There are some people who should not be vaccinated without first consulting a physician. These include the following:

- People who have a severe allergy to chicken eggs

- People who have had a severe reaction to an influenza vaccination in the past

- People who developed Guillain-Barré syndrome (GBS) within six weeks of getting an influenza vaccine previously

- Children less than six months of age

- People who have a moderate or severe illness with a fever (these people should wait to get vaccinated until their symptoms lessen)

Vaccine Effectiveness

The ability of flu vaccine to protect a person depends on the age and health status of the person getting the vaccine, and the similarity or "match" between the virus strains in the vaccine and those in circulation. Testing has shown that both the flu shot and the nasal-spray vaccine are effective at preventing the flu.

Vaccine Side Effects (What to Expect)

Different side effects can be associated with the flu shot and LAIV.

The flu shot: The viruses in the flu shot are killed (inactivated), so you cannot get the flu from a flu shot. Some minor side effects that could occur are as follows:

- Soreness, redness, or swelling where the shot was given
- Fever (low grade)
- Aches

If these problems occur, they begin soon after the shot and usually last one to two days. Almost all people who receive influenza vaccine have no serious problems from it. However, on rare occasions, flu vaccination can cause serious problems, such as severe allergic reactions. As of July 1, 2005, people who think that they have been injured by the flu shot can file a claim for compensation from the National Vaccine Injury Compensation Program (VICP).

LAIV (FluMist®): The viruses in the nasal-spray vaccine are weakened and do not cause severe symptoms often associated with influenza illness. (In clinical studies, transmission of vaccine viruses to close contacts has occurred only rarely.)

In children, side effects from LAIV (FluMist®) can include the following:

- Runny nose
- Wheezing
- Headache
- Vomiting
- Muscle aches
- Fever

In adults, side effects from LAIV (FluMist®) can include the following:

- Runny nose
- Headache
- Sore throat
- Cough

Section 6.3

Antiviral Drugs to Prevent Influenza

Excerpted from "Key Facts about Antiviral Drugs and Influenza (Flu),"
Centers for Disease Control and Prevention, September 18, 2007.

While getting a flu vaccine each year is the best way to protect you from the flu, there also are drugs that can fight against influenza viruses, offering a second line of defense against the flu. These are called "influenza antiviral drugs" and they must be prescribed by a health care professional. These drugs can be used to treat the flu or to prevent infection with flu viruses. Influenza antiviral drugs work against only influenza viruses—they will not help treat or prevent symptoms caused by infection from other viruses that can cause symptoms similar to the flu.

Antiviral drugs are used in different settings and circumstances to treat the flu and to prevent people from getting the flu:

- Antiviral drugs are used to help control flu outbreaks in places where a lot of people at high risk of serious flu complications live in close contact with each other, like nursing homes or hospital wards, for example.

- Antiviral drugs are used in the community setting to treat people with the flu to reduce severity of symptoms and reduce the number of days that people are sick.

- Antiviral drugs are used to prevent the flu:
  - For people who have been close to someone with the flu; or
  - For people that need protection from the flu but they either don't get protection after vaccination, or the vaccine is unavailable or they can't get the vaccine because of allergies, for example.

While most healthy people recover from the flu and don't have serious complications, some people—such as older people, young children, and people with certain health conditions—are at higher risk for serious flu-related complications. It's especially important that these people are protected from the flu.

Remember, a flu vaccine is the first and best defense against the flu, but antiviral drugs can be an important second line of defense to treat the flu or prevent flu infection.

Use of Antiviral Drugs for Treatment

For treatment, influenza antiviral drugs should be started within two days after becoming sick and taken for five days. When used this way, these drugs can reduce flu symptoms and shorten the time you are sick by one or two days. They also may make you less contagious to other people.

If you become sick with flu-like symptoms this season, your doctor will consider the likelihood of influenza being the cause of your illness, the number of days you have been sick, side effects of the medication, etc. before making a recommendation about using antivirals. He or she may test you for influenza, but testing is not required in order for a physician to recommend influenza antiviral medications for you.

Use of Antiviral Drugs for Prevention

Influenza antiviral drugs can also be used to prevent influenza when they are given to a person who is not ill, but who has been or may be near a person with influenza. When used to prevent the flu, antiviral drugs are about 70 to 90 percent effective. It's important to remember that flu antiviral drugs are not a substitute for getting a flu vaccine. When used for prevention, the number of days that they should be used will vary depending on a person's particular situation.

In some instances, your doctor may choose to prescribe antiviral drugs to you as a preventive measure, especially if you are at high risk for serious flu complications and either did not get the flu vaccine or may still be at risk of illness even after vaccination. Also, if you are in close contact with someone who is considered at high risk for complications, you may be given antiviral drugs to reduce the chances of catching the flu and passing it on to the high-risk person.

Who Should Get Antiviral Drugs?

In general, antiviral drugs can be offered to anyone one year of age or older who wants to avoid and/or treat the flu. People who are at high risk of serious complications from the flu may benefit most from these drugs.

Antiviral drugs can also be used to prevent influenza among people with weak immune systems who may not be protected after getting a flu vaccine or who haven't been vaccinated.

Remember, a flu vaccine is the first and best defense against seasonal flu, but antiviral drugs can be an important second line of defense to treat the flu or prevent flu infection.

Notes

This information is summarized from Prevention & Control of Influenza—Recommendations of the Advisory Committee on Immunization Practices (ACIP). *MMWR* 2007 Jul 13; 56(RR06):1–54.

Section 6.4

Pneumococcus and the Pneumococcal Vaccine: Questions and Answers

"Pneumococcus: Questions and Answers," © 2007 Immunization Action Coalition (www.immunize.org). Reprinted with permission.

What causes pneumococcal disease?

Pneumococcal disease is caused by *Streptococcus pneumoniae,* a bacterium. There are more than ninety subtypes. Most subtypes can cause disease, but only a few produce the majority of invasive pneumococcal infections. The ten most common subtypes cause 62 percent of invasive disease worldwide.

How does pneumococcal disease spread?

The disease is spread from person to person by droplets in the air. The pneumococci bacteria are common inhabitants of the human respiratory tract. They may be isolated from the nasopharynx of 5 to 70 percent of normal, healthy adults.

How long does it take to show signs of pneumococcal disease after being exposed?

As noted above, many people carry the bacteria in their nose and throat without ever developing invasive disease. The incubation period for specific diseases caused by an invasive pneumococcal infection is noted below.

What diseases can pneumococci bacteria cause?

There are three major conditions caused by invasive pneumococcal disease: pneumonia, bacteremia, and meningitis. They are all caused by infection with the same bacteria, but have different symptoms.

Pneumococcal pneumonia (lung disease) is the most common disease caused by pneumococcal bacteria. It is estimated that 175,000 hospitalizations due to pneumococcal pneumonia occur each year in the United States. The incubation period is short (one to three days). Symptoms include abrupt onset of fever, shaking chills or rigors, chest pain, cough, shortness of breath, rapid breathing and heart rate, and weakness. The fatality rate is 5 to 7 percent and may be much higher in the elderly.

Pneumococcal bacteremia (blood infection) occurs in about 25 to 30 percent of patients with pneumococcal pneumonia. More than fifty thousand cases of pneumococcal bacteremia occur each year in the United States. Bacteremia is the most common clinical presentation among children younger than age two years, accounting for 70 percent of invasive disease in this group.

Pneumococci cause 13 to 19 percent of all cases of bacterial meningitis (infection of the covering of the brain or spinal cord) in the United States. There are three thousand to six thousand cases of pneumococcal meningitis each year.

Symptoms may include headache, tiredness, vomiting, irritability, fever, seizures, and coma. Children younger than age one year have the highest rate of pneumococcal meningitis, approximately ten cases per 100,000 population. The case fatality rate is high (30 percent overall, up to 80 percent in the elderly).

Pneumococci are also a common cause of acute otitis media (middle ear infection). Approximately 28 to 55 percent of such ear infections are caused by *S. pneumoniae*. In the United States., there are 4.9 million cases of otitis media each year in children younger than age five years. Middle ear infections are the most frequent reason for pediatric office visits in the United States, resulting in more than twenty million visits annually.

How serious is pneumococcal disease?

Pneumococcal disease is a serious disease that causes much sickness and death. In fact, pneumococcal disease kills more people in the United States each year than all other vaccine-preventable diseases combined. More than fifty thousand cases and more than ten thousand deaths from invasive pneumococcal diseases (bacteremia and meningitis) are estimated to have occurred in the United States in 2002. More than half of these cases occurred in adults for whom pneumococcal polysaccharide vaccine was recommended. Young children and the elderly (individuals younger than age five years as well as those older than age sixty-five years) have the highest incidence of serious disease.

Case-fatality rates are highest for meningitis and bacteremia, and the highest mortality occurs among the elderly and patients who have underlying medical conditions. Despite appropriate antimicrobial therapy and intensive medical care, the overall case fatality rate for pneumococcal bacteremia is about 20 percent among adults. Among elderly patients, this rate may be as high as 60 percent.

Before a vaccine was available in the United States, pneumococcal disease caused serious disease in children younger than age five years. Each year it was responsible for causing seven hundred cases of meningitis, seventeen thousand blood infections, five million ear infections, and two hundred deaths. Children younger than age two years are at the highest risk for serious pneumococcal disease.

Is there a treatment for pneumococcal disease?

Penicillin is the drug of choice for treatment of pneumococcal disease; however, resistance to penicillin and other antibiotics has been on the rise. Studies indicate that in some areas of the United States up to 40 percent of invasive pneumococci are resistant to common antibiotics. Treating patients infected with resistant organisms requires expensive alternative antimicrobial agents and may result in prolonged hospital stays.

The increased difficulty of treating this serious bacterial infection makes prevention through vaccination even more important.

How long is a person with pneumococcal disease contagious?

The exact period of communicability is not known. It appears that transmission can occur as long as the organism remains in respiratory secretions.

How common is pneumococcal disease in the United States?

Healthcare providers are not required by law to report pneumococcal disease to health authorities, so exact numbers are not known. Estimates have been made from a variety of population studies, however, and it is believed that forty-five thousand cases of invasive pneumococcal disease (meningitis and blood infections) occur each year in the United States. (Pneumonia and middle ear infections are most common but are not considered "invasive" diseases.) The incidence of the disease varies greatly by age group. The highest rate of invasive pneumococcal disease occurs in young children, especially those younger than age two years. Children with certain chronic diseases (e.g., sickle cell disease or human immunodeficiency virus [HIV] infection) are at very high risk of invasive disease.

Can you get pneumococcal disease more than once?

Yes. There are more than ninety known subtypes of pneumococcus bacteria, with twenty-three subtypes included in the current pneumococcal polysaccharide (adult) vaccine and seven subtypes included in the current conjugate (child) vaccine. Having been infected with one type does not always make the patient immune to other types. Even if an individual has had one or more episodes of invasive pneumococcal disease, he or she needs to be vaccinated.

When did pneumococcal vaccine become available?

There are two types of pneumococcal vaccine, pneumococcal polysaccharide vaccine and pneumococcal conjugate vaccine.

The first pneumococcal polysaccharide vaccine was licensed in the United States in 1977. In 1983, an improved pneumococcal polysaccharide vaccine was licensed, containing purified protein from twenty-three types of pneumococcal bacteria (the old formulation contained fourteen types). This pneumococcal polysaccharide vaccine is commonly known as PPV23 or PPV. The PPV vaccine is licensed for use in adults and persons with certain risk factors who are age two years and older.

The pneumococcal conjugate vaccine was licensed in early 2000. It is recommended for use in preventing pneumococcal disease in infants and young children (from age six weeks to the fifth birthday). It is commonly known as PCV7 or PCV.

What kind of vaccines are they?

Both pneumococcal vaccines are made from inactivated (killed) bacteria. The pneumococcal polysaccharide vaccine (PPV) contains long chains of polysaccharide (sugar) molecules that make up the surface capsule of the bacteria. The twenty-three types of pneumococci that are included cause 88 percent of invasive pneumococcal disease.

The pneumococcal conjugate vaccine (PCV) includes purified capsular polysaccharide of seven types of the bacteria "conjugated" (or joined) to a harmless variety of diphtheria toxin. The seven types of purified bacteria included account for 86 percent of bacteremia, 83 percent of meningitis, and 65 percent of acute otitis media (ear infection) among children younger than age six years in the United States.

How is this vaccine given?

The polysaccharide vaccine (PPV) can be given as a shot in either the muscle or the fatty tissue of the arm or leg. The conjugate vaccine (PCV) is given as a shot in the muscle.

Who should get the pneumococcal polysaccharide vaccine (PPV)?

- All adults age sixty-five years or older

- Anyone age two years or older who has a long-term health problem such as cardiovascular disease, sickle cell anemia, alcoholism, lung disease, diabetes, cirrhosis, or leaks of cerebrospinal fluid

- Anyone who has or is getting a cochlear implant

- Anyone age two years or older who has a disease or condition that lowers the body's resistance to infection, such as Hodgkin disease, kidney failure, nephrotic syndrome, lymphoma, leukemia, multiple myeloma, HIV infection or AIDS, damaged spleen or no spleen, or organ transplant

- Anyone age two years or older who is taking any drug or treatment that lowers the body's resistance to infection, such as long-term steroids, certain cancer drugs, or radiation therapy

- Alaska natives and certain Native American populations

Who should get the pneumococcal conjugate vaccine (PCV)?

All infants beginning at two months of age should receive a four-dose series of vaccine; catch-up vaccination is recommended for children younger than age five years who did not receive PCV vaccine on schedule.

What is the schedule for the routine doses of PCV for children?

All infants and toddlers should get four doses of PCV vaccine, usually given at ages two, four, six, and twelve to fifteen months.

What if my three-year-old child never got his PCV shots?

The number of doses a child needs to complete the series depends on his or her current age. Older children need fewer doses. For example, you should consider giving a healthy unvaccinated child age twenty-four to fifty-nine months a single dose of PCV. Your healthcare provider can tell you how many doses are needed to complete the series at a certain age. PCV is not routinely recommended for individuals who are age five years or older.

Do some children need to get both PCV and PPV?

Yes, children at high risk of invasive pneumococcal disease should receive PCV and then also receive PPV when age two years or older. PPV is not given routinely to healthy children (or adults younger than age sixty-five years).

If influenza vaccine is recommended for healthcare workers to protect high-risk patients from getting influenza, why isn't pneumococcal vaccine also recommended?

Influenza virus is easily spread from healthcare workers to their patients, and infection usually leads to clinical illness. Pneumococcus is probably not spread from healthcare workers to their patients as easily as is influenza, and infection with pneumococcus does not necessarily lead to clinical illness. Host factors (such as age, underlying illness) are more important in the development of invasive pneumococcal disease than just having the bacteria in one's nose or throat.

My elderly neighbor got a second pneumococcal shot. I thought just one was required.

Revaccination is not done routinely, but a single revaccination dose is recommended for groups of people at highest risk of serious infection. No one should receive more than two doses of PPV.

For example, persons who received a first dose when they were younger than age sixty-five years should receive a second dose at age sixty-five years if at least five years have elapsed since the previous dose. Likewise, persons age two years or older who are at high risk for pneumococcal disease due to certain long-term health problems, in particular immunosuppression, HIV infection, and not having a functional spleen (or having no spleen) should get a second dose five or more years after the first dose.

High-risk children (e.g., who have sickle cell disease, HIV/AIDS, or diabetes) who received the full PCV series as young children should receive one dose of PPV at age two years or older (at least two months following the last PCV dose).

Who recommends pneumococcal vaccines?

The Centers for Disease Control and Prevention, the American Academy of Pediatrics, and the American Academy of Family Physicians have all recommended routine vaccination for infants and young children with PCV vaccine. The Centers for Disease Control and Prevention, the American College of Obstetricians and Gynecologists, the American Academy of Family Physicians, and the American College of Physicians all recommend the PPV vaccine.

Should all nursing home patients ages sixty-five years and older be vaccinated against pneumococcal disease?

Yes.

Can pregnant women get this vaccine?

The safety of PPV vaccine for pregnant women has not been studied, although no adverse consequences have been reported among newborns whose mothers were vaccinated with PPV during pregnancy. Women who are at high risk of pneumococcal disease should be vaccinated before becoming pregnant, if possible. Unvaccinated pregnant women who are in a high-risk group should consult with a healthcare professional about getting the vaccination during pregnancy.

How safe is this vaccine?

PPV and PCV are both very safe vaccines.

For PPV, about 30 to 50 percent of the people who get the vaccine have very mild side effects, such as redness or pain where the shot was given. Fewer than 1 percent of recipients develop a fever, muscle aches, or more severe local reactions. Serious allergic reactions have been reported very rarely. For PCV, about 10 to 20 percent of children develop redness, tenderness, or swelling where the shot was given. About 11 percent may have a mild fever.

How effective is pneumococcal polysaccharide vaccine (PPV)?

Overall, PPV is 60 to 70 percent effective in preventing invasive disease. Older adults (e.g., older than age sixty-five years) and persons with significant underlying illnesses do not respond as well, but vaccination with PPV is still recommended because such persons are at high risk of developing severe pneumococcal disease.

How effective is pneumococcal conjugate vaccine (PCV)?

In a large clinical trial, PCV was shown to be 97 percent effective in preventing invasive disease caused by the pneumococci contained in the vaccine and 89 percent effective against all types of *S. pneumoniae*, including those not found in the vaccine. Children with chronic diseases such as sickle cell disease and HIV infection also seem to respond well to PCV.

Who should not receive pneumococcal vaccine?

For both PPV and PCV, persons who had a severe allergic reaction to one dose should not receive another (such reactions are rare).

Persons who are moderately or severely ill should wait until their condition improves to be vaccinated.

Can the vaccine cause pneumococcal disease?

No. Both PPV and PCV are inactivated vaccines containing only a portion of the microbe; therefore the vaccines cannot possibly cause pneumococcal disease.

Part Two

Symptoms, Diagnosis, and Treatment of Respiratory Disorders

Chapter 7

Symptoms of Lung Disorders

Chapter Contents

Section 7.1

Cough

Is coughing normal or abnormal?

It is normal to cough occasionally. Excessive coughing or coughing that brings up blood or thick, discolored mucus is abnormal. Abnormal coughing can also leave you feeling exhausted or light-headed, cause chest or abdominal discomfort, or even cause you to "wet" yourself.

What causes cough?

Whether coughing is normal or abnormal, it has a purpose. Coughing is the body's way of keeping foreign matter from getting down into your lungs—like when you swallow a piece of food "the wrong way" and immediately cough it up. Coughing also helps to clear excessive mucus from your air passages. You may have excessive mucus in your air passages if you are a smoker, if you have a cold or other respiratory infection, or if your normal mucus-clearing mechanisms do not work properly. Even if your coughing is not productive, it is a signal that something is wrong and that you need to see your doctor.

How does the body know when to make you cough?

The body has a cough "trigger." Foreign matter or excessive mucus in your air passages irritates special nerve endings in your respiratory tract. When these nerve endings are irritated, they signal the body to cough.

What is the cause if a person cannot stop coughing?

Doctors divide coughing into three different categories, based on how long the cough has gone on. They call these categories acute (for coughing of less than three weeks), subacute (for coughing of three to eight weeks), and chronic (for coughing of more than eight weeks).

Acute cough (less than three weeks): Most often, caused by a "common cold." It is usually worse for the first few days of a cold, then gradually goes away in one or two weeks, as you get over the cold.

Subacute cough (three to eight weeks): Often, a cough that lingers after a cold or other respiratory tract infection is over. A subacute cough may eventually go away without treatment but may need to be treated by a doctor after its cause is diagnosed. An example of a subacute cough that requires treatment is one that persists after whooping cough.

Chronic cough (more than eight weeks): Due to one or more of the conditions described in more detail below. The most common causes are upper airway cough syndrome (UACS), asthma, and gastroesophageal reflux disease (GERD). Chronic cough is also common in smokers.

Why is whooping cough (pertussis) a common cause of subacute cough in adults? Isn't whooping cough a childhood disease of the past?

Most of us think of whooping cough as a disease of childhood, and most of us were vaccinated against it when we were children. However, the commonly used whooping cough vaccine gives protection for less than ten years. Unless you were revaccinated as an adult, you can probably get whooping cough. U.S. government health authorities say that 28 percent of whooping cough cases are in adults.

Whooping cough gets its name from the loud noise that patients make when they cough. A fit of coughing ends with a loud noise when the patient takes a breath. This coughing can cause frequent vomiting.

There is a new safe and effective whooping cough vaccine that is recommended for adults up to sixty-five years old. You should ask your physician if you should receive it. Antibiotics are effective in whooping cough only when given early in the infection. A vaccine prevents the disease.

What about the causes of chronic cough?

The most common causes are UACS, asthma, and GERD.

Upper airway cough syndrome (UACS): UACS includes conditions that cause cough by affecting the nose, sinuses, or throat. They stimulate cough nerve endings by a combination of postnasal drip, irritation, or inflammation of the tissues. Upper respiratory tract infection, allergies, and exposure to environmental irritants, such as dusts and gases, are the usual cause of UACS.

Asthma: Asthma is a disease in which the air passages of the lungs are inflamed and narrowed. This happens in response to "triggers," such as allergens (pollen, dust mites, many others), cold air, or infections. Airway narrowing and increased "twitchiness" (or responsiveness to a "trigger") can make the airway narrow and cause coughing.

Gastroesophageal reflux disease (GERD): GERD is caused when stomach juice backs up from the stomach into the esophagus, the tube that carries food from your mouth and throat down into your stomach. Stomach juice contains acid and enzymes that help to digest the food you swallow. If it backs up (refluxes) into your throat, it can cause burning pain and cause you to cough. The burning pain is sometimes called "heartburn." However, most people who have chronic cough from GERD do not have heartburn. This is called "silent GERD."

What about smoking as a cause of cough?

"Smoker's cough" is often due to a lung disease called chronic bronchitis, a disease most commonly caused by cigarette smoking. Irritation from the smoke causes increased mucus production and inflammation of the large air passages of the lungs. Most smokers do not seek medical attention for this cough, because they assume it is from smoking. Sometimes, however, a smoker is coughing from another cause. Just as in nonsmokers, the cough could be from UACS, asthma, or GERD, but it also could be a warning of an even more serious disorder, like lung cancer.

If you are coughing from cigarette smoking and chronic bronchitis, will the cough go away if you stop smoking?

Typically, it will, but it can take four weeks to as long as a few months. If the cough seems different from your usual "smoker's cough," or if it persists despite stopping smoking for a month or longer, it definitely should be checked out by your doctor.

What other conditions cause chronic cough?

There are many other causes, but only a few occur often enough to discuss in this overview. The following are some of these more frequent causes:

- Nonasthmatic eosinophilic bronchitis has some similarities to asthma, but its only significant symptom is cough. It is seen more frequently in countries outside the United States but should be considered, especially if UACS, asthma, GERD, and cigarette smoking have been eliminated as causes of the coughing.

- An important cause of chronic cough is related to a class of medication often used to treat high blood pressure or heart problems. This group of drugs is known as angiotensin-converting enzyme inhibitors, or ACE inhibitors. They can produce a very annoying cough, often associated with throat irritation. The cough may not occur until a person has been on the medication for many months. It will always go away within days to weeks once the medication is stopped.

- Bronchiectasis is a disease in which parts of the lower air passages are damaged, dilated, and prone to recurrent infection. It can cause a cough that persists after a respiratory tract infection, lung cancer, and inflammatory or scarring diseases of the lungs.

- Chronic cough can also be due to heart failure.

Can you have more than one cause of chronic cough at the same time?

Absolutely. In fact, it is common for two causes to be present simultaneously, and, sometimes, even three or more will be present.

Is it important to determine the specific cause(s) of a chronic cough?

Yes. Chronic coughing can be more than annoying. It can lead to complications, such as fatigue, sweating, and even broken ribs from really hard coughing. It can make you worry that something may be seriously wrong with your health. The best way to get rid of your cough and these complications is to treat the underlying cause(s).

What is the best way for a doctor to determine the cause(s) of a cough?

A combination of selected tests and targeted treatments allow the specific cause(s) of a chronic cough to be determined in the vast majority of cases. A lung specialist (pulmonologist) should be able to determine the cause(s) in about 90 percent of cases. When a cause cannot be determined, a referral and visit to a cough specialist (pulmonologist with particular expertise in cough) will usually result in an answer in the majority of these more difficult cases.

Does treatment for chronic cough usually work?

Yes. In over 90 percent of cases, the cough will be greatly improved or disappear entirely with treatment. The key is to use the correct medications at the right dose for each cause of the cough. The length of treatment is also very important. Whether the cause is a UACS, asthma, GERD, or one of the less common causes, it is not unusual for treatment to take weeks, to even months, to be completely successful. This is particularly true for GERD.

What are the main treatments for causes of chronic cough?

The best treatment for UACS is antihistamines. It is important that the correct antihistamine is used when treating the UACS. This is because all antihistamines are not equal. The older antihistamines are the sedating type—they make you sleepy. The newer antihistamines are the nonsedating type—they do not make you sleepy. A common error is to use one of the newer nonsedating-type antihistamines as part of the treatment of UACS. Unless the cause of the UACS is an allergy (only a small percentage of cases), the old-fashioned, more sedating, antihistamines work much better. If the dose is gradually increased, and you stay on the medication consistently, the sedating effect is not a significant problem, in most cases.

The cough from asthma responds best to treatment with inhaled corticosteroids.

An important part of the treatment of GERD is a medication called proton-pump inhibitors that reduce or eliminate acid production in the stomach. However, GERD can cause cough even if the acid in your stomach is eliminated. Use of proton-pump inhibitors does not guarantee that the cough will improve or disappear. Changes in diet or elevating the head of your bed on eight-inch blocks may be needed for successful treatment of GERD.

Factors in treatment of other causes include completely stopping smoking, withdrawing ACE inhibitors, if they are found at fault, and eliminating environmental irritants or allergens.

If there is more than one cause of cough, it is critical to treat all the causes with the right medications at the same time.

Can a chronic cough be due to psychological problems or a habit?

Both "psychogenic" and habit cough can occur, but both are quite uncommon. In most cases, some specific abnormality is causing the chronic cough. A diagnosis of psychogenic or habit cough should usually only be made when other, more common, causes have been eliminated and the psychological (or habit) explanation seems to make sense to both the physician and the patient.

When the cause of chronic coughing is not determined, patients can become anxious and depressed. Because of this, patients and doctors need to understand that anxiety and depression may be due to the coughing, rather than causing it.

Is cough contagious?

There are causes of cough due to infections, such as tuberculosis or whooping cough, that can be contagious. In the overwhelming majority of cases, however, a cough is not a risk to anyone else.

What about the use of cough medications?

Most so-called cough medications are not very effective. Although it is usually most effective to treat the specific cause of the cough, cough medications can be helpful. When cough is not due to the common cold, most effective cough medications, by far, are narcotics, such as codeine. They should be used only when there is no effective treatment for the cause of the cough (such as some cancers involving the lung) and the cough is causing the patient a lot of distress (such as inability to sleep).

What tests are done to diagnose the cause(s) of chronic cough?

A chest x-ray is recommended for all patients with chronic cough. If the x-ray has negative results, your doctor may decide not to order additional tests until he or she has seen your response to therapy. If you do not respond to treatment as expected, your doctor may also order a variety of other tests. These may include breathing tests, blood studies, sputum studies, other x-rays (such as those of the sinuses), barium swallow, and other gastrointestinal tests, such as 24-hour monitoring of the function of the esophagus, a computed axial tomography (CAT) scan of the lungs, or a bronchoscopy.

Breathing tests are done primarily to see if you might have asthma as a cause of cough. If the initial test shows you have normal lung function, then a test may be done to detect overactivity of the air passages of the lungs. This test is called a bronchoprovocation challenge, and it should be done before asthma is ruled out as the cause of your cough. This test involves breathing a medication (most often one called methacholine). You breathe this medication in, and then the breathing test is repeated. If you have asthma, your lung function will decrease at least 20 percent for a short period of time. The decrease can usually be reversed quickly by inhaling a common asthma medication.

A bronchoscopy involves putting a thin, flexible tube, containing a tiny video camera, through the nose or mouth, down into the air passages of the lungs. This is a relatively painless and safe test when done by a lung specialist. This test can detect tumors, infections, foreign bodies, or other abnormalities of the lower air passages that could be causing chronic cough. It is only needed in a small number of patients who usually have a significant abnormality on the initial chest x-ray. When the initial chest x-ray has normal results, a bronchoscopy result will also typically be normal, and, therefore, it should not be one of the first tests done. However, later in the workup, if the common causes have been eliminated, a bronchoscopy test should be done, because, occasionally, an uncommon cause of the chronic cough is discovered by this test.

Section 7.2

Hemoptysis

Hemoptysis is simply a medical term for coughing up blood. The blood can appear as flecks, streaks, or can be quite massive in amount. Hemoptysis can be caused by many things, but it is important to make sure that the blood really is from the lungs and not from other structures like the nose or the gastrointestinal system. If you ever cough up blood, it is important to see your doctor so that they can investigate the possible cause.

What Is Hemoptysis?

While it may seem simple enough, coughing up blood (also known as hemoptysis) has a very specific definition as it means that the blood is coming from the lungs, below the vocal cords. Hemoptysis can result in coughing up blood as small flecks, streaks or even as a massive bleed. Sometimes it can accompany mucus or sputum. To make sure that it is really hemoptysis then other sources of the blood such as the nose, throat, or the gastrointestinal system have to be excluded.

What Causes Hemoptysis?

There are many different causes of hemoptysis. Some of the causes are:

- The most common cause is an acute infection, especially in exacerbations of chronic obstructive pulmonary disease (COPD), usually secondary to smoking

- Chronic bronchitis

- Bronchiectasis, where the blood is often mixed with thick, smelly sputum

- Pulmonary embolism (a blood clot in the lungs)

- Lobar pneumonia, usually described as having "rust colored" sputum

- Pulmonary edema (fluid in the lungs): pink, frothy sputum secondary to heart conditions such as mitral stenosis or left ventricular failure

- Lung cancer

- Tuberculosis

- Inhaled foreign body

- Rupture of a blood vessel after vigorous coughing

In about one quarter of cases, even after thorough investigation the cause of the bleeding is never found.

When to See a Doctor about Hemoptysis

Many, if not all of the causes of hemoptysis require looking into by a doctor and there are many very serious conditions that can lead to it. If you ever have an episode of hemoptysis it is important to see your doctor so that he or she can decide whether it is worth worrying about or not.

Tests and Examinations for Hemoptysis

Your doctor will want to examine your heart and your lungs for any signs of diseases that can cause you to cough up blood. He or she will probably also want to look in your nose to make sure that the blood is not coming from there (it can sometimes be hard to tell!). He or she will also want to take your temperature, as a fever can be a sign of infection.

Your doctor will usually want to do a chest x-ray and may want to do a computed tomography (CT) scan or bronchoscopy (where a tube is inserted into the airway allowing the doctor to see what is inside) depending on how severe the hemoptysis is, or what they find after taking your history and doing an examination.

Section 7.3

Dyspnea

Why Do I Have Shortness of Breath?

Shortness of breath (dyspnea)—the feeling like you cannot get enough air—has many causes. Many people experience shortness of breath once in a while. However, call your doctor if it is severe, limits your activities, or does not go away. This information is designed to help you understand what causes shortness of breath. There is also information about some of the tests your doctor may use to discover what is causing your breathing problem.

First Tests

In order to find the cause of your shortness of breath, your doctor will start by asking you questions about your medical history and, then, will do a physical examination. Next, your doctor will check the amount of oxygen in your blood. This is a simple test done by placing a sensor on your finger or earlobe while you are sitting and walking. Once those tests are done, your doctor may then perform one or more of the following screening tests:

- **Chest x-ray:** To look at the lungs.

- **Breathing tests (called pulmonary function tests):** To see how well the lungs get air in and out. These tests can help identify problems of the airways or bronchial tubes, such as COPD (chronic obstructive pulmonary disease), asthma, scarring of the lungs (fibrosis), or other breathing problems.

- **Blood tests:** To check for anemia or low blood count.

- **Heart tracing (called an electrocardiogram or ECG):** To see if there is any heart damage.

Additional Tests

Sometimes, even after the first tests, the cause of the shortness of breath is still not known. Other common tests for patients with shortness of breath include the following:

- **Computed tomography (CT) scan of the chest:** Shows more detail than a chest x-ray and may show scarring in the lungs (interstitial lung disease). Sometimes CT scans are done with contrast. This means a dye is injected into a vein to give an even more detailed view. This may be done if your doctor thinks there may be a blood clot in your lungs.

- If your doctor suspects you may have asthma, you may be given a medication that affects the bronchial tubes while breathing tests are done.

- **Bronchoscopy:** If the breathing tests show that something is blocking your airway, your doctor may need to look into your airways with a lighted scope. This procedure is called a bronchoscopy. This test may also be necessary, along with a biopsy of the lung, if the CT scan shows areas which are not normal.

- **Muscle and nerve testing:** To see if your muscles or nerves are causing weak breathing muscles (this is rare).

- **Heart tests:** Many times, shortness of breath is not caused by a lung problem but by a heart problem instead. The most common heart tests for patients with shortness of breath include:

  - *Echocardiogram:* Ultrasound waves are used to get a detailed look at the heart valves and how well the heart pumps.

  - *Stress test:* Walking on a treadmill to check the heart during exercise.

  - *Nuclear medicine testing:* Another way to get a look at how well the heart is working.

  - *Maximum cardiopulmonary exercise test:* This means exercising on a treadmill or bicycle until you cannot go any further. This test helps your doctor see how well your whole body is working during activity.

More Causes of Shortness of Breath

The heart tests help your doctor to identify problems, such as the following:

- Leaky heart valves.

- Stiff heart muscles (diastolic dysfunction).

- Heart muscles that do not get enough blood during exercise (ischemic heart disease).

- An opening in the heart that should not be there (patent foramen ovale or atrial septal defect). This condition makes it difficult for the lungs to get enough oxygen into the blood.

- A connection between veins and arteries in the lungs or somewhere else in the body that should not be there (arteriovenous malformation or AVM).

- High pressure on the right side of the heart. This can be from a lung problem or from blood clots or other blockages in the lungs (chronic pulmonary embolism or pulmonary vasculitis). High pressures in the right side of the heart can also be from an unknown cause (primary pulmonary hypertension).

Other possible causes of shortness of breath include the following:

- **Postnasal discharge:** When sinus drainage collects in the back of your throat.

- **Gastroesophageal reflux (GER):** When stomach acids "splash" up into your throat.

- **Deconditioning:** When you have a low level of physical fitness.

- **Hyperventilation:** When breathing is too fast, often as a result of anxiety or feelings of panic.

Shortness of Breath: Common Causes

- Brain (psychological):
  - Stress/anxiety
- Heart (cardiac):
  - Leaky heart valves
  - Fluid in lungs
  - Holes between heart chambers
- Lungs (pulmonary):
  - Asthma
  - Emphysema

- Blood clots in lungs
- High blood pressure in lungs
- Other causes:
  - Out of shape
  - Rapid weight gain

Remember, shortness of breath should not be ignored. Since it has many causes, it may take awhile for your doctor to find the exact reason for your breathing trouble. You may even need to repeat certain tests. Once a cause has been determined, your doctor will talk to you about how best to treat your condition.

Section 7.4

Stridor

"Stridor," by Steven D. Handler, M.D., M.B.E., February 2006.
Reprinted with permission from The Children's Hospital of Philadelphia (www.chop.edu), © 2006.

What is stridor?

Stridor is a high-pitched sound that is usually heard when a child breathes in (inspiration). It is usually caused by an obstruction or narrowing in your child's upper airway. The upper airway consists of the following structures in the upper respiratory system:

- **Nose.**
- **Mouth.**
- **Throat (pharynx and larynx).**
- **Pharynx:** The muscle-lined space that connects the nose and mouth to the larynx and esophagus (eating tube).
- **Larynx:** Also known as the voice box, the larynx is a cylindrical grouping of cartilage, muscles, and soft tissue which contains

the vocal cords. The larynx is the upper opening into the windpipe (trachea), the passageway to the lungs. The subglottic space is immediately below the vocal cords. It is the narrowest part of the upper airway. The epiglottis is a flap of soft tissue and cartilage that folds over the vocal cords to prevent food and irritants from entering the lungs.

- **Trachea (windpipe):** A tube that extends from the voice box to the bronchi in the lungs.

The sound of stridor depends on location of the obstruction in the upper respiratory tract. Sometimes, the stridor is heard when the child breathes in (inspiration) and can also be heard when the child breathes out (expiration).

What are the causes of stridor?

There are many different causes of stridor. Some of the causes are diseases, while others are problems with the anatomical structure of the child's airway. The upper airway in children is narrower than that of an adult and therefore more susceptible to problems with obstruction.

The following are some of the more common causes of stridor in children.

- Congenital causes (problems present at birth), including:
  - **Laryngomalacia:** Parts of the larynx (voice box) are floppy and collapse causing partial airway obstruction. The child will usually outgrow this condition by the time he or she is eighteen months old. In rare instances, some children may need surgery.
  - **Subglottic stenosis:** The subglottis is the space in the larynx (voice box) right below the vocal cords. If the area is too small, this is referred to as subglottic stenosis. A child can be born with this problem (congenital subglottic stenosis) or it can result from trauma such as prolonged tracheal intubation—placing a tube into the trachea, or "windpipe" (acquired subglottic stenosis). Subglottic stenosis can prevent adequate movement of air into the child's lungs and cause stridor. Symptoms often worsen with upper respiratory infection or colds. The child may outgrow mild subglottic stenosis, but more severe cases will require surgical intervention.

- **Subglottic hemangioma:** A hemangioma is a mass made of blood vessels; it is similar to a strawberry birthmark or "stork bite." Hemangiomas usually grow rapidly for six to twelve months and then shrink. If a hemangioma in the subglottic space causes airway obstruction, the child may need medical and/or surgical treatment.

- **Vascular rings:** The trachea, or windpipe, may be compressed by an artery inside the chest. Surgery may be required to alleviate this condition.

- Infectious causes:

  - **Croup:** Croup is an infection caused by a virus that leads to swelling in the subglottic space (the area below the vocal cords.) It causes breathing problems. Croup is caused by a variety of different viruses, most commonly the parainfluenza virus. Treatment includes breathing humidified air and the occasional use of oral steroids.

  - **Epiglottitis:** Epiglottitis is an acute life-threatening bacterial infection that results in swelling and inflammation of the epiglottis. (The epiglottis is an elastic cartilage structure at the back of the tongue that helps to prevent food from entering the windpipe when swallowing.) This causes breathing problems that can progressively worsen and may, ultimately, lead to airway obstruction. There is so much swelling that air cannot get in or out of the lungs, resulting in a medical emergency. Epiglottitis is usually caused by the bacteria *Haemophilus influenzae*, and now is rare because children are routinely vaccinated against this bacteria.

  - **Bronchitis:** Bronchitis is an inflammation of the breathing tubes (airways), called bronchi, that causes increased production of mucus and other changes. Acute bronchitis is usually caused by infectious agents such as bacteria or viruses. It may also be caused by physical or chemical agents—dusts, allergens, strong fumes—and those from chemical cleaning compounds or tobacco smoke.

  - **Severe tonsillitis:** The tonsils are small, oval pieces of tissue that are located in the back of the mouth on the side of the throat. Tonsils help fight infections by producing antibodies. Tonsillitis is an inflammation of the tonsils. When the inflamed tonsils get very large, airway obstruction can occur.

- **Abscess in the throat:** An abscess in the throat is a collection of pus surrounded by inflamed tissue. If the abscess is large enough, it may narrow the airway to a critically small opening. These abscesses may occur next to the tonsil or in the soft tissue of the neck surrounding the airway.

- Traumatic causes:
  - **Foreign bodies:** Foreign bodies in the breathing tract may cause severe airway symptoms. Foreign bodies are any objects placed in the mouth that do not belong there. For example, a peanut in the trachea (windpipe) may close off the breathing passages and result in suffocation and death.

- Other causes:
  - **Trauma (injury) to the neck:** Trauma to the neck may cause a fracture to the larynx or bleeding into the airway.
  - **Swallowing a harmful substance:** Swallowing a harmful substance (acid, lye) may cause damage to the airways.

How is stridor diagnosed?

Stridor is usually diagnosed relying on the medical history and physical examination of your child. It is important to remember that stridor is a symptom of some underlying problem or condition. If your child has stridor, your child's physician may order some of the following tests to help determine the cause of the stridor:

- **Blood tests.**
- **X-ray of the chest and/or neck.**
- **Pulse oximetry:** An oximeter is a small machine that measures the amount of oxygen in the blood. To obtain this measurement, a small sensor (like an adhesive bandage) is taped onto a finger or toe. When the machine is on, a small red light can be seen in the sensor. The sensor is painless and the red light does not get hot.
- **Culture:** Sputum culture is a diagnostic test performed on the material that is coughed up from the lungs and into the mouth. A sputum culture is often performed to determine if an infection is present. A nose or throat culture may also be obtained.
- **Endoscopic evaluation of the airway:** Visualization of the upper airway that is obtained by inserting a small, flexible,

lighted instrument into the child's nose to examine the nose, pharynx, and larynx. Topical anesthesia may be required for this procedure.

The specific treatment for this condition depends on many factors and is tailored for each child. Please discuss your child's condition, treatment options and your preferences with your child's physician or healthcare provider.

Treatment may include:

- Referral to an ear, nose and throat specialist (otolaryngologist) for further evaluation (if your child has a history of stridor);

- Surgery;

- Medications by mouth or injection (to help decrease the swelling in the airways);

- Hospitalization and emergency surgery may be necessary depending on the severity of the stridor.

Section 7.5

Wheezing

Alternative Names

Sibilant rhonchi

Definition

Wheezing is a high-pitched whistling sound during breathing. It occurs when air flows through narrowed breathing tubes.

Considerations

Wheezing is a sign that a person may be having breathing problems. The sound of wheezing is most obvious when exhaling (breathing out), but may be heard when taking a breath (inhaling).

Wheezing most often comes from the small bronchial tubes (breathing tubes deep in the chest), but it may be due to a blockage in larger airways or in those with certain vocal cord problems.

Causes

- Asthma
- Bronchiectasis
- Bronchiolitis
- Bronchitis
- Gastroesophageal reflux disease
- Viral infection, especially in infants younger than two years old
- Pneumonia
- Emphysema (COPD), especially when a respiratory infection is present

- Smoking
- Insect sting which causes an allergic reaction
- Medications (particularly aspirin)
- Breathing a foreign object into the lungs
- Heart failure (cardiac asthma)

Home Care

Take all of your medications, especially respiratory inhalers, as directed.

Sitting in an area where there is moist, heated air may help relieve some symptoms. This can be done running a hot shower or by using a vaporizer.

When to Contact a Medical Professional

- Wheezing is occurring for the first time
- Wheezing is associated with significant shortness of breath, bluish skin color, or mental status changes
- Wheezing is a recurrent, unexplained problem
- Wheezing is caused by an allergic reaction to a bite or medication

If wheezing is severe or is accompanied by severe shortness of breath, you may have to go directly to the nearest emergency department.

What to Expect at Your Office Visit

Your doctor will perform a physical examination and ask questions, such as:

- When did the wheezing begin?
- How long does it last?
- Does it occur often? Daily?
- At what time of day does it occur?
- Is it worse at night or in the early morning?
- What does the wheezing sound like?
- Does it make breathing difficult?
- Does it require stopping all physical activity?

- Does it go away without treatment?
- What seems to cause it?
  - Eating certain foods?
  - Taking certain medications?
- Do any of the following things make it worse?
  - Exercise
  - Stress
  - Being around pollens, insects, dust, chemicals (perfumes, cosmetics)
  - Being in cold air
  - A cold or flu
- What helps relieve it?
  - Rest?
  - Medications such as bronchodilators?
- Are any of the other symptoms present?
  - Fever
  - Coughing
  - Swelling of the lips or tongue
  - Panic or confusion
  - Loss of voice
  - Loss of consciousness
  - Bluish color to lips or nails
  - Stuffy nose
  - Puffy, red eyes
  - Insect bite
- Did you have an episode of choking?
- Is there a history of asthma or allergies?
- What medications do you take?
- Have you been around tobacco smoke?
- Have you recently been sick?

The physical examination may include listening to the lung sounds (auscultation). If your child is the one with symptoms, the doctor will make sure he or she did not swallow a foreign object.

Tests that may be done include:

- Chest x-ray;

- Pulmonary function tests;

- Blood studies, possibly including arterial blood gases.

Your doctor may prescribe drugs to relieve narrowing of the airways, such as albuterol.

A hospital stay may be needed if:

- Breathing is particularly difficult;

- The person needs to be closely watched by medical personnel;

- Medicines need to be given by IV (intravenous line);

- Supplemental oxygen is required.

Section 7.6

Cyanosis

What Is Cyanosis?

Cyanosis refers to a blue or purple hue to the skin. It is most easily observed on the lips, tongue, and fingernails.

Cyanosis indicates there may be decreased oxygen in the bloodstream. It may suggest a problem with the lungs, but most often is a result of mixing blue and red blood due to defects of the heart or great vessels. Cyanosis is a finding based on observation, not a laboratory test.

Cyanosis Types

"Acrocyanosis" refers to the presence of cyanosis in the extremities, particularly the palms of the hands and the soles of the feet. It can also be seen on the skin around the lips. Acrocyanosis is often normal in babies, provided it is not accompanied by central cyanosis.

"Central cyanosis" refers to the presence of cyanosis on "central" parts of the body, including lips, mouth, head, and torso. Central cyanosis is never normal, and is almost always associated with a decrease in blood oxygen.

Why Cyanosis Occurs

Central cyanosis occurs because blood changes color in the presence (or absence) of oxygen. Red blood has ample oxygen whereas blood with decreased oxygen turns blue or purple. Red blood flowing through capillaries in the skin produces a healthy red-pink color.

Blue blood causes a blue-purple (or cyan) tint to the skin.

What Conditions Cause Cyanosis?

Cyanosis is usually caused by abnormalities of the heart, the lungs, or the blood. Under normal conditions the red (oxygenated) blood delivers oxygen. The returning (blue) blood is shipped to the lungs to collect more oxygen.

Abnormalities in the lungs can cause some blood to flow through them without collecting oxygen.

Heart abnormalities can cause some blood to bypass the lungs altogether.

Abnormalities in the blood can decrease its ability to absorb oxygen. The common denominator is that blue blood is pumped to the body.

Finally, having far too many oxygen carrying cells (polycythemia) can also cause cyanosis.

Does All Heart Disease Cause Cyanosis in Children?

Not all heart or lung disease is associated with cyanosis. The absence of cyanosis may be reassuring, but it does not exclude the possibility of a heart defect.

Common Questions and Answers

1. Can I tell if my child has cyanosis? Parents can usually recognize cyanosis, but it is not always easy (even for physicians). This is especially true in children of darker complexions. The best way to look for cyanosis is to look at the nail beds, lips,

and tongue, and to compare them to someone with a similar complexion. Usually a parent or sibling serves as a good comparison.

2. What if I think my child has cyanosis? First, don't panic. Second, examine your child. Cyanosis limited exclusively to the hands, the feet, and the area around the lips is known as acrocyanosis and is a normal finding in babies. Cyanosis on the lips, tongue, head, or torso is central cyanosis, and should be promptly evaluated by a physician.

3. What will my physician do if cyanosis is present? It depends. First, your doctor will likely gather more historical information and perform a physical examination. Depending on the findings your physician may be able to provide reassurance, or he/she may determine that additional evaluation or a consultation is necessary. Laboratory evaluation may include blood work or oximetry. Oximetry painlessly "measures" the color of blood (without needles) to determine how much oxygen it contains. The test is performed by placing a special lighted probe on the finger. Alternatively, your doctor may decide that a consultation with a specialist is in order. Depending on his findings, he may request the services of a heart or lung specialist, the emergency room, or doctors specialized in intensive care.

Section 7.7

Clubbing of the Fingers or Toes

Clubbing is a thickening of the flesh under the toenails and fingernails. The nail curves downward, similar to the shape of the round part of an upside-down spoon.

Considerations

Clubbing is associated with a wide number of diseases. It is most often noted in heart and lung diseases that cause a lower-than-normal amount of oxygen in the blood.

Clubbing may also be due to lung cancer, and diseases of the liver and gastrointestinal tract.

Clubbing may also occur in families. In this case it may not be due to an underlying disease.

Causes

- Bronchiectasis
- Celiac disease
- Cirrhosis
- Congenital heart disease (cyanotic type)
  - Tetralogy of Fallot
  - Total anomalous venous return
  - Transposition of the great vessels
  - Tricuspid atresia
  - Truncus arteriosus
- Crohn disease
- Cystic fibrosis
- Lung abscess

- Lung cancer
- Pulmonary fibrosis

Home Care

There is no specific treatment for the clubbing itself. Home care depends on the diagnosis.

When to Contact a Medical Professional

If you notice clubbing, call your health care provider.

What to Expect at Your Office Visit

A person with clubbing generally has other symptoms and signs that define a specific condition. Diagnosis of that condition is based on:

- Family history
- Medical history
- Physical exam that looks at the lungs and chest

Medical history questions may include:

- Do you have any breathing difficulty?
- Does it affect the fingers, toes, or both?
- Is it becoming more noticeable?
- Is the skin ever bluish colored?
- What other symptoms are also present?
- When did you first notice this?

The following tests may be done:

- Arterial blood gas
- Chest computed tomography (CT) scan
- Chest x-ray
- Echocardiogram
- Electrocardiogram (EKG)
- Pulmonary function tests

References

Zipes DP, Libby P, Bonow RO, Braunwald E, eds. *Braunwald's Heart Disease: A Textbook of Cardiovascular Medicine*, 7th ed. St. Louis, Mo.: WB Saunders; 2005:78–79.

Murray J, Nadel J. *Textbook of Respiratory Medicine*. 3rd ed. Philadelphia, Pa.: WB Saunders; 2000:506.

Spicknall KE. Clubbing: an update on diagnosis, differential diagnosis, pathophysiology, and clinical relevance. *J Am Acad Dermatol*. 2005; 52(6): 1020–28.

Section 7.8

Chest Pain

Chest pain is one of the most commonly presented problems to the doctor. It is both a common and threatening problem because in many instances the cause is potentially serious, especially in chest pain of sudden onset. The main causes of acute chest pain include heart, gut, respiratory, and muscular causes. As heart disease is the leading cause of death in Western nations it is important for patients at risk to seek medical advice if they do experience chest pain.

Causes of Chest Pain

Chest pain is discomfort or pain that you feel anywhere along the front of your body between your neck and upper abdomen and can be considered in terms of whether it is caused by a heart problem or a problem in another part of the body. Many people with chest pain fear a heart attack. However, there are many possible causes of chest pain. Some causes are mildly inconvenient, while other causes are serious, even life-threatening. Any organ or tissue in the chest can be the source of pain, including the heart, lungs, esophagus, muscles, ribs, tendons, or nerves.

Angina is a type of heart-related chest pain. This pain occurs because your heart is not getting enough blood and oxygen. Angina pain can be similar to the pain of a heart attack, but is generally less severe and shorter in duration. Angina is called stable angina when chest pain begins at a predictable level of activity, for instance, when you walk up a steep hill. However, if chest pain happens unexpectedly after light activity or during rest, this is called unstable angina. This is a more dangerous form of angina—if this occurs, you should seek medical attention as soon as possible.

Heart-related chest pain can also be caused by a problem with the heart valves, or can occur due to irritation of the lining around the heart after a person has had an infection.

Other causes of chest pain include:

- Pneumonia (infection in the lung), pulmonary embolism (caused by a blood clot to the lung), pneumothorax (the collapse of a small area of a lung), or inflammation of the lining around the lung (pleurisy). In these cases, the chest pain often worsens when you take a deep breath.

- Strain or inflammation of the muscles and tendons between the ribs.

- Referred pain from back/spine problems which goes to the chest.

- Anxiety and rapid breathing.

- Problems with the digestive system, such as indigestion or heartburn and gallstones.

- Shingles can also cause chest pain (usually accompanied by a rash a few days later).

Patients should seek medical attention if they experience any of the following:

- Sudden crushing, squeezing, tightening, or pressure in your chest

- Nausea, dizziness, sweating, a racing heart, or shortness of breath.

- They know they have angina and their chest discomfort is suddenly more intense, brought on by lighter activity, or lasts longer than usual.

- Angina symptoms occur at rest.

- They have sudden sharp chest pain with shortness of breath, especially after a long trip, a stretch of bed rest (for example, following an operation), or other lack of movement that can lead to formation of a blood clot in the leg.

- Chest-wall pain persists for longer than three to five days.

A person's risk of heart attack is higher if they have a family history of heart disease, smoke or use cocaine, have high cholesterol, high blood pressure, or diabetes.

Treatment of Chest Pain

Emergency measures will be taken, if necessary. Hospitalization may be required in difficult or serious cases, or when the cause of the pain is unclear. Normally, the doctor will ask some questions about the pain and the patient's past health, perform a physical examination, and monitor their vital signs (temperature, pulse, rate of breathing, blood pressure). Following this, the patient will normally be put on oxygen, and have some tests done (blood tests, chest x-ray, and electrocardiogram (ECG) of the heart). If the pain is severe, medications are given to control it. Treatment will depend on the results of the tests and the doctor's findings. Sometimes, further tests are necessary, or the patient may be started on some new medications. The use of spinal cord stimulation is currently being investigated for treatment of chest pain in patients with angina pectoris.

If the chest pain was caused by a heart problem, the patient may be advised on ways to improve their health and hopefully prevent more heart problems in the future.

Measures include:

- Achieve and maintain normal weight;

- Control high blood pressure, high cholesterol, and diabetes;

- Avoid cigarette smoking and second-hand smoke;

- Eat a diet low in saturated and hydrogenated fats and cholesterol, and high in starches, fiber, fruits, and vegetables;

- Exercise three hours per week or more (such as thirty minutes per day, six days per week);

- Reduce stress.

Drugs used in the treatment of chest pain:

• Morphine sulfate;

• Aspirin.

Diseases presenting with chest pain include:

• Mitral regurgitation (MR);

• Aortic stenosis (AS);

• Cardiomyopathy;

• Pericarditis and pericardial disease;

• Angina pectoris and unstable angina;

• Myocarditis;

• Congestive heart failure;

• Arrhythmia;

• Adenocarcinoma of the lung;

• Heart disease;

• Chronic heart failure;

• Coronary heart disease (CHD);

• Myocardial infarction (MI)—heart attack.

Chapter 8

Tests to Assess Lung Function

Chapter Contents

Section 8.1

Arterial Blood Gases

Reprinted from "Blood Gases," © 2008 A.D.A.M., Inc.
Reprinted with permission. Updated March 1, 2007.

Blood gases is a test done to measure how much oxygen and carbon dioxide is in your blood. It also looks at the acidity (pH) of the blood. Usually, blood gases look at blood from an artery. In rarer cases, blood from a vein may be used.

How the Test is Performed

The test is performed using a small needle to collect a sample of blood from an artery. The sample may be collected from the radial artery in the wrist, the femoral artery in the groin, or the brachial artery in the arm.

Before blood is drawn, the health care provider may test circulation to the hand (if the wrist is the site). After the blood is drawn, pressure applied to the puncture site for a few minutes stops the bleeding.

The test must be sent to the laboratory for analysis quickly to ensure accurate results.

How to Prepare for the Test

There is no special preparation. If the person having the test is on oxygen, the oxygen concentration must remain constant for twenty minutes before the test. If the test is done without oxygen, the oxygen must be turned off for twenty minutes before the sample is taken to ensure accurate test results.

How the Test Will Feel

The health care provider will insert a needle through the skin into the artery. You can choose to have anesthesia at the site. You may feel brief cramping or throbbing at the puncture site. The needle will be withdrawn after the sample is collected.

Pressure applied over the site for five to ten minutes helps prevent bleeding. A bandage will be placed over the puncture site. The health care provider will watch the site for signs of bleeding or circulation problems.

Why the Test is Performed

The test is used to evaluate respiratory diseases and conditions that affect the lungs. It helps determine the effectiveness of oxygen therapy. The acid-base component of the test also gives information about kidney function.

Normal Results

Values at sea level:

- Partial pressure of oxygen (PaO_2): 75–100 mm Hg;
- Partial pressure of carbon dioxide ($PaCO_2$): 35–45 mm Hg;
- A pH of 7.35–7.45;
- Oxygen saturation (SaO_2): 94–100%;
- Bicarbonate (HCO_3): 22–26 mEq/liter.

Note: mEq/liter = milliequivalents per liter; mm Hg = millimeters of mercury

At altitudes of three thousand feet and above, the oxygen values are lower.

What Abnormal Results Mean

Abnormal results may indicate respiratory, metabolic, or renal diseases. The results may also be abnormal with head or neck injuries, or other traumas that affect breathing.

Risks

In general, there is a very low risk when the procedure is done correctly. There may be bleeding or bruising at the puncture site, or delayed bleeding from the site. Circulatory impairment in the area of the puncture may occur, although it is rare.

Considerations

Tell your health care provider if you notice bleeding, bruising, numbness, tingling, or discoloration at the puncture site. Also let your doctor know if you are taking any blood-thinning medications (anti-coagulants) or aspirin.

References

Ford M, Delaney KA, Ling L, Erickson T. *Clinical Toxicology*. 1st ed. Philadelphia, Pa.: Saunders, 2000.

Mason RJ, Broaddus VC, Murray JF, Nadel JA. *Murray and Nadel's Textbook of Respiratory Medicine*. 4th ed. Philadelphia, Pa.: Saunders, 2005.

Section 8.2

Pulmonary Function Tests

Alternative Names

PFTs; spirometry; spirogram; lung function tests

Definition

Pulmonary function tests are a group of tests that measure how well the lungs take in and release air and how well they move oxygen into the blood.

How the Test Is Performed

In a spirometry test, you breathe into a mouthpiece that is connected to an instrument called a spirometer. The spirometer records the amount and the rate of air that you breathe in and out over a period of time.

For some of the test measurements, you can breathe normally and quietly. Other tests require forced inhalation or exhalation after a deep breath.

Lung volume measurement can be done in two ways:

- The most accurate way is to sit in a sealed, clear box that looks like a telephone booth (body plethysmograph) while breathing in and out into a mouthpiece. Changes in pressure inside the box help determine the lung volume.

- Lung volume can also be measured when you breathe nitrogen or helium gas through a tube for a certain period of time. The concentration of the gas in a chamber attached to the tube is measured to estimate the lung volume.

To measure diffusion capacity, you breathe a harmless gas for a very short time, often one breath. The concentration of the gas in the air you breathe out is then measured. The difference in the amount of gas inhaled and exhaled can help estimate how quickly gas can travel from the lungs into the blood.

How to Prepare for the Test

Do not eat a heavy meal before the test. Do not smoke for four to six hours before the test. You'll get specific instructions if you need to stop using bronchodilators or inhaler medications. You may have to breathe in medication before the test.

How the Test Will Feel

Since the test involves some forced breathing and rapid breathing, you may have some temporary shortness of breath or light-headedness. You breathe through a tight fitting mouthpiece, and you'll have nose clips.

Why the Test Is Performed

Pulmonary function tests are done to:

- Diagnose certain types of lung disease (especially asthma, bronchitis, and emphysema);

- Find the cause of shortness of breath;

- Measure whether exposure to contaminants at work affects lung function.

It also can be done to:

115

- Assess the effect of medication;
- Measure progress in disease treatment.

Spirometry measures airflow. By measuring how much air you exhale, and how quickly, spirometry can evaluate a broad range of lung diseases.

Lung volume measures the amount of air in the lungs without forcibly blowing out. Some lung diseases (such as emphysema and chronic bronchitis) can make the lungs contain too much air. Other lung diseases (such as fibrosis of the lungs and asbestosis) make the lungs scarred and smaller so that they contain too little air.

Testing the diffusion capacity (also called the diffusing capacity of the lung for carbon monoxide, or DLCO) allows the doctor to estimate how well the lungs move oxygen from the air into the bloodstream.

Normal Results

Normal values are based upon your age, height, ethnicity, and sex. Normal results are expressed as a percentage. A value is usually considered abnormal if it is less than 80 percent of your predicted value.

Normal value ranges may vary slightly among different laboratories. Talk to your doctor about the meaning of your specific test results.

What Abnormal Results Mean

Abnormal results usually mean that you may have some chest or lung disease.

Risks

The risk is minimal for most people. There is a small risk of collapsed lung in people with a certain type of lung disease. The test should not be given to a person who has experienced a recent heart attack, or who has certain other types of heart disease.

Considerations

Your cooperation while performing the test is crucial in order to get accurate results. A poor seal around the mouthpiece of the spirometer can give poor results that can't be interpreted. Do not smoke before the test.

References

Mason RJ, Broaddus VC, Murray JF, Nadel JA. *Murray and Nadel's Textbook of Respiratory Medicine*. 4th ed. Philadelphia, Pa.: Saunders, 2005.

Section 8.3

Peak Flow Monitoring

What Is a Peak Flow Meter?

A peak flow meter is a portable, inexpensive, hand-held device used to measure how air flows from your lungs in one "fast blast." In other words, the meter measures your ability to push air out of your lungs.

Peak flow meters may be provided in two ranges to measure the air pushed out of your lungs. A low range peak flow meter is for small children, and a standard range meter is for older children, teenagers, and adults. An adult has much larger airways than a child and needs the larger range.

There are several types of peak flow meters available. Talk to your doctor or pharmacist about which type to use.

Who can Benefit from Using a Peak Flow Meter?

Many doctors believe that people who have asthma can benefit from the use of a peak flow meter. If you need to adjust your daily medication for asthma, a peak flow meter can be an important part of your asthma management plan.

Children as young as three years have been able to use a meter to help manage their asthma. In addition, some people with chronic bronchitis and emphysema may also benefit from the use of a peak flow meter.

Not all physicians use peak flow meters in their management of children and adults with asthma. Many doctors believe a peak flow meter may be of most help for people with moderate and severe asthma. If your asthma is mild or you do not use daily medication, a peak flow meter may not be useful for asthma management.

Why Should I Measure My Peak Flow Rate?

Measurements with a peak flow meter can help you and your doctor monitor your asthma. These measurements can be important and help your doctor prescribe medicines to keep your asthma in control.

A peak flow meter can show you that you may need to change the way you are using your medicines. For example, peak flow readings may help be a signal for you to implement the medication plan you and your doctor have developed for worsening asthma.

On the other hand, if you are doing well, then measuring your peak flow may be helpful as you and your doctor try to lower the level of your medicines.

A peak flow meter can help you when your asthma is getting worse. Asthma sometimes changes gradually. Your peak flow may show changes before you feel them. It can allow your doctor to adjust your treatment to prevent urgent calls to the doctor, emergency room visits, or hospitalizations.

A peak flow meter may help you and your doctor identify causes of your asthma at work, home, or play. It may help parents to determine what might be triggering their child's asthma.

A peak flow meter can also be used during an asthma episode. It can help you determine the severity of the episode, decide when to use your rescue medication, and decide when to seek emergency care.

Knowing your "personal" peak flow rate allows you to elevate your readings. Being at your "best" can provide reassurance and make you feel more self-confident.

How Do You Use a Peak Flow Meter?

Step 1: Before each use, make sure the sliding marker or arrow on the peak flow meter is at the bottom of the numbered scale (zero or the lowest number on the scale).

Step 2: Stand up straight. Remove gum or any food from your mouth. Take a deep breath (as deep as you can). Put the mouthpiece of the peak flow meter into your mouth. Close your lips tightly around the mouthpiece. Be sure to keep your tongue away from the mouthpiece. In one breath blow out as hard and as quickly as possible. Blow a "fast hard blast" rather than "slowly blowing" until you have emptied out nearly all of the air from your lungs.

Step 3: The force of the air coming out of your lungs causes the marker to move along the numbered scale. Note the number on a piece of paper.

Step 4: Repeat the entire routine three times. (You know you have done the routine correctly when the numbers from all three tries are very close together.)

Step 5: Record the highest of the three ratings. Do not calculate an average. This is very important.

You can't breathe out too much when using your peak flow meter but you can breathe out too little. Record your highest reading.

Step 6: Measure your peak flow rate close to the same time each day. You and your doctor can determine the best times. One suggestion is to measure your peak flow rate twice daily, between 7 and 9 a.m. and between 6 and 8 p.m.

You may want to measure your peak flow rate before or after using your medicine. Some people measure peak flow both before and after taking medication. Try to do it the same way each time.

Step 7: Keep a chart of your peak flow rates. Discuss the readings with your doctor.

How Do I Chart My Peak Flow Rates?

Chart the *highest* of the three readings. The chart could include the date at the top of the page with a.m. and p.m. listed. The left margin could list a scale, starting with zero (0) liters per minute (L/min) at the bottom of the page and ending with 600 L/min at the top.

You could leave room at the bottom of the page for notes to describe how you are feeling or to list any other thoughts you may have.

What Is a "Normal" Peak Flow Rate?

A "normal" peak flow rate is based on a person's age, height, sex, and race. A standardized "normal" may be obtained from a chart comparing the patient with a population without breathing problems.

A personal best normal may be obtained from measuring the patient's own peak flow rate. Therefore, it is important for you and your doctor to discuss what is considered "normal" for you.

Once you have learned your usual and expected peak flow rate, you will be able to better recognize changes or trends.

How Can I Determine a "Normal" Peak Flow Rate for Me?

Three zones of measurement are commonly used to interpret peak flow rates. It is easy to relate the three zones to the traffic light colors: green, yellow, and red. In general, a normal peak flow rate can vary as much as 20 percent.

Be aware of the following general guidelines. Keep in mind that recognizing changes from "normal" is important. Your doctor may suggest other zones to follow.

Green zone: 80 to 100 percent of your usual or "normal" peak flow rate signals all clear. A reading in this zone means that your asthma is under reasonably good control. It would be advisable to continue your prescribed program of management.

Yellow zone: 50 to 80 percent of your usual or "normal" peak flow rate signals caution. It is a time for decisions. Your airways are narrowing and may require extra treatment. Your symptoms can get better or worse depending on what you do, or how and when you use your prescribed medication. You and your doctor should have a plan for yellow zone readings.

Red zone: Less than 50 percent of your usual or "normal" peak flow rate signals a medical alert. Immediate decisions and actions need to be taken. Severe airway narrowing may be occurring. Take your rescue medications right away. Contact your doctor now and follow the plan he has given you for red zone readings.

Some doctors may suggest zones with a smaller range such as 90 to 100 percent. Always follow your doctor's suggestions about your peak flow rate.

Management Plan Based on Peak Flow Readings

It is important to know your peak flow reading, but it is even more important to know what you will do based upon that reading. Work with your doctor to develop an asthma management plan that follows your green-yellow-red zone guidelines.

Record the peak flow readings that your doctor recommends for your green zone, yellow zone, and red zone. Then work out with your doctor what you plan to do when your peak flow falls in each of those zones.

When Should I Use My Peak Flow Meter?

Use of the peak flow meter depends on a number of things. Its use should be discussed with your doctor.

If your asthma is well controlled and you know the "normal" rate for you, you may decide to measure your peak flow rate only when you sense that your asthma is getting worse. More severe asthma may require several measurements daily.

Don't forget that your peak flow meter needs care and cleaning. Dirt collected in the meter may make your peak flow measurements inaccurate. If you have a cold or other respiratory infection, germs or mucus may also collect in the meter.

Proper cleaning with mild detergent in hot water will keep your peak flow meter working accurately and may keep you healthier.

Does Using a Peak Flow Meter Have Any Side Effects?

A peak flow meter is not a medicine. It has no major side effects. Sometimes pushing the air out of your lungs in a "fast blast" may cause you to cough or wheeze.

Check with your doctor before you start using a peak flow meter.

Using the meter is as simple as taking a deep breath and blowing out a candle. If used properly, it can only help.

You must realize that measuring peak flow is only one step in a program to manage asthma. Its importance must not be exaggerated or over-interpreted.

Using a peak flow meter is not a substitute for regular medical care. Ask your doctor to help you understand your peak flow measurements.

Ideas to Review

Now you are aware of some of the techniques for using and caring for peak flow meters. You also know how meters may help manage asthma and other breathing problems.

Discuss the use of a peak flow meter with your doctor. Make measuring your peak flow rate a part of your personal asthma management program.

Section 8.4

Spirometry

Spirometry Tests Your Lung Function

Pulmonary function testing measures how well you are breathing.
There are different types of pulmonary function tests that can be done.
Spirometry is one type of pulmonary function test. Spirometry is a
simple test to measure how much (volume) and how fast (flow) you
can move air into and out of your lungs.

Why Test My Lung Function?

Through routine spirometry, lung diseases can often be diagnosed
in the early stages when treatment is most effective. Once a lung disease is diagnosed and treated, routine spirometry tests can monitor
changes in lung functions with specific treatment. This will help your
doctor find the best treatment plan for you.

What Happens During the Spirometry Test?

You will be instructed how to perform spirometry. Basically, you
will take in a deep breath and blow into a mouthpiece attached to the
spirometer. You will blow out as hard and as fast as you can until your
lungs feel absolutely empty. You will be asked to repeat the test several more times until there are two to three good efforts. You will be
coached and encouraged to do your best during the test. A good effort
during the test is important to get good results.

A computerized sensor (which is part of the spirometer) calculates
and graphs the results. The results demonstrate a person's airflow
rates or the volume forced out within the first second. This is the forced
expiratory volume in the first second (FEV1). This indicates whether
or not there is airway obstruction. Spirometry also records the total

volume of air forced out of the lungs. This is the forced vital capacity (FVC).

"The spirometry test is really analogous to the blood pressure measurement," says National Jewish pulmonologist Dr. Reuben M. Cherniack. "Both should be given every time a physician sees a patient, since both tests show changes that can be recognized immediately."

Chapter 9

Lung Imaging Tests

Chapter Contents

Section 9.1

Chest X-Ray

A chest x-ray is a radiology procedure that involves exposing the chest briefly to minimal amounts of radiation. The image produced can be used to define heart abnormalities, including fluid around the heart, an enlarged heart, heart failure, or abnormal anatomy of the heart.

A chest x-ray (or chest radiography) provides your doctor with an image of your heart, lungs, and surrounding organs. Getting an x-ray is really just having a picture taken, so the procedure is painless. An x-ray is usually performed in a hospital radiology department or in a doctor's office by a technician. It may be ordered by your physician if you have a persistent cough or chest pain, as it is used to diagnose abnormalities in the heart and lungs. It is routinely ordered immediately prior to surgery.

What to Expect Before

Before the procedure, you will be asked to remove your clothing and to put on a hospital gown. You may be asked to remove any jewelry as well. Women must inform their doctor or the technician if there is a possibility they are pregnant, as x-rays are usually not recommended during the first and second trimesters of pregnancy.

Complications and Risks

Because the x-ray procedure involves the use of radiation, there is a very low risk of radiation exposure. The procedures are strictly regulated, though, to ensure that the minimum amount of radiation necessary to provide an image is used. Most doctors agree that the benefits of having the image far outweigh the risks. Pregnant women and children, however, are most susceptible to the risks of radiation exposure.

What to Expect During

You may be asked to stand with your chest against a photographic plate. The technician will tell you how to stand (i.e., hands on hips, elbows out). Or, you may lie down on a table with the x-ray equipment suspended above you. In both cases, the technician will tell you to remain as still as possible and to take a deep breath and hold it. He or she will not be in the room with you, but will step outside the room or to a booth for the actual x-ray. Once the picture is taken, you will be told to breathe. A front-to-back image will probably be taken (medically called the posteroanterior view), and a side-view may also be taken (called the lateral view).

What to Expect After

Once the images have been taken, you are free to get dressed. Your health care provider will let you know whether you need to wait for results.

Frequently Asked Questions

Why would I need a chest x-ray?

Your doctor would order a chest x-ray if you are having certain symptoms, including shortness of breath, persistent coughing, or chest pain, or if you've had an injury to your chest. Sometimes, it is used as a screening test or to provide a baseline should a problem develop in the future. Also, most people having surgery are asked to get a chest x-ray immediately before the operation.

What types of things would a chest x-ray show?

A chest x-ray would show your doctor if there was a change in the shape of your heart (as in the case of heart failure, which causes the heart to become enlarged) or a problem with your lungs, such as pneumonia, pleurisy, or lung cancer. It also is used to verify that your lungs are healthy for surgery.

Why would my doctor order a series of chest x-rays?

Your doctor would order a series of chest x-rays if he or she sees an abnormality on the initial x-ray and wants to monitor any changes over time (for example, to see if an enlarged heart is becoming more enlarged). Repeated x-rays are sometimes taken because the first x-rays were not clear or could not be read easily.

Section 9.2

Computed Tomography (CT) Scan

Reprinted from "Thoracic CT," © 2008 A.D.A.M., Inc. Reprinted with permission. Updated July 18, 2007.

Alternative Names

Chest CT; CT scan—lungs; CT scan—chest

Definition

Thoracic CT is a computed tomography scan of the chest and upper abdomen.

How the Test Is Performed

You will be asked to lie on a narrow table (gantry) that slides into the center of the scanner. Depending on what is being scanned, you may lie on the stomach, back, or side. If contrast media (dye) is to be given, an IV (intravenous needle or tube) will be placed in a small vein of your hand or arm.

As with standard photography, if you move while the CT image is being taken, it will blur. Because of this, the operator of the scanner will tell you when to hold your breath and not move.

As the exam takes place, the gantry will advance small intervals through the scanner. Modern spiral scanners can perform the examination in one continuous motion of the gantry. Generally, complete scans will only take a few minutes. However, additional contrast-enhanced or higher-resolution scans will add to the scan time. The newest multi-detector scanners can image the entire body, head-to-toe, in under thirty seconds.

How to Prepare for the Test

The health care provider may advise you to avoid eating or drinking for four to six hours prior to the scan, if contrast dye is to be used.

The CT scanner has a weight limit to prevent damage to the mechanized gantry. Have the health care provider contact the scanner operator if you weigh more than three hundred pounds.

Metal interferes with the x-rays, so you may be asked to remove jewelry and wear a hospital gown during the study.

How the Test Will Feel

The x-rays are painless. The primary discomfort may be from the need to lie still on the table.

If intravenous contrast dye is given, you may feel a slight burning sensation in the injected arm, a metallic taste in the mouth, and a warm flushing of the body. These sensations are normal and usually go away within a few seconds.

Why the Test Is Performed

Thoracic CT may be recommended when there is a need for examination of the structures inside the chest. It is noninvasive and poses less risk than invasive procedures (such as angiography or exploratory surgery).

Common indications for thoracic CT include:

- When there is a chest injury;

- When a tumor or mass (clump of cells) is suspected;

- To determine the size, shape, and position of internal organs;

- To look for bleeding or fluid collections in the lungs or other areas.

What Abnormal Results Mean

Thoracic CT may show many disorders of the heart, lungs, or chest area, including:

- Enlarged lymph nodes (lymphadenopathy);
- Abnormalities of the structure or position of the heart, lungs, or blood vessels;
- Bronchiectasis;

- Tumors, nodules, or cysts within the chest;
- The stage of some lung tumors or esophageal cancer;
- Aortic aneurysm (thoracic);
- Pleural effusion;
- Pneumonia;
- Accumulations of blood or fluid.

Additional conditions under which the test may be performed:

- Alcoholic cardiomyopathy;
- Asbestosis;
- Atrial myxoma;
- Cardiac tamponade;
- Coarctation of the aorta;
- Dilated cardiomyopathy;
- Echinococcus;
- Heart failure;
- Histoplasmosis;
- Hypertensive heart disease;
- Idiopathic cardiomyopathy;
- Infective endocarditis;
- Ischemic cardiomyopathy;
- Left-sided heart failure;
- Mesothelioma (malignant);
- Metastatic cancer to the lung;
- Mitral regurgitation, acute;
- Mitral regurgitation, chronic;
- Mitral valve prolapse;
- Pericarditis, bacterial;
- Pericarditis, constrictive;
- Pericarditis, post-myocardial infarction (MI);
- Peripartum cardiomyopathy;
- Pulmonary edema;
- Restrictive cardiomyopathy;

- Senile cardiac amyloid;
- Superior vena cava (SVC) obstruction.

Risks

CT scans and other x-rays are regulated to provide the minimum amount of radiation exposure needed to produce the image. During pregnancy, a thoracic CT scan is not recommended unless the benefits outweigh the risk of radiation exposure to the fetus. CT scans provide low levels of radiation.

The most common dye used is iodine-based. A person who is allergic to iodine may experience nausea, vomiting, sneezing, itching, or hives, and occasionally anaphylaxis (life-threatening allergic response). In people with kidney problems, the dye may have toxic effects on the kidneys.

Considerations

The benefits of a CT scan usually far outweigh the risks. A CT scan is one of the best ways of looking at soft tissues such as the heart and lungs.

Section 9.3

Gallium Scan

Reprinted from "Lung Gallium Scan," © 2008 A.D.A.M., Inc. Reprinted with permission. Updated July 17, 2007.

Alternative Names

Gallium 67 lung scan; Lung scan; Gallium scan—lung; Scan—lung

Definition

Lung gallium scan is a type of nuclear scan involving radioactive gallium (Ga). The test helps determine whether a patient has inflammation in the lungs.

How the Test Is Performed

Gallium is injected into a vein. The scan will be taken six to twenty-four hours after the gallium is injected. (Test time depends on whether your condition is acute or chronic).

During the test, you lie on a table that moves underneath a scanner called a gamma camera. The camera detects the rays emitted by the gallium. Images display on a computer screen.

During the scan, it is important that you remain still to get a clear image. The technologist can help make you comfortable before the scan begins. The test will take about thirty to sixty minutes.

How to Prepare for the Test

You must sign an informed consent form. Several hours to one day before the scan, the injection of gallium will be administered to you at the hospital or doctor's office.

Just before the scan, remove jewelry, dentures, or other metal objects that can affect the scan. Replace the clothing on the upper half of your body with a hospital gown.

How the Test Will Feel

The injection of gallium will sting, and the puncture site may hurt when touched for several hours or days. The scan is painless. However, you must remain still. This may cause discomfort for some patients. The wait between the injection and scan can cause some patients to become agitated.

Why the Test Is Performed

This test is most often performed when there is evidence of inflammation in the lungs (sarcoidosis).

Normal Results

The lungs should appear of normal size and texture with little uptake of gallium.

What Abnormal Results Mean

- Sarcoidosis
- Other respiratory infections

Additional conditions under which the test may be performed:

- Primary pulmonary hypertension;
- Pulmonary embolus.

Risks

There is some risk to children or fetuses. Because a pregnant or nursing woman may pass on radiation, special precautions will be made for these women.

For women who are not pregnant or nursing, and for men, there is very little risk from the radiation in gallium, because the amount is very small. There are increased risks with numerous exposures to radiation (such as x-rays, and scans), which you should discuss with the health care provider who recommends the test.

Considerations

Usually a chest x-ray will indicate the need for this scan. Small defects may not be visible.

Section 9.4

Magnetic Resonance Imaging

Reprinted from "Chest MRI," National Heart, Lung, and Blood Institute, National Institutes of Health, March 2008.

What Is Chest MRI?

Chest magnetic resonance imaging (MRI) is a safe, noninvasive test. "Noninvasive" means that no surgery is done and no instruments are inserted into your body. This test creates detailed pictures of the structures in your chest, like your chest wall, heart, and blood vessels.

Chest MRI uses radio waves, magnets, and a computer to create these pictures. The test is used to:

- Look for tumors in the chest;

- Look at blood vessels, lymph nodes, and other structures in the chest;

- Help explain results of other tests, such as chest x-rays or chest CT scans (also called computed tomography scans).

As part of some chest MRIs, a special substance (called contrast dye) is injected into a vein in your arm. This dye allows the MRI to take more detailed pictures of the structures in your chest.

Chest MRI has few risks. Unlike a CT scan or standard x-ray, MRI doesn't use radiation or have any risk of causing cancer. Rarely, the contrast dye used for some chest MRIs may cause an allergic reaction.

Other Names for Chest MRI

Chest MRI also may be called chest nuclear magnetic resonance.

Who Needs a Chest MRI?

You may need a chest MRI if your doctor suspects you have a chest condition, such as:

- A tumor;

- Problems in the blood vessels, such as an aneurysm or blood clot;

- Abnormal lymph nodes;

- Other chest conditions.

A chest MRI also may be used to explain the results of other tests, such as chest x-ray and chest CT scan.

What to Expect before Chest MRI

Your doctor or the MRI technician will ask you some questions before a chest MRI, including:

- Are you pregnant or do you think you could be?

- Have you had any surgery? If so, what kind?

- Do you have any metal objects in your body, like metal screws or pins in a bone?

- Do you have any medical devices in your body, such as a pace-maker, an implantable cardioverter defibrillator, cochlear (inner-ear) implants, or brain aneurysm clips? The strong magnets in the MRI machine can damage these devices.

Your answers will help your doctor decide whether you should have a chest MRI.

Items Not Allowed in the MRI Room

Your doctor or technician will ask you to not wear or bring metal or electronic objects into the MRI room. These include:

- Hearing aids;
- Credit cards;
- Jewelry and watches;
- Eyeglasses;
- Pens;
- Removable dental work;
- Any other magnetic objects.

MRI magnets can damage these objects, and they can interfere with the MRI machine.

The MRI Machine

An MRI machine looks like a long, narrow tunnel. During the MRI, you lie on your back on a sliding table. The table passes through the scanner as it takes pictures of your chest. Newer machines are shorter and wider and don't completely surround you; others are open on all sides.

Tell your doctor if you're afraid of tight or closed spaces. He or she may give you medicine to help you relax or find you a place that has an open MRI machine.

If you do receive medicine to relax you, your doctor may ask you to stop eating about six hours before you take it. This medicine may make you tired, so you'll need to arrange for a ride home after the test.

Contrast Dye

Your doctor may give you a special substance (called contrast dye) before the MRI. This dye allows the MRI to take more detailed pictures of the structures in your chest.

The contrast dye will be injected into a vein in your arm. You may feel some discomfort where the needle is inserted. You also may have a cool feeling as the dye is injected.

The contrast dye used in a chest MRI doesn't contain iodine, so it won't create problems for people who are allergic to iodine. Rarely, people develop allergic symptoms from the dye, such as hives and itchy eyes. If this happens, your doctor will give you medicine to relieve the symptoms.

If you're breast-feeding, ask your doctor how long you need to wait after the test before you breast-feed. The contrast dye can be passed to your baby through your breast milk.

You may want to prepare for the test by pumping and saving milk for twenty-four to forty-eight hours in advance. You can bottle-feed your baby in the hours after the test.

What to Expect during Chest MRI

A chest MRI usually is done at a hospital or at a special medical imaging facility. A radiologist or other doctor with special training in this type of test oversees the testing.

A chest MRI usually takes forty-five to ninety minutes, depending on how many pictures are needed. The test may take less time with some newer MRI machines.

How the Test Is Done

A chest MRI is painless and has few risks. During the test, you lie on your back on a sliding table as it passes through the MRI machine. The technician will control the machine from the next room. He or she will be able to see you through a glass window and talk to you through a speaker. Tell the technician if you have a hearing problem.

You will hear loud humming, tapping, and buzzing noises from the MRI machine. You may be able to use earplugs or listen to music during the test.

Moving your body can cause the pictures to blur. The technician will ask you to remain very still during the test. If you can't lie still, you may be given medicine to help you relax. The technician also may ask you to hold your breath for ten to fifteen seconds at a time, while he or she takes pictures of the structures in your chest.

What to Expect after Chest MRI

You usually can return to your normal routine right after a chest MRI.

If you got medicine to help you relax during the MRI, your doctor will tell you when you can return to your normal routine. The medicine may make you tired, so you'll need someone to drive you home.

If contrast dye was used during the test, you may have a bruise where the needle was inserted. Also, if you're breast-feeding, you'll need to bottle-feed your baby for a short time after the test. The contrast dye can be passed to your baby through your breast milk.

Ask your doctor how long you need to wait before you breast-feed. You may want to prepare for the test by pumping and saving milk for twenty-four to forty-eight hours in advance.

What Does a Chest MRI Show?

A chest MRI may show a tumor, problems in the blood vessels (such as an aneurysm or blood clot), abnormal lymph nodes, and other chest conditions.

What Are the Risks of Chest MRI?

There are no risks from the magnetic fields or radio waves used during a chest MRI.

Serious reactions to the contrast dye used for some MRIs are very rare. However, side effects are possible and include the following:

• Headache;

• Nausea (feeling sick to your stomach);

• Dizziness;

• Changes in taste;

• Allergic reactions, such a hives and itchy eyes.

Rarely, contrast dye is harmful to people who have severe kidney disease.

Key Points

Chest MRI is a safe, noninvasive test. It creates detailed pictures of the structures in your chest, like your chest wall, heart, and blood vessels. Radio waves, magnets, and a computer are used to make these pictures.

Chest MRI is used to look for tumors in the chest; look at blood vessels, lymph nodes, and other structures in the chest; and help explain results from other tests, such as chest x-ray and chest CT scan.

You may need a chest MRI if your doctor suspects you have a chest condition, such as a tumor, a problem in the blood vessels (such as an aneurysm or blood clot), abnormal lymph nodes, or other chest conditions.

Before a chest MRI, your doctor or the MRI technician will ask you questions about your health to make sure an MRI is safe for you. You should not wear or bring metal or electronic objects into the MRI room. The MRI can damage these items, and they can interfere with the MRI machine.

An MRI machine looks like a long, narrow tunnel. New machines are shorter and wider and don't completely surround you; others are open on all sides. Tell your doctor if you're afraid of tight or closed spaces. He or she may give you medicine to help you relax or find you a place that has an open MRI machine.

Before the test, your doctor may inject a special substance (called contrast dye) into a vein in your arm. This dye allows the MRI to take more detailed pictures of the structures in your chest.

If you're breast-feeding, ask your doctor how long you should wait after the test before you breast-feed. The contrast dye can be passed through your breast milk. You may want to prepare for the test by pumping and saving milk for twenty-four to forty-eight hours in advance. You can bottle-feed your baby in the hours after the MRI.

A chest MRI is painless. During the test, you lie on your back on a sliding table as it passes through the MRI machine. The machine takes pictures of your chest. Moving your body can cause the pictures to blur. You will be asked to remain very still during the test.

You usually can return to your normal routine right after a chest MRI. If you got medicine to help you relax, your doctor will tell you when you can return to your normal routine. The medicine may make you tired, so you'll need someone to drive you home.

Chest MRI has few risks. Rarely, the contrast dye used for some chest MRIs may cause an allergic reaction.

Chapter 10

Invasive and Surgical Diagnostic Tests

Chapter Contents

Section 10.1

Bronchoscopy

Reprinted from "Bronchoscopy: Pulmonary Branch Protocols,"
Warren Grant Magnuson Clinical Center, National Institutes of Health,
June 2001. Reviewed by David A. Cooke, M.D., April 2008.

What is a bronchoscopy?

Bronchoscopy is a routine diagnostic procedure that lets your doctor see inside your lungs and possibly get tissue to examine. The procedure uses a bronchoscope: a small, narrow tube with a light and lens at the tip.

Who might have a bronchoscopy?

People who have symptoms of a lung problem may have a bronchoscopy to help make an exact diagnosis. Patients with known lung disease may need this test to check the status of their disease. For comparison, bronchoscopy may also be done on people with normal lungs.

How do I prepare for it?

Before the procedure, you will have a chest x-ray, pulmonary function test, physical exam, blood work, and an electrocardiogram. Also, you will be asked to sign an informed consent, which will be signed by your doctor.

Do not eat or drink anything eight hours before the procedure.

The morning of the procedure, a small, intravenous tube (catheter) will be put into one of your arm veins. This will be used to give you fluids and medication to help you relax. You may get an injection of medications into your muscle to help control coughing and secretions in your mouth.

What happens during a bronchoscopy?

When you are in the bronchoscopy suite, the nurse will attach patches to your chest to monitor your heart, a blood pressure cuff to monitor your blood pressure, and a clip on your finger to check how much oxygen is in your blood.

After this, you will breathe a mist of topical anesthesia (numbing medication) through your mouth. You will breathe this mist from a tube attached to an oxygen flow meter. You will be asked to breathe through your mouth until this mist is gone.

The nurse will give you a topical anesthetic to gargle, or the back of your throat will be sprayed with anesthetic. A small amount of lidocaine (numbing medication) will be put into one of your nostrils to let the bronchoscopy tube pass through.

What are the side effects?

Because of the sedatives you may have received, you may feel groggy for several hours. Your mouth may feel dry during, and shortly after, the procedure. Some people also have a slight sore throat, blood-tinged saliva, or a low fever.

What happens afterward?

When the procedure is over, the nurse will take you back to your room. Your vital signs (temperature, heartbeat, blood pressure) will be monitored. Your nurse will also ask you to take deep breaths and cough gently. This helps clear your lungs of the fluid used during the procedure.

Because your throat and gag reflex will be numb, do not eat or drink for at least two hours after the bronchoscopy. In two hours, your nurse will check your gag reflex. If it has returned, you may try to drink; then eat.

Are there special instructions to follow after the procedure?

If you develop a fever higher than 100 degrees Fahrenheit, take Tylenol every four hours as recommended by your doctor or nurse practitioner. If your fever lasts longer than twenty-four hours, call your doctor.

If you have a sore throat, take throat lozenges as needed. If you have any of the following, go to the nearest emergency room:

- Difficulty catching your breath
- Bleeding from your nose
- Coughing up blood
- Chest pain or chest discomfort

Section 10.2

Mediastinoscopy

"Mediastinoscopy," reprinted with permission from
CNY Thoracic Surgery, PC (www.cnythoracic.org), © 2006.

What is it?

Mediastinoscopy is a surgical procedure to examine and biopsy lymph nodes or abnormal tissue in the center of the chest (mediastinum).

Why is it done?

Mediastinoscopy is done to collect biopsy specimens from the center of the chest. Frequently, these nodes are near the outside of the trachea and large bronchi. This procedure allows your doctor to get good samples of the abnormal tissue, so the pathologist can examine the tissue and make a diagnosis.

Mediastinoscopy is a diagnostic procedure. This means that your doctor is not trying to remove all of the abnormal tissue, only to get a good sample.

This procedure is frequently combined with other procedures like bronchoscopy or thoracotomy.

How is it done?

Mediastinoscopy requires a general anesthetic. Once asleep, a breathing tube is placed in the airway. Sterile prep solution (DuraPrep®) is spread on the skin from the chin to the bellybutton. A small amount of long-lasting local anesthetic is injected in the skin and a small incision is made in the notch at the base of the neck. The neck tissue is separated in the midline down to the level of the trachea. The mediastinoscope is then advanced into the chest along the trachea. The mediastinal tissue is examined for lymph nodes and abnormal tissue.

When tissue is found that needs a biopsy, a small needle is inserted into the tissue to make sure it is not a blood vessel. Small bites of the tissue are then taken and submitted for pathology.

Any bleeding is controlled, and then the wound is closed with absorbable sutures. Sterile tape (Steri-Strips®) are placed on the wound and then a waterproof dressing.

Is there any preparation?

The usual preparation is nothing to eat after midnight. You may take your medicines with a sip of water. Alert your doctor if you are taking blood thinners like Coumadin® or Plavix®. Aspirin is fine to take.

It is a good idea, before any surgery, to shower for a two or three days with 4 percent chlorhexidine soap. This can be obtained from a pharmacy without a prescription.

You should also expect to receive a preoperative antibiotic an hour before the surgery begins. Only one dose is required. Your doctor may hold the dose if the biopsy is for cultures. In that case, antibiotics will be given after the specimen is collected.

How long does it take?

A mediastinoscopy takes about an hour.

When can I expect results?

Most mediastinoscopies are done with an immediate frozen section. A frozen section is where the pathologist examines the tissue with a microscope. The frozen section is used to get an idea of what type of disease has caused the abnormal tissue. Your doctor will tell you and your family the frozen section results after the procedure. Occasionally, the frozen section will be inconclusive, and you will have to wait for the final results.

Any results based on frozen section are preliminary and based on a limited set of tests. The final results allow for finer diagnostic evaluation and may verify or change the frozen section results.

Cultures take from two days to two months to get results.

What will I feel like afterwards?

You may have a sore throat. It is fine to take throat lozenges. The front of your neck may be sore as well. You may shower with the waterproof dressing in place. Two days after surgery, remove the waterproof dressing (i.e., for a procedure on Monday, remove the dressing Wednesday). The Steri-Strips should be left in place until the edges curl up. This takes about a week. Once the edges curl up, remove the strips.

It is all right to place ice on the wound for comfort. Expect a slight amount of swelling at the site that will last for a month or so. The prep solution takes about five showers to remove.

Tylenol (acetaminophen) or Advil (ibuprofen) can be used as needed for pain. Your doctor will give you a prescription for something like Tylenol #3, Lortab®, or Darvon® for more severe pain.

You will need someone to drive you home.

What are the risks?

The risks include, but are not limited to:

- Having a reaction to the anesthetic, heart attack, stroke, death, or other devastating complications. This would be exceedingly rare, but still possible.

- Hoarseness (rare). This may develop for a variable period of time due to swelling or injury to the nerve to the vocal cord. The nerve runs along the backside of the trachea and sometimes near the lymph nodes.

- Bleeding (rare). This may develop from the close proximity of the large blood vessels near the lymph nodes and trachea. Usually your body will stop any bleeding due to normal blood clotting. Very rarely the doctor may have to make a larger incision to directly repair the blood vessel. Bleeding could also require a blood transfusion if enough blood is lost.

- There is a small risk of developing an infection.

Section 10.3

Pleural Needle Biopsy

Alternative Names: Closed pleural biopsy; Needle biopsy of the pleura

Definition: A pleural biopsy is a procedure to remove a sample of the tissue lining the lungs and the inside of the chest wall to check for disease or infection.

How the Test Is Performed: This test does not have to be done in the hospital. It may be done at a clinic or doctor's office.

You will be sitting up for the biopsy. The health care provider will cleanse the skin at the biopsy site, and inject a local numbing drug (anesthetic) through the skin and into the lining of the lungs and chest wall (pleural membrane).

A larger, hollow needle is then placed through the skin and into the chest cavity. The doctor rotates the needle. At various times during the procedure, you will be asked to sing, hum, or say "eee." This helps prevent air from getting into the chest cavity, which can cause a lung collapse (pneumothorax).

The doctor removes the needle to collect tissue samples. Usually, three biopsy samples are taken. When the test is completed, a bandage is placed over the biopsy site.

How to Prepare for the Test: You will have blood tests before the biopsy, and you may have a chest x-ray taken. You must sign consent forms.

How the Test Will Feel: With the injection of the local anesthetic, you may feel a brief prick and a burning sensation. When the biopsy needle is inserted, you may feel pressure. As the needle is being removed, you may feel a tugging sensation.

Why the Test Is Performed: Pleural biopsy is usually done to determine the cause of a collection of fluid around the lung (persistent pleural effusion) or other abnormality of the pleural membrane. Pleural biopsy can diagnose tuberculosis, cancer, and other diseases.

Normal Results: The pleural tissues appear normal, without signs of inflammation, infection, or cancer.

Normal value ranges may vary slightly among different laboratories. Talk to your doctor about the meaning of your specific test results.

What Abnormal Results Mean: Abnormal results may reveal cancer, tuberculosis, a viral disease, a fungal disease, a parasitic disease, or collagen vascular disease.

Other conditions under which the test may be done include:

- Metastatic pleural tumor;
- Primary lung cancer.

Risks: There is a slight chance of the needle puncturing the wall of the lung, which can partially collapse the lung. This usually gets better on its own. There is a chance of excessive blood loss.

Considerations: If a closed pleural biopsy is not enough to make a diagnosis, you may need a surgical biopsy of the pleura.

References

Mason RJ, Murray J, Broaddus VC, Nadel JA. *Textbook of Respiratory Medicine*. 4th ed. Philadelphia, Pa.: WB Saunders, 2005.

Noble J. *Textbook of Primary Care Medicine*. 3rd ed. St. Louis, Mo.: Mosby; 2001, 725.

Section 10.4

Thoracentesis

Excerpted from National Heart, Lung, and Blood
Institute, National Institutes of Health, December 2007.

What Is Thoracentesis?

Thoracentesis is a procedure to remove excess fluid in the space between the lungs and the chest wall. This space is called the pleural space.

Normally, the pleural space is filled with a small amount of fluid—about four teaspoons full. But some conditions, such as heart failure, lung infections, and tumors, can cause more fluid to build up. When this happens, it's called a pleural effusion. A lot of extra fluid can press on the lungs, making it hard to breathe.

Overview

Thoracentesis is done to find the cause of a pleural effusion. It also may be done to help you breathe easier.

During the procedure, your doctor inserts a thin needle or plastic tube into the pleural space and draws out the excess fluid. Usually, doctors take only the amount of fluid needed to find the cause of the pleural effusion. However, if there's a lot of fluid, they may take more. This helps the lungs expand and take in more air, which allows you to breathe easier.

After the fluid is removed from your chest, it's sent for testing. Once the cause of the pleural effusion is known, your doctor will plan treatment. For example, if an infection is causing the excess fluid, you may be given antibiotics to fight the infection. If the cause is heart failure, you will be treated for that condition.

Thoracentesis usually takes ten to fifteen minutes. It may take longer if there's a lot of fluid in the pleural space. You will be watched for up to a few hours after the procedure for complications.

Outlook

The procedure usually doesn't cause serious problems, but some risks are involved. These include pneumothorax, or collapsed lung; pain, bleeding, bruising, or infection where the needle or tube was inserted; and liver or spleen injury (very rare).

Most of these complications get better on their own, or they're easily treated.

Who Needs Thoracentesis?

You may need thoracentesis if you have a pleural effusion. A pleural effusion is the buildup of excess fluid in the pleural space (the space between the lungs and chest wall).

Thoracentesis helps find the cause of the pleural effusion. It also may be done to help you breathe easier, if there's a lot of fluid in the pleural space.

The most common cause of a pleural effusion is heart failure. This is a condition in which the heart can't pump enough blood to the body.

Other causes include lung cancer, tumors, pneumonia, tuberculosis, pulmonary embolism, and other lung infections. Asbestosis, sarcoidosis, and reactions to some drugs also can lead to a pleural effusion.

What to Expect before Thoracentesis

Before thoracentesis, your doctor will talk to you about the procedure and how to prepare for it. Tell your doctor what medicines you're taking, about any previous bleeding problems, and about allergies to medicines or latex.

No special preparations are needed before thoracentesis.

What to Expect during Thoracentesis

Thoracentesis is done at a doctor's office or hospital. The entire procedure (including preparation) usually takes ten to fifteen minutes, but the needle or tube is in your chest for only a few minutes during that time. If there's a lot of fluid, the procedure may take up to forty-five minutes.

You will sit on the edge of a chair or exam table, lean forward, and rest your arms on a table. Your doctor will tell you not to move, cough, or breathe deeply once the procedure begins.

He or she cleans the area of your skin where the needle or tube will be inserted and injects medicine to numb the area. You may feel some stinging at this time.

Your doctor then inserts the needle or tube between your ribs and into the pleural space (the area between the lungs and chest wall). You may feel some discomfort and pressure at this time. Your doctor may use ultrasound to find the right place to insert the needle or tube. (Ultrasound uses sound waves to create images of your lungs.)

He or she then draws out the excess fluid around your lungs using the needle or tube. You may feel like coughing, and you may feel some chest pain. If a lot of fluid is removed, your lungs will have more room to fill with air as the fluid is drawn out. This can make it easier to breathe.

Once the fluid is removed, your doctor takes out the needle or tube. A small bandage is placed on the site where the needle or tube was inserted.

What to Expect after Thoracentesis

After thoracentesis, you may need a chest x-ray to check for any lung problems. Your blood pressure and breathing will be checked for up to a few hours to make sure you don't have complications.

Your doctor will let you know when you can return to your normal activities, such as driving, physical activity, and working.

Once at home, call your doctor right away if you have any breathing problems.

What Does Thoracentesis Show?

Your doctor will send the fluid removed during thoracentesis for testing. It will be looked at for signs of heart failure, infection, cancer, or other conditions that may be causing the pleural effusion (the buildup of fluid between the lungs and chest wall).

Once the cause of the pleural effusion is known, your doctor will talk to you about a treatment plan. For example, if an infection is causing the excess fluid, you may need antibiotics to fight the infection. If the cause is heart failure, you will be treated for that condition.

What Are the Risks of Thoracentesis?

The risks of thoracentesis are usually minor and will get better on their own, or they're easily treated. Your doctor may do a chest x-ray after the procedure to check for lung problems.

The risks of thoracentesis include:

- **Pneumothorax:** This is a condition in which air collects in the pleural space (the area between the lungs and chest wall). Sometimes air comes in through the needle, or the needle makes a hole in a lung. Usually, a hole will seal itself. If enough air gets into the pleural space, however, the lung can collapse. Your doctor may need to put a tube in your chest to remove the air and let the lung expand again.

- **Pain, bleeding, bruising, or infection where the needle or tube was inserted:** In rare cases, bleeding may occur in or around the lungs. Your doctor may need to put a tube in the chest to drain the blood. In some cases, surgery may be needed.

- **Liver or spleen injury:** These complications are very rare.

Section 10.5

Thoracoscopy

The Thoracoscopy Procedure

A thoracoscopy uses an endoscope to visually examine the pleura, lungs, and mediastinum and to obtain tissue for testing purposes. An endoscope is an illuminated optic instrument that is inserted through an incision.

The anesthesiologist gives you general anesthesia, which lets you sleep and keeps you free from pain during surgery. Once you're asleep, you're positioned comfortably on your side.

Several small incisions are made in your side.

The surgeon inserts a thin, tubelike instrument containing a tiny camera through one of the incisions. This camera allows the surgeon to view your lungs on a video monitor. Surgical instruments are inserted through the other incisions.

When the procedure is finished, one or more tubes may be temporarily placed in the chest to drain fluid and air. The incisions are then closed with sutures or staples.

Risks and Complications

The risks of thoracoscopy include the following:

- Wound infection

- Bleeding
- Air leak through the lung wall, requiring a longer hospital stay
- Pain or numbness at the incision site
- Inflammation of the lungs (pneumonia)

Recovering in the Hospital

After surgery, you'll wake up in a recovery area. At first you'll probably feel groggy and thirsty. An intravenous (IV) line provides you with fluids and medications to relieve pain, and monitors keep track of your breathing and heartbeat.

To help keep your lungs clear and prevent inflammation, a respiratory therapist will teach you breathing exercises to do every hour or so. Depending on your condition, a nurse or therapist will help you get up and walk soon after your surgery to keep your blood moving and improve your healing.

The hospital stay after a thoracoscopy is generally one to four days. If you have chest tubes, you won't go home until they're removed.

Recovering at Home

When you return home, follow your doctor's instructions about how to care for your healing skin and lungs. These instructions may include the following:

- Walk to keep your blood moving and strengthen your muscles, but avoid strenuous activity, heavy lifting, and driving for several weeks.
- Continue to do the breathing exercises taught to you by your therapist.
- Resume sexual relations when you feel ready.
- Ask your doctor when you can go back to work.
- Take your pain medications as prescribed to help relieve soreness and make activity and deep breathing easier.
- Follow up with your doctor, who'll monitor your healing and discuss the results of the procedure.

When to Call Your Doctor

Call your doctor if you have any of the following symptoms after your procedure:

- Shortness of breath
- Very red or draining incision
- Sudden, sharp chest pain
- Fever over 101°F
- Coughing up bright red blood

Section 10.6

Diagnostic Thoracotomy

"Patient Guide to Testing—Thoracotomy," © Todd Demmy, M.D. Reprinted with permission. The text of this document is available online at http://www.ellisfischel.org/thoracic/testing/thoracotomy.shtml; accessed September 21, 2007.

This procedure involves your physician making a six- to seven-inch incision from your upper back, under your arm, to around the front of your rib cage (following the rib cage). This procedure involves parting of the muscles and ribs, exposing the lung, and taking the biopsy. A thoracotomy requires a possible hospital stay of five to seven days. You will have a chest tube, require pain medication, and possibly require a urinary catheter.

Advantages

Advantages to a thoracotomy include possible removal of the lung mass at the same time as the biopsy and knowing if the results are positive for cancer the day of the procedure.

Side Effects

This procedure does involve a small risk for bleeding and infection, like pneumonia. There is also a small risk of chronic pain related to the disruption of nerves that follow the chest wall along the rib cage.

What to Expect after the Procedure

You may be in intensive care for the first twenty-four to forty-eight hours, then you will be moved to the general surgery floor. You will probably have a chest tube in as long as forty-eight to seventy-two hours, possibly longer if necessary. For pain management, an epidural can be offered which will be put in during surgery and stay in for about three days. This epidural will require placement of a urinary catheter which can be removed after the epidural pain catheter is removed. The incision will be painful and will require pain medication management for one to two weeks, at a minimum. You will have an intravenous line (IV) for three to five days and will require chest x-rays to monitor your lung.

What to Report to Your Physician

- Increased shortness of breath
- Chest pain
- Fever more than 101 degrees
- Heart palpitations
- Swelling of an extremity, or leg pain

Chapter 11

Tests for Cystic Fibrosis and Tuberculosis

Chapter Contents

Section 11.1

Sweat Test

The sweat test has been the "gold standard" for diagnosing cystic fibrosis (CF) for more than forty years. When it is performed by trained technicians, and evaluated in an experienced, reliable laboratory, the sweat test is still the best test to diagnose CF.

It is recommended that the sweat test be performed in a Cystic Fibrosis Foundation–accredited care center where strict guidelines are followed to ensure the accuracy of the results. The test can be performed on individuals of any age. However, some infants may not make enough sweat for the laboratory to analyze. If an infant does not produce enough sweat on the first sweat test, the test should be repeated.

What happens during a sweat test?

The sweat test determines the amount of chloride in the sweat. There are no needles involved in the procedure. In the first part of the test, a colorless, odorless chemical, known to cause sweating, is applied to a small area on an arm or leg. An electrode is then attached to the arm or leg, which allows the technician to apply a weak electrical current to the area to stimulate sweating. Individuals may feel a tingling sensation in the area, or a feeling of warmth. This part of the procedure lasts approximately five minutes.

The second part of the test consists of cleaning the stimulated area and collecting the sweat on a piece of filter paper or gauze or in a plastic coil. Thirty minutes later, the collected sweat is sent to a hospital laboratory for analysis. The entire collection procedure takes approximately one hour.

What does the sweat test reveal?

Your doctor has asked that this test be performed to rule out the presence of CF, an inherited disorder of the lungs, intestines, and sweat glands. Children and adults with CF have an increased amount of chloride (salt) in their sweat. In general, sweat chloride concentrations less than 40 mmol/L are normal (does not have CF); values between 40 to 60 mmol/L are borderline; and sweat chloride concentrations greater than 60 mmol/L are consistent with the diagnosis of CF.

For individuals who have CF, the sweat chloride test will be positive from birth. Once a test result is positive, it is always positive. Sweat test values do not change from positive to negative or negative to positive as a person grows older. Sweat test values also do not vary when individuals have colds or other temporary illnesses.

Is there any preparation for the sweat test?

There are no restrictions on activity or diet or special preparations before the test. However, one should not apply creams or lotions to the skin twenty-four hours before the test. All regular medications may be continued and will have no effect on the test results.

When are sweat test results made available?

Sweat test results are usually available to your doctor on the next working day after the test is performed. In a small number of cases, the quantity of sweat obtained is not sufficient to give an accurate result, and the test may need to be repeated.

Can the test results be inconclusive?

Yes. In a small number of cases, the test results fall into "borderline" range between not having CF and indicative of CF. In these situations, repeat sweat tests, as well as other diagnostic procedures, may need to be carried out. These will only be done after consultation with a doctor.

Section 11.2

Tuberculosis Skin Test

"The TB (Tuberculosis) Skin Test (Mantoux)," reprinted
with permission from the Minnesota Department of Health
(www.health.state.mn.us). Copyright June 2007.

The tuberculosis (TB) skin test, sometimes called a "Mantoux," is
a simple, harmless way to find out if you have latent TB infection.

What is latent TB infection?

There are two phases of TB. Both phases can be treated with medicine. When TB germs first enter your body, they cause latent TB infection. Without treatment, latent TB infection can become active TB disease. Anyone can get TB because it spreads from one person to another through the air.

How can I tell if I have latent TB infection?

A TB skin test ("Mantoux") can show if you have latent TB infection. You could have latent TB infection if you have ever spent time

Table 11.1. Phases of Tuberculosis Infection

Phase 1: Latent TB Infection	Phase 2: Active TB Disease
TB germs are "asleep" in your body. This phase can last for a very long time—even many years.	TB germs are active and spreading. They are damaging tissue in your body.
You don't look or feel sick. Your chest x-ray is usually normal.	You usually feel sick. Your doctor will do special tests to find where TB is harming your body.
You can't spread TB to other people.	If the TB germs are in your lungs, you can spread TB to other people by coughing, sneezing, talking, or singing.
Usually treated by taking one medicine for nine months.	Treated by taking three or four medicines for at least six months.

158

close to someone with active TB disease (even if you didn't know they were sick). Your health care provider will use a small needle to inject some harmless testing fluid (called "tuberculin") under the skin on your arm.

Your health care provider must check your arm two or three days after the TB skin test, even if your arm looks ok to you.

If you have a reaction to the test, it will look like a raised bump. Your health care provider will measure the size of the reaction. If there is a bump, it will go away in a few weeks.

How do I take care of my arm after the TB skin test?

- Don't cover the spot with a bandage or tape.
- Be careful not to rub it or scratch it.
- If the spot itches, put a cold cloth on it.
- You can wash your arm and dry it gently.

Don't be afraid to be tested. TB can be cured!

What if my TB skin test is negative?

The test is "negative" if there is no bump (or only a very small bump) at the spot where the fluid was injected. A negative TB skin test usually means that you don't have TB.

In some situations, you may need to have another TB skin test later.

What if my TB skin test is positive?

The test is "positive" if there is a bump of a certain size where the fluid was injected. This means you probably have TB germs in your body. Most people with a positive TB skin test have latent TB infection. To be sure, your doctor will examine you and give you a chest x-ray. You may need other tests to see if you have active TB disease.

Protect your health and the health of your family—get a TB skin test!

To get a TB skin test, contact your doctor or your public health department.

You should have a TB skin test if:

- You have had frequent close contact with someone who has active TB disease;
- You have lived in a country where many people have TB;

159

- You work or live in a nursing home, clinic, hospital, prison, or homeless shelter; or

- You have human immunodeficiency virus (HIV) infection or certain other health problems.

What if I've had Bacille Calmette-Guérin (BCG) vaccine?

Even if you have had BCG vaccine, you can have a TB skin test:

- People who have had BCG vaccine still can get latent TB infection and active TB disease.

- BCG vaccine may help protect young children from getting very sick with TB. This protection goes away as people get older.

- BCG vaccine sometimes causes a positive TB skin test reaction. But if you have a positive reaction to the TB skin test, it probably is from TB germs in your body—not from your BCG vaccine.

Section 11.3

Routine Sputum Culture

"Instructions for Collecting Sputum for TB (Tuberculosis),"
reprinted with permission from the Minnesota Department of Health
(www.health.state.mn.us). Copyright September 2006.

Why Is a Sputum Test Necessary?

Your doctor wants to collect some of the sputum ("phlegm") that you cough up from your lungs. The laboratory will test the sputum for tuberculosis (TB) germs.

Checking your sputum is the best way to find out if you have TB disease. If you are already taking medicine for TB, checking your sputum is the best way to tell if the medicine is working.

To be sure the test is accurate, you must cough up sputum from deep inside your lungs. Sputum from your lungs is usually thick and sticky. Saliva comes from your mouth and is watery and thin. Do not collect saliva.

Tip: If you cannot cough up sputum, try breathing steam from a hot shower or a pan of boiling water.

How to Collect a Sputum Sample

Your doctor or nurse will give you a special plastic cup for collecting your sputum. Follow these steps carefully:

1. The cup is very clean. Don't open it until you are ready to use it.

2. As soon as you wake up in the morning (before you eat or drink anything), brush your teeth and rinse your mouth with water. Do not use mouthwash.

3. If possible, go outside or open a window before collecting the sputum sample. This helps protect other people from TB germs when you cough.

4. Take a very deep breath and hold the air for five seconds. Slowly breathe out. Take another deep breath and cough hard until some sputum comes up into your mouth.

5. Spit the sputum into the plastic cup.

6. Keep doing this until the sputum reaches the 5 ml line (or more) on the plastic cup. This is about one teaspoon of sputum.

7. Screw the cap on the cup tightly so it doesn't leak.

8. Wash and dry the outside of the cup.

9. Write on the cup the date you collected the sputum.

10. Put the cup into the box or bag the nurse gave you.

11. Give the cup to your clinic or nurse. You can store the cup in the refrigerator overnight if necessary. Do not put it in the freezer or leave it at room temperature.

Chapter 12

Medication for the Treatment of Respiratory Disorders

Chapter Contents

Section 12.1

Antihistamines, Decongestants, and Cold Remedies

Drugs for stuffy nose, sinus trouble, congestion, and the common cold constitute the largest segment of the over-the-counter market for America's pharmaceutical industry. When used wisely, they provide welcome relief for at least some of the discomforts that affect almost everyone occasionally and that affect many people chronically. Drugs in these categories are useful for relief of symptoms from allergies, upper respiratory infections (i.e., sinusitis, colds, flu), and vasomotor rhinitis (a chronic stuffy nose caused by such unrelated conditions as emotional stress, thyroid disease, pregnancy, and others). These drugs do not cure the allergies, infections, etc.; they only relieve the symptoms, thereby making the patient more comfortable.

Antihistamines

Histamine is an important body chemical that is responsible for the congestion, sneezing, and runny nose that a patient suffers with an allergic attack or an infection. Antihistamine drugs block the action of histamine, therefore reducing the allergy symptoms. For the best result, antihistamines should be taken before allergic symptoms get well established.

The most annoying side effect that antihistamines produce is drowsiness. Though desirable at bedtime, it is a nuisance to many people who need to use antihistamines in the daytime. To some people, it is even hazardous. These drugs are not recommended for daytime use for people who may be driving an automobile or operating equipment that could be dangerous. Newer nonsedating antihistamines, available by prescription only, do not have this effect. The first few doses cause the most sleepiness; subsequent doses are usually less troublesome.

Typical antihistamines include Allegra®, Benadryl®, Chlor-Trimeton®, Claritin®, Clarinex®, Teldrin®, Zyrtec®, etc.

Decongestants

Congestion in the nose, sinuses, and chest is due to swollen, expanded, or dilated blood vessels in the membranes of the nose and air passages. These membranes have an abundant supply of blood vessels with a great capacity for expansion (swelling and congestion). Histamine stimulates these blood vessels to expand as described previously.

Decongestants, on the other hand, cause constriction or tightening of the blood vessels in those membranes, which then forces much of the blood out of the membranes so that they shrink, and the air passages open up again.

Decongestants are chemically related to adrenalin, the natural decongestant, which is also a type of stimulant. Therefore, the side effect of decongestants is a jittery or nervous feeling. They can cause difficulty in going to sleep, and they can elevate blood pressure and pulse rate. Decongestants should not be used by a patient who has an irregular heart rhythm (pulse), high blood pressure, heart disease, or glaucoma. Some patients taking decongestants experience difficulty with urination. Furthermore, decongestants are often used as ingredients in diet pills. To avoid excessively stimulating effects, patients taking diet pills should not take decongestants.

Typical decongestants are phenylephrine (Neo-Synephrine®*), and pseudoephedrine (Sudafed®, etc.).

Combination Remedies

Theoretically, if the side effects could be properly balanced, the sleepiness sometimes caused by antihistamines could be cancelled by the stimulation of decongestants. Numerous combinations of antihistamines with decongestants are available: Actifed®*, Allegra-D®, Chlor-Trimeton D®*, Claritin D®, Contac®*, Co-Pyronil 2®*, Deconamine®, Demazin®*, Dimetapp®*, Drixoral®*, Isoclor®*, Nolamine®, Novafed A®, Ornade®, Sudafed Plus®, Tavist D®*, Triaminic®*, and Trinalin®, to name just a few.

A patient may find one preparation quite helpful for several months or years but may need to switch to another one when the first loses its effectiveness. Since no one reacts exactly the same as another to the side effects of these drugs, a patient may wish to try his own ideas on adjusting the dosages. One might take the antihistamine only at night and take the decongestant alone in the daytime. Or take them together, increasing the dosage of antihistamine at night (while decreasing the decongestant dose) and then doing the opposite for daytime use.

For example: Antihistamine (Chlor-Trimeton®*, 4 mg)—one tablet three times daily and two tablets at bedtime. *Plus:* Decongestant (Sudafed®*, 30 mg)—two tablets three times daily and one tablet at bedtime.

"Cold" Remedies

Decongestants and/or antihistamines are the principal ingredients in "cold" remedies, but drying agents, aspirin (or aspirin substitutes), and cough suppressants may also be added. The patient should choose the remedy with ingredients best suited to combat his own symptoms. If the label does not clearly state the ingredients and their functions, the consumer should ask the pharmacist to explain them.

Nose Sprays

The types of nose sprays that can be purchased without a prescription usually contain decongestants for direct application to nasal membranes. They can give prompt relief from congestion by constricting blood vessels. However, direct application creates a stronger stimulation than decongestants taken by mouth. It also impairs the circulation in the nose, which, after a few hours, stimulates the vessels to expand to improve the blood flow again. This results in a "bounce-back" effect. The congestion recurs. If the patient uses the spray again, it

Table 12.1. Medicines for Respiratory Disorders

Medicine	Symptoms Relieved	Possible Side Effects
Antihistamines	Sneezing	Drowsiness
	Runny nose	Dry mouth and nose
	Stuffy nose	
	Itchy eyes	
	Congestion	
Decongestants	Stuffy nose	Stimulation
	Congestion	Insomnia
		Rapid heart beat
Combinations of above	All of above	Any of above (more or less)

starts the cycle again. Spray—decongestion—rebound—and more congestion.

In infants, this rebound rhinitis can develop in two days, whereas in adults, it often takes several more days to become established. An infant taken off the drops for twelve to twenty-four hours is cured, but well-established cases in adults often require more than a simple "cold turkey" withdrawal. They need decongestants by mouth, sometimes corticosteroids, and possibly (in patients who continuously have used the sprays for months and years) a surgical procedure to the inside of the nose. For this reason, the labels on these types of nose sprays contain the warning "Do not use this product for more than three days." Nose sprays should be reserved for emergency and short-term use. (The above description and advice does not apply to the type of prescription anti-allergy nose sprays that may be ordered by your physician.)

Note

*May be available over-the-counter without a prescription. Read labels carefully, and use only as directed.

Section 12.2

Asthma Medicines

"About Asthma Medicines," © 2005 American Lung Association. Reprinted with permission. For more information about the American Lung Association or to support the work it does, call 1-800-LUNG-USA (1-800-586-4872) or log on to http://www.lungusa.org.

Asthma medicines keep the air tubes in your lungs open. There are two groups of asthma medicines:

• Bronchodilators are medicines that help to stop asthma attacks after they've started and can help prevent expected attacks, as from exercise.

• Anti-inflammatories are medicines that help to control the airway inflammation and prevent asthma attacks from starting.

These medicines are sold under many brand names. They come in different forms, too. They can include sprays, pills, powders, liquids, and shots. The doctor chooses the medicine and form that will work best for you.

Let's take a closer look at how these medicines can help you.

Bronchodilators give you relief during an asthma attack. These medicines work to relax the muscles in your air tubes. As this happens, your air tubes open up, making it easier for you to breathe.

Anti-inflammatories, on the other hand, work to keep your air tubes open all of the time so that you don't have an asthma attack in the first place. These medicines reduce the swelling in your air tubes and decrease the mucus. Cromolyn and nedocromil are two examples of anti-inflammatory medicines.

Another example is corticosteroids. When you hear the word "steroid" you might think of the steroids used by athletes. This may worry you if you have heard about the problems and side effects athletes have when taking steroids. But corticosteroids are not the steroids used by athletes. Those steroids are called "anabolic steroids."

Remember that corticosteroids are used to help prevent asthma attacks from starting. When you take this medicine in a spray form, the risk of serious side effects is very little.

The chance of serious side effects increases when these medicines are taken in a pill or liquid form over a long period. In that case, you need to get regular check-ups by a doctor to make sure that the medicine works the best way for you.

Let's talk about side effects for a moment. Every kind of medicine, even aspirin, can have some side effects. But a doctor can help you by finding ways to control side effects.

When it comes to asthma medicines, it is important to check regularly with a doctor to make sure that these medicines are helping you.

Sometimes you may have some side effects, such as a sore throat, nervousness, nausea, rapid heartbeat, loss of appetite, or staying awake. Tell a doctor if you feel this way. The doctor may want to change your dose, or try a different asthma medicine.

The purpose of asthma medicines is to help you feel better and control your asthma so that you can do what you want to do without asthma getting in your way.

One final note on medicines. There is another kind of treatment that may be helpful to you if your asthma attacks get started by allergies. This treatment is called hyposensitization therapy or allergy shots. These shots may be helpful to you in preventing your asthma attacks. Not all experts agree about the usefulness of allergy shots.

On the other hand, the kinds of things that you do are just as important as the kinds of medicines that you take. You can help yourself when you try to avoid or get rid of the things that make you allergic, such as dust, feathers, or animal fur. By doing this, you really take control and make it possible for your asthma medicines to work successfully.

Section 12.3

Bronchodilators

Bronchodilators help open the airways in the lungs by relaxing smooth muscle around the airways. There are three types of bronchodilators: beta-agonists, anticholinergics, and theophyllines.

Combination medications contain more than one type of medicine and are sometimes more beneficial than either medicine used alone.

Beta-Agonists

Beta-agonists can be short acting or long acting.

Short-acting beta-agonists work quickly (within fifteen to twenty minutes) to relieve shortness of breath. They are sometimes described as "rescue" or "quick-reliever" medications. Your doctor may prescribe a short-acting beta-agonist to use regularly or as needed to relieve shortness of breath.

Common short-acting inhaled beta-agonists include:

- Proventil® and Ventolin® (albuterol);
- Maxair® (pirbuterol);
- Alupent® (metaproterenol).

Long-acting beta-agonists do not begin working immediately, but their effects last for a long time (about twelve hours). Therefore, these medicines should not be used for acute attacks of breathlessness or in an emergency. Long-acting beta-agonists are used regularly, usually twice a day, to open the airways and keep them open.

Common long-acting inhaled beta-agonists include:

• Serevent® (salmeterol);

• Foradil® (formoterol).

Anticholinergics

Anticholinergics do not act right away. They should not be taken for quick relief or in emergencies. These medications are inhaled regularly to open the airways, and keep them open.

Common anticholinergics are:

• Atrovent® (ipratropium);

• Spiriva ® (tiotropium).

A combination medication, Combivent® contains a short-acting beta-agonist (albuterol) and an anticholinergic (ipratropium). When these medications are combined, their effects are greater than if each medication were taken alone.

Theophylline

Theophylline is available in pills and is taken regularly. A theophylline blood level between five and fifteen micrograms/milliliter usually gives relief of symptoms while avoiding side effects. Theophylline can interact with other medications, herbals, and dietary supplements, so it is important to tell your doctor and pharmacist that you are on this medication.

Common theophylline brand names include:

• Theo-Dur®;

• Slo-bid®;

• Uniphyl®;

• Uni-Dur®.

Section 12.4

Anti-Inflammatories

Anti-inflammatories help reduce airway inflammation and decrease mucus production. Inhaled corticosteroids and corticosteroid pills are two types of anti-inflammatories frequently used to treat chronic obstructive pulmonary disease (COPD).

What about Inhaled Corticosteroids?

Some people with COPD benefit from the use of inhaled corticosteroids. Inhaled corticosteroids are usually taken regularly. Long-term use at high doses can be associated with side effects, such as loss of bone mineral density, so you should discuss the risks and benefits of these medications with your physician. Using a spacer with inhaled corticosteroids and rinsing your mouth after inhaling the medication reduces the risk of thrush. Thrush, a possible side effect, is a yeast infection causing a white discoloration of the tongue.

Inhaled corticosteroids include:

- Vanceril® and Beclovent® (beclomethasone);
- Azmacort® (triamcinolone);
- AeroBid® (flunisolide);
- Flovent® (fluticasone);
- Pulmicort® (budesonide).

Inhaled Corticosteroid and Long Acting Beta-Agonists

Advair® is a combination medication. Flovent® and Serevent® are the medications combined in Advair ®. Advair® is used regularly.

171

What about Corticosteroid Pills?

Most people with COPD show little or no improvement when corticosteroid pills are given over a long period of time. They are, however, used in special circumstances, such as when your symptoms are getting worse or you need to be hospitalized. Long-term use of corticosteroid pills can result in serious side effects.

Corticosteroid pills include:

- Deltasone® (prednisone);
- Medrol® (methylprednisolone).

Section 12.5

Leukotriene Receptor Antagonists

"Leukotriene Receptor Antagonists for Asthma Treatment," reprinted with permission from www.mydr.com.au © 2007 CMPMedica Australia. The material provided by CMPMedica Australia Pty Ltd is intended for Australian residents, is of a general nature and is provided for information purposes only. The material is not a substitute for independent professional medical advice from a qualified health care professional. It is not intended to be used by anyone to diagnose, treat, cure, or prevent any disease or medical condition. No person should act in reliance solely on any statement contained in the material provided, and at all times should obtain specific advice from a qualified health care professional. CMPMedica Australia Pty Ltd, its servants and agents are not responsible for the continued currency of the material or for any errors, omissions or inaccuracies in the material, whether arising from negligence or otherwise, or from any other consequence arising there from. [Editor's Note: Australian spellings for drug names have been retained; please talk to your physician if you have questions about equivalent spellings in other countries.]

In the past few years, a class of medicines known as leukotriene receptor antagonists has been developed for the treatment of asthma.

Leukotriene receptor antagonists, such as montelukast sodium (e.g., Singulair® tablets) or zafirlukast (e.g., Accolate® tablets), treat asthma via a totally different pathway to other available medicines. They work by blocking substances in your lungs called leukotrienes, which cause narrowing and swelling of the airways. Blocking leukotrienes can improve asthma symptoms, including nighttime symptoms, and can help prevent asthma attacks.

Research has shown that leukotriene receptor antagonists may offer some protection against asthma which is allergen-induced, as well as from asthma which is exercise-induced. They have also been found to be effective for those people with asthma who are sensitive to aspirin.

The most common side effects of leukotriene receptor antagonists are headache and gastrointestinal upsets.

Because they come in tablet form, leukotriene antagonists can be a helpful preventive therapy for people who would rather not use an inhaled medicine, or who have difficulty using their inhaler properly. Even children can take them; for example, children two years of age and above can take Singulair as it comes in a chewable tablet form.

A leukotriene receptor antagonist can be used instead of inhaled steroids to help prevent asthma, or in conjunction with your other asthma medicines if you need extra help to keep your asthma under control.

Leukotriene receptor antagonists are not used to treat an acute attack of asthma. They are preventers and should be taken daily, as prescribed by your doctor.

Your doctor can advise if a leukotriene receptor antagonist is suitable for you or your child.

Chapter 13

Respiratory Assist Devices

Chapter Contents

Section 13.1

Inhalers

Inhaled asthma medications are generally inhaled through either a metered dose inhaler (MDI), with or without a spacer, or a dry powder device.

There is also another type of inhaler device, the nebulizer, a device that pumps pressurized air through liquid medication to convert it into a fine vapor, which is then breathed in through a mask or mouthpiece. Nebulizers are useful for giving high doses of medication, but are generally prescribed only for people with severe, life-threatening asthma.

Selection of Your Device

Selection of the type of device is often a personal preference. Some people prefer a MDI to a breath-activated dry powder device and vice versa. However, the individual device you use can depend on the medication you're taking, as medication manufacturers often present their medicine in their own type of device. It is important that you feel comfortable with the inhaler chosen, and that you can use it properly. If you're unsure about your inhaler technique, ask your doctor or pharmacist for advice.

Metered Dose Inhalers

A common inhaler device is the pressurized metered dose inhaler, also known as an aerosol inhaler.

Aerosol inhalers contain an aerosol canister that dispenses the medication in a fine mist that you can then breathe in.

Some of the chlorofluorocarbon (CFC)–free formulations of asthma medications are stickier than the older formulations. This means that your inhaler could become clogged with medication. Clean your inhaler regularly, as instructed by the manufacturer or your doctor.

Some of the medications available in aerosol inhalers include:

- Relievers such as salbutamol (e.g., Airomir®, Ventolin®) and ipratropium bromide (e.g., Atrovent®);

- Preventers such as beclomethasone (e.g., Qvar®), fluticasone (e.g., Flixotide®), sodium cromoglycate (e.g., Intal®, Intal Forte®) and nedocromil sodium (e.g., Tilade®);

- Symptom controllers such as salmeterol (e.g., Serevent®); and

- Combination products such as the combination of fluticasone (a preventer) and salmeterol (a symptom controller) in Seretide®.

Aerosol inhalers require coordination and good timing between activation (pressing down on the inhaler) and inhalation. Most adults and children older than about seven years can be taught to use pressurized MDIs correctly, but MDIs can be difficult to coordinate. People with arthritis or poor strength in their hands may also have difficulty operating a MDI.

Overcoming Coordination Problems

To aid coordination, your doctor might recommend using a spacer with the MDI. A spacer is a large, plastic device which acts as a holding chamber for medication for the few seconds that might elapse between activating your MDI and breathing in the medication. By putting one end of the spacer in your mouth and attaching your MDI to the other end of the spacer, you can inhale your medication effectively without having to press the MDI and breathe at exactly the same time. Most children under seven years old will probably need to use a spacer to help deliver their medication correctly.

Another type of MDI that can help coordination is the Autohaler, a breath-activated metered-dose inhaler that delivers medications such as salbutamol (e.g., Airomir®), and beclomethasone (e.g., Qvar®). You use it by flicking a switch, and then breathing in through the mouthpiece. However, it is usually not recommended for children under seven years old.

Dry Powder Inhalers

There are a number of different types of dry powder inhalers. The type of dry powder device you receive will depend on the type and brand of medication your doctor prescribes, since medication manufacturers often present their medicine in their own type of device.

Dry powder inhalers require you to take a deep breath to activate the device and get the powder into your lungs. It is important not to exhale into the mouthpiece before inhaling as the moisture from your breath can stop the inhaler from working properly.

Some children aged five to seven years may be able to use dry powder devices effectively. However, often a MDI and spacer are recommended for children under the age of seven years.

Dry powder inhalers include the Accuhaler, Aerolizer, Rotahaler, Diskhaler and Turbuhaler. There are also other inhalers available so ask your doctor for advice.

The Accuhaler is a breath-activated, multi-dose, dry powder inhaler that delivers the medications salmeterol (Serevent®) or fluticasone (Flixotide®), or a combination of both (Seretide®).

The Aerolizer is a breath-activated, single-dose, dry powder inhaler which comes with capsules of medication that must be loaded into the device before use. The Aerolizer delivers eformoterol (Foradile®).

The Rotahaler delivers capsules of medication called Rotacaps, which must be loaded into the device before use. A Rotahaler can be used to administer salbutamol (Ventolin Rotacaps).

The Diskhaler is a multi-dose dry powder inhaler that can deliver salbutamol (Ventolin Disks).

The Turbuhaler is a breath-activated inhaler that can deliver terbutaline (Bricanyl®), budesonide (Pulmicort®) or eformoterol (Oxis®), or a combination of both budesonide and eformoterol (Symbicort®).

There are many types of asthma medications and different methods of delivery. Your doctor can advise you about the inhaler that's best for you.

Section 13.2

Nebulizers

What Is a Nebulizer?

A nebulizer is a device that pumps pressurized air through liquid medication to convert it into a fine vapor, which is then breathed in through a mask or mouthpiece.

Asthma medication solution should be 80 percent vaporized within about eight minutes; the liquid left in the nebulizer bowl is mostly saline, used to dilute the medication.

Who Needs a Nebulizer?

Nebulizers are useful for giving high doses of medication, but are generally prescribed only for people with severe, life-threatening asthma. In the case of an asthma attack, most people with asthma— even children—do not need to have a nebulizer, as they can use a metered dose inhaler with a valved spacer to deliver their reliever medication just as effectively. Your doctor will recommend the medication delivery method that is best for you.

Types of Nebulizers

If your doctor has recommended that you use a nebulizer, make sure you use the type that best suits your needs.

For example, you can get nebulizers that are plugged in directly to the main power supply, but you can also get battery-operated pumps, and pumps that plug into car cigarette lighters.

There are different types of nebulizer pumps, including low-flow pumps, for delivering one type of medication for occasional use, and heavy-duty high-flow pumps, for delivering more than one medication, or for inhaled corticosteroids (preventer medication) or antibiotics, or for use by more than one person.

Cleaning and Maintenance

Nebulizers must be well maintained and cleaned after each use to prevent respiratory infection and ensure they operate at their best.

Nebulizer bowls and face masks should be washed in warm soapy water, allowed to air dry, and then stored in airtight containers.

The bowl and tubes should be checked regularly for cracks and replaced frequently as they deteriorate with repeated use. The nebulizer pump itself should also be serviced every six to twelve months, and its filters changed in the same time frame, to ensure that it delivers enough air to turn the liquid medication into a vapor.

Because they require so much maintenance, nebulizers are not as convenient as a spacer and inhaler used together.

Section 13.3

Home Oxygen Therapy

"Home Oxygen Therapy," © 2005 American Association for Respiratory Care. Reprinted with permission. For additional information, visit www.yourlunghealth.org.

More and more people are using oxygen therapy outside the hospital, permitting them to lead active, productive lives. People with asthma, emphysema, chronic bronchitis, occupational lung disease, lung cancer, cystic fibrosis, or congestive heart failure may use oxygen therapy at home.

The Prescription

A physician must write a prescription for oxygen therapy. The prescription will spell out the flow rate, how much oxygen you need per minute—referred to as liters per minute (LPM or L/M)—and when you need to use oxygen. Some people use oxygen therapy only while exercising, others only while sleeping, and still others need oxygen continuously. Your physician will order a blood test that will indicate what your oxygen level is and help determine what your needs are.

The Equipment

There are three common ways of providing oxygen therapy. Oxygen can be delivered to your home in the form of a gas in various-sized cylinders or as a liquid in a vessel. The third way to provide oxygen therapy is by using an oxygen concentrator. Each method is examined in more detail below.

Compressed gas: Oxygen is stored under pressure in a cylinder equipped with a regulator that controls the flow rate. Because the flow of oxygen out of the cylinder is constant, an oxygen-conserving device may be attached to the system to avoid waste. This device releases the gas only when you inhale and cuts it off when you exhale. Oxygen can be provided in a small cylinder that can be carried with you, but the large tanks are heavy and are only suitable for stationary use.

Liquid oxygen: Oxygen is stored as a very cold liquid in a vessel very similar to a thermos. When released, the liquid converts to a gas and you breathe it in just like the compressed gas. This storage method takes up less space than the compressed gas cylinder, and you can transfer the liquid to a small, portable vessel at home. Liquid oxygen is more expensive than the compressed gas, and the vessel vents when not in use. An oxygen-conserving device may be built into the vessel to conserve the oxygen.

Oxygen concentrator: This is an electrically powered device that separates the oxygen out of the air, concentrates it, and stores it. This system has a number of advantages because it doesn't have to be re-supplied and it is not as costly as liquid oxygen. Extra tubing permits the user to move around with minimal difficulty. Small, portable systems have been developed that afford even greater mobility. You must have a cylinder of oxygen as a backup in the event of a power failure. You should advise your electric power company in order to get priority service when there is a power failure.

Oxygen Delivery Devices

There are three common means of oxygen delivery. A nasal cannula is a two-pronged device inserted in the nostrils that is connected to tubing carrying the oxygen. The tubing can rest on the ears or be attached to the frame of eyeglasses.

People who need a high flow of oxygen generally use a mask. Some people who use a nasal cannula during the day prefer a mask at night or when their noses are irritated or clogged by a cold.

Transtracheal oxygen therapy requires the insertion of a small flexible catheter in the trachea or windpipe. The transtracheal catheter is held in place by a necklace. Since transtracheal oxygen bypasses the mouth, nose, and throat, a humidifier is absolutely required at flow rates of 1 LPM or greater.

Safety

You should never smoke while using oxygen. Warn visitors not to smoke near you when you are using oxygen. Put up no-smoking signs in your home where you most often use the oxygen. When you go to a restaurant with your portable oxygen source, ask to be seated in the non-smoking section. Stay at least five feet away from gas stoves, candles, lighted fireplaces, or other heat sources. Don't use any flammable products like cleaning fluid, paint thinner, or aerosol sprays while using your oxygen.

If you use an oxygen cylinder, make sure it is secured to some fixed object or in a stand. If you use liquid oxygen, make sure the vessel is kept upright to keep the oxygen from pouring out; the liquid oxygen is so cold it can hurt your skin. Keep a fire extinguisher close by, and let your fire department know that you have oxygen in your home. If you use an oxygen concentrator, notify your electric company so you will be given priority if there is a power failure. Also, avoid using extension cords if possible.

Care of Equipment

The home medical equipment and services company that provides the oxygen therapy equipment you use should provide you with instructions on user care and maintenance of your particular equipment. Here are some general guidelines for your cleaning procedures. You should wash your nasal prongs with a liquid soap and thoroughly rinse them once or twice a week. Replace them every two to four weeks. If you have a cold, change them when your cold symptoms have passed.

Check with your health care provider to learn how to clean your transtracheal catheter. The humidifier bottle should be washed with soap and warm water and rinsed thoroughly between each refill. Air dry the bottle before filling with sterile or distilled water. The bottle and its top should be disinfected after they are cleaned.

If you use an oxygen concentrator, unplug the unit, then wipe down the cabinet with a damp cloth and dry it daily. The air filter should be cleaned at least twice a week. Follow your home medical equipment and services company's directions for cleaning the compressor filter.

Dos and Don'ts

- Don't ever change the flow of oxygen unless directed by your physician.

- Don't use alcohol or take any other sedating drugs because they will slow your breathing rate.

- Make sure you order more oxygen from your dealer in a timely manner.

- Use water-based lubricants on your lips or nostrils. Don't use an oil-based product like petroleum jelly.

- To prevent your cheeks or the skin behind your ears from becoming irritated, tuck some gauze under the tubing. If you have persistent redness under your nose, call your physician.

Trouble

Call your physician if you experience frequent headaches, anxiety, blue lips or fingernails, drowsiness, confusion, restlessness, anxiety, or slow, shallow, difficult, or irregular breathing. Also, call your physician if you feel any symptoms of illness.

Medicare, Medicaid, and Commercial Insurance

Certain insurance policies may pay for all your oxygen, but payment is based on laboratory results, diagnosis, and other information. Your physician or medical equipment and services provider may be able to answer your questions about coverage.

Section 13.4

Mechanical Ventilation

Mechanical Ventilation: What Is It?

Mechanical ventilation is a method for using machines to help patients breathe when they are unable to breathe sufficiently on their own.

Most often, mechanical ventilation is used for a few days to help a
patient breathe during a serious illness. This type of breathing support is usually done in an intensive care unit—an ICU for short.

Sometimes patients still can't breathe on their own after the acute
illness is over, despite efforts to restore spontaneous breathing. Patients
may no longer need to be in the ICU but still require mechanical ventilation because of an extended need for the breathing assistance of
the ventilator.

Other patients may have stable, longer-term (chronic) conditions
that make them unable to breathe on their own.

Due to a variety of reasons, including the cost of hospital care and
the patient's quality of life, for the patient who is dependent on a ventilator for breathing assistance, it may be better to receive mechanical
ventilation at home or at a nonhospital institution offering specialized
nursing or rehabilitation services.

Over time, with the professional support of physicians and respiratory therapists, some ventilator-assisted individuals are able to
become less dependent on the ventilator and breathe on their own for
substantial portions of every day. Other patients have medical conditions that require twenty-four-hour mechanical ventilation for many
months or years, or even for a lifetime.

Ventilator Dependence

"Weaning" is the word used to describe the process of gradually removing the patient from the ventilator and restoring spontaneous

breathing after a period of mechanical ventilation. Physicians and the ICU respiratory care specialists help patients to wean when weaning is determined to be medically appropriate. While patients with some conditions can be weaned from mechanical ventilation after a few days to a week in the ICU, patients with other conditions cannot or should not be taken off the ventilator. Patients with stable chronic medical conditions are more likely to require long-term mechanical ventilation, for example, patients with neuromuscular disorders or chest wall deformities.

Mechanical ventilation is required when a patient's spontaneous efforts are unable to sustain adequate ventilation of the lungs.

Conditions such as stroke and spinal cord injury damage the nerves that control breathing and make spontaneous breathing impossible for an extended period or for life.

Chronic stable illnesses, such as neuromuscular disorders and chest wall deformities, and/or advanced age, may make long-term mechanical ventilation necessary for extended periods or for life.

Chronic illness that requires recurrent ICU hospitalization may require frequent repeated treatments with mechanical ventilation and repeated attempts to wean from mechanical ventilation.

Long-Term Mechanical Ventilation: Who, When, and Where

Who

The patient's physician and respiratory care team determine (1) the need for long-term ventilatory assistance, and (2) the type of mechanical ventilation, both technique and equipment, best for the patient after discharge from the ICU.

These determinations are based on (1) the patient's current illness and past medical history, (2) complete medical assessment, and (3) tests of daytime, and sometimes of nighttime, breathing efficiency and ability to breathe without help.

Patients who benefit from long-term mechanical ventilation are those whose medical conditions would become unstable if they were removed from mechanical ventilation. They might have recurrent or chronic conditions that make it more difficult for the patient to carry out activities of daily living.

When

Medical criteria determine when a patient can be discharged from the ICU on long-term mechanical ventilation to a site outside the ICU.

However, other considerations also are important. Successful discharge on long-term mechanical ventilation is more likely when:

- the patient is highly motivated to accept the responsibility to make long-term ventilation work;

- the patient may be able to independently do some activities of daily living;

- the patient is able to communicate with caregivers and give them direction;

- the patient and his or her family understand all available options for long-term ventilation;

- the family is able and willing to participate in long-term care;

- financial resources are available for mechanical ventilation equipment and caregiver assistance such as nursing services; and

- medical and respiratory care professionals are available to monitor and supervise long-term care.

Where

The optimal location for long-term ventilator-assisted individuals may be with the family in the home. In the home, the patient's quality of life is likely to be better than at any other location. Costs of care are usually lower when the patient is at home, but insurance coverage of home-care costs must be evaluated on an individual basis to determine if adequate reimbursement is available. Usually, the cost of home care must be less than the cost of a long-term care facility in order for benefits to apply.

Home is not the only site for patients to receive long-term mechanical ventilation. Other nonhospital sites may be appropriate for the patient's needs and resources. The appropriate site for long-term mechanical ventilation is one in which all of the patient's needs—medical care, respiratory care, psychological support, and rehabilitation—can be met by available resources. A site other than the home may be more appropriate for some patients.

The choice of a site for long-term mechanical ventilation is a joint responsibility of the patient, patient's family, and patient's physician, with consultation from other members of the respiratory care team—respiratory therapist, nurse, social worker, case manager, and benefits manager.

187

Types of Facilities That May Be Considered

For patients who can leave the ICU but still require hospitalization:

- Specialized respiratory care unit of the hospital
- General medical/surgical unit of the hospital

For patients who can leave the hospital but have special needs for care, monitoring, or rehabilitation:

- Subacute care unit of the hospital
- Long-term care hospital
- Rehabilitation hospital

For patients capable of some degree of independent living:

- Skilled nursing facility
- Congregate living center
- Home

Mechanical Ventilation: Methods

The method of long-term mechanical ventilation that is best for the patient will be determined by the physician, respiratory therapist, and the patient. A patient capable of some independent activities and several hours a day off the ventilator will have different requirements than the patient who needs ventilator assistance twenty-four hours a day.

Invasive methods use a tracheostomy—a surgical hole in the windpipe through which a tube is channeled to assist breathing.

Noninvasive methods use masks, nasal tubes, and other techniques that do not require surgical entry into the respiratory tract. Some apply positive pressure to the mouth and/or nose. Others apply negative pressure to the chest or body by lowering the pressure outside the body.

All methods of ventilation require an initial assessment of comfort and efficacy and follow-up monitoring of daytime and nighttime breathing. The patient and caregivers should be educated in use and maintenance of the equipment needed to provide the support.

Noninvasive Methods

Positive pressure ventilation—mouth and/or nose: Positive pressure ventilation delivers air (and sometimes extra oxygen when medically necessary) to the patient through a facemask, mouthpiece, or nasal mask. Patients who can be independent of the ventilator for portions of the day may use noninvasive positive-pressure ventilation to assist nighttime breathing.

Negative pressure ventilation: Entry of air into the lungs is assisted by applying intermittent negative pressure (like a vacuum) to the chest and abdomen by means of a body tank (iron lung), a chest shell, or a body jacket.

Rocking bed: A bed with rocking motion assists ventilation by intermittently causing the diaphragm to move up and down, creating a "pumping" motion in the chest, and thus, helping air to go in and out of the lungs.

Pneumobelt: An inflatable band around the abdomen presses on the abdomen and forces air in and out of the lungs. The pneumobelt may be used in combination with other noninvasive methods of ventilation. It may not be suitable for some patients—for example, patients who are excessively underweight or overweight. The patient must be sitting up for this device to work. It is often used by patients in a wheelchair.

Diaphragm pacing: An electronic pacer stimulates the diaphragm to contract, thus assisting breathing by "bellows" motion of the diaphragm. This method is used by patients who have high (C1–C2) spinal cord injury, and with tracheostomy in some children who cannot breathe spontaneously because of a problem with central control of breathing.

Glossopharyngeal breathing: Sometimes called "frog" breathing—a technique in which the patient learns to "gulp" air into the lungs. Some patients use this technique in order to spend more time off the ventilator and to have "free" time in case of ventilator failure.

Manually assisted coughing: A caregiver helps the patient to exhale and clear mucus from the lungs by delivering a thrust similar to a Heimlich maneuver. Thorough training of the patient and caregivers is required to make this technique effective and to avoid injury to the patient.

Invasive Methods

Invasive methods may be needed for patients who are unable to use noninvasive methods. Invasive mechanical ventilation requires a tracheostomy for placement of a tracheostomy tube into the wind-pipe to deliver air directly into the lungs. The patient and caregivers are trained in care of the tracheostomy and tube to prevent compli-cations such as infection around the tracheostomy tube or clogging of the tube.

Chapter 14

Respiratory Disease Management

Chapter Contents

Section 14.1

Pulmonary Rehabilitation

Excerpted from "Pulmonary Rehabilitation: A Team Approach to Improving Quality of Life." Reprinted with permission from The American College of Chest Physicians (www.chestnet.org), © 2005. All rights reserved.

What is pulmonary rehabilitation?

Pulmonary rehabilitation combines exercise training and behavioral and educational programs designed to help patients with chronic lung disease control symptoms and improve day-to-day activities. It is a team approach—patients work closely with their doctors; nurses; respiratory, physical, and occupational therapists; psychologists; exercise specialists; and dietitians.

The main goals of pulmonary rehabilitation are to help patients improve their day-to-day lives and restore their ability to function independently. If your illness has affected your daily living, pulmonary rehabilitation can help you:

- Reduce and control breathing difficulties and other symptoms;

- Learn more about your disease, treatment options, and coping strategies;

- Learn to manage your disease and reduce your dependence on health professionals and costly medical resources;

- Maintain healthy behaviors such as smoking cessation, good nutrition, and exercise.

In addition, pulmonary rehabilitation can help reduce the number and length of hospital stays and increase your chances of living longer.

Who benefits from pulmonary rehabilitation?

In the past, pulmonary rehabilitation was used primarily for patients with chronic obstructive pulmonary disease (COPD). However, it can also be helpful to people with other chronic lung conditions such as:

- Interstitial diseases;

- Cystic fibrosis;

- Bronchiectasis;

- Thoracic cage abnormalities;

- Neuromuscular disorders.

Pulmonary rehabilitation can also be helpful to those who need lung transplants or other lung surgeries. Whether you have a chronic respiratory system disease or are experiencing disabling symptoms, such as shortness of breath, cough, and/or mucus production, pulmonary rehabilitation can help. Even patients with severe disease can benefit.

What is involved in pulmonary rehabilitation?

Pulmonary rehabilitation involves these components:

- Exercise training: lower body, upper body, ventilatory muscle training (for some patients)

- Psychosocial support

- Educational programs

Lower body training: Lower body exercises like walking or riding a stationary bicycle will help strengthen your leg muscles and increase muscle tone and flexibility. These exercises will help you move about more easily, often for longer periods of time. They can also make certain tasks, like walking up stairs, easier to do.

Many patients find that as their technique improves, their motivation to continue with the exercise program increases as well. As a result, many patients report feeling better about themselves and their ability to control symptoms such as breathing difficulties.

Upper body training: Upper body training increases the strength and endurance of arm and shoulder muscles. Strengthening these muscles is important because they provide support to the ribcage and can improve breathing. These exercises can also help in tasks that require arm work such as carrying groceries, cooking dinner, lifting items, making the bed, vacuuming, taking a bath or shower, and combing hair. They can also decrease the amount of oxygen needed for these activities. This may be due to less worry about breathing difficulties and better coordination of the muscles involved in raising the arms.

Many patients with lung diseases are not in very good physical condition or have never exercised on a regular basis. Don't worry. Your pulmonary rehabilitation team will meet with you to assess your needs and will work with you to develop an exercise program designed specifically for you. They will advise you about which exercises will give you the best results, how often you should do them, for how long, and at what level. They will give you information on how to maintain your exercise abilities on a regular basis.

Ventilatory muscle training: Weakness of the respiratory muscles can contribute to breathing problems and make exercising difficult. For some patients, ventilatory muscle training (VMT) may improve respiratory muscle function, help reduce the severity of breathlessness, and improve the ability to exercise.

Research at this time does not support the use of VMT for everyone. However, it may be helpful for some patients with chronic lung disease who have respiratory muscle weakness and breathlessness. Your pulmonary rehabilitation team will let you know if you are a candidate for VMT.

Psychosocial support and education: In addition to exercise training, many pulmonary rehabilitation programs provide help with the emotional stresses common to chronic lung disease. Some patients never experience any significant emotional distress as a result of their disease. But for many, chronic lung disease can cause depression, anxiety, or other emotional problems. These might include concerns about:

- Body image;
- Increased loneliness;
- Relationships with family and friends;
- Lack of social support;
- Negative self-concept and low self-esteem.

Support may be provided through patient education programs, or as part of support or stress management groups. Patients are counseled about depression and anxiety, taught relaxation skills, encouraged to talk about their feelings, and learn the importance of giving and receiving emotional support from others.

It is important to remember that support for psychological or emotional difficulties is most beneficial over a longer period of time—there is no such thing as a "quick fix." If you are experiencing any of the above feelings, make sure you discuss them with your pulmonary rehabilitation team.

Since smoking is well known to be the primary risk factor for the onset and working of COPD, many pulmonary rehabilitation programs provide educational sessions and counseling to help patients stop smoking. Most patients with COPD have quit smoking by the time they begin a pulmonary rehabilitation program. Others may continue to smoke as a way to cope with depression, anxiety, and loneliness.

Other patient education classes often cover a wide variety of topics. These might include:

- How the lungs work;

- Information about COPD and other chronic lung diseases;

- Information about medications, including drug action, side effects, using an inhaler, and self-care techniques;

- Understanding and using oxygen therapy;

- Diet, nutrition, and weight management;

- Breathing retraining;

- Importance of exercise;

- Strategies for managing breathing problems;

- Symptom assessment and knowledge about when to seek medical treatment;

- Travel.

Information may be provided through lectures, printed handouts, demonstrations, or one-on-one instruction.

In summary, much has been learned about the effectiveness and benefits of pulmonary rehabilitation. Patients with chronic lung disease greatly benefit from the combination of physical training and behavioral and emotional support. Pulmonary rehabilitation helps patients with chronic lung disease improve their quality of life and their ability to function independently. Talk to your physician about pulmonary rehabilitation and how it can help you.

Section 14.2

Breathing Techniques

"Managing COPD: Breathing Techniques," © American Lung Association of San Diego and Imperial Counties. Reprinted with permission. The text of this document is available online at http://www.lunsandiego.org/copd/adults_manage_breathe.asp; accessed September 24, 2007.

Two techniques can be beneficial to people with chronic obstructive pulmonary disease (COPD) and some other chronic lung conditions.

Pursed Lip Breathing (PLB)

What is PLB?

PLB is a technique that helps people gain control of breathing while exercising or while experiencing breathing distress. It helps increase oxygen levels in the blood. Regular use of PLB trains one to use the proper breathing muscles, and to exhale as much air as possible before drawing in a new breath.

To do PLB, inhale through your nose, keeping your the mouth closed. Then merely purse your lips as if kissing or whistling and exhale softly against them. The key to PLB is to exhale at least twice as long as you inhale.

How does PLB work?

People with COPD commonly have a problem with air trapping in the lungs. Airways become floppier, and tend to collapse during exhalation, trapping the air in the air sacs (alveoli) at the end of the airways. When you breathe out against pursed lips, it builds a resistance in your airways. This resistance creates a back pressure extending down your airways, helping to keep them open during exhalation. By prolonging your exhalation at least twice as long as your inhalation, you help ensure that more air has a chance to escape the alveoli. More fully emptying your lungs means that, with the next inhalation, more oxygen will get into your lungs and your bloodstream.

When should I use PLB?

PLB should be used anytime you feel short of breath. It should be used in conjunction with diaphragmatic breathing (discussed next) when you exercise. Coordinating PLB with body movements will help you feel less short of breath exercising or when performing any activity (e.g., stair climbing) which causes you shortness of breath.

Diaphragmatic Breathing

What is diaphragmatic breathing?

Diaphragmatic breathing is an exercise to better use and to strengthen the diaphragm, the major and most efficient muscle of breathing. Regular practice of diaphragmatic breathing can help restore function to your diaphragm, and return you to a more efficient breathing pattern.

The diaphragm sits under the lungs and is dome-shaped if lungs are normal. During exhalation, the normally functioning diaphragm recoils upward, helping to expel air from the chest.

Because of the air trapping that can occur in COPD, it becomes harder for the diaphragm to function, and it can become flattened and less useful in breathing. The flattened diaphragm forces more of the work of breathing onto other muscles in the chest. These other muscles are less suited for this task and have to work harder, burning more energy and tiring you out faster.

Practicing a deeper, diaphragmatic style of breathing can help ease the work of breathing and expel more stale air.

When starting to practice diaphragmatic breathing, it helps to lie down. Put one pillow under your head and another behind your knees. Place one hand on your upper chest, and the other on the center of your stomach, below the rib cage. The key to diaphragmatic breathing is to use your diaphragm for breathing, and not your upper chest muscles.

Inhale through your nose while expanding, or pushing out, your stomach muscles. Your upper chest should not move outward. When exhaling, exhale slowly through pursed lips while pulling in your stomach muscles. At first, you will have to force your abdomen to move in this way. But with practice and regular use, it should become more natural. If you can, work your way toward using diaphragmatic breathing all the time.

Section 14.3

Airway Clearance Techniques

"Airway Clearance Techniques," © Cystic Fibrosis Foundation. Reprinted with permission. The text of this document is available online at http://www.cff.org/treatments/Therapies/Respiratory/AirwayClearance/; accessed September 21, 2007.

Airway clearance techniques (ACTs) are treatments that help people with cystic fibrosis (CF) stay healthy and breathe easier. ACTs loosen thick, sticky lung mucus so it can be cleared by coughing or huffing. Clearing the airways reduces lung infections and improves lung function. There are many ACTs. Most are easy to do. For infants and toddlers, ACTs can be done by almost anyone. Older kids and adults can do their own ACTs.

ACTs are often used with other treatments, like inhaled bronchodilators and antibiotics. Bronchodilators should be taken before or with ACTs to open airways. Inhaled antibiotics should be taken after ACTs to treat opened airways. Your CF care team will help you choose the best ACT and other treatments. Each year, review and update your routine with your CF care team.

The Lungs

Learning about breathing and the lungs can help you to see how ACTs work. ACTs move mucus from small to large (more central) airways to be coughed or huffed out. The right lung has three lobes: the upper, middle, and lower lobes. The left lung has two lobes: the upper and lower lobes. Lobes divide into smaller segments. ACTs clear these segments. Each segment has airways (bronchi), air sacs (alveoli), and blood vessels (arteries, veins, and capillaries). Oxygen and carbon dioxide flow between the blood and air through the air sacs.

Mucus

The lungs make mucus to help defend against germs. CF changes the mucus, making it thick and hard to clear. This mucus is where infections can occur. Infections cause inflammation or swelling of the lungs. Both infections and inflammation cause more mucus to be made. More mucus in the lungs can lead to more infections. This cycle of infection, inflammation, and more mucus can hurt the lungs and lower lung function. Antibiotics treat infections. They make you feel better but, over time, the damage builds. This is why your CF care team may say to do ACTs even when you are well. When you get sick, do them more often.

How Does Mucus Move out of the Lungs?

Mucus moves three ways:

- Tiny hairs, called cilia, line bronchi. Cilia move back and forth. Mucus is carried on top of cilia. Cilia cannot carry thick, extra mucus as well.

- Mucus builds and lines the bronchi walls. ACTs increase airflow through the bronchi. As air rushes over the mucus in the bronchi, the mucus is pulled toward the large airways. This is like wind on the water making a crest on waves, or wind across a dry plain blowing dust. The faster the air flows, the better it moves mucus.

- If air gets behind thick mucus, it can push it into larger airways. More air behind mucus means more air flowing over it, pulling the mucus along. If air does not get behind mucus, mucus is hard to move.

Airway Clearance Techniques

Coughing is the most basic ACT. It is a reflex. It clears mucus with high-speed airflow. But sometimes mucus cannot be cleared just with a lot of coughing. Coughing a lot can make you feel more short of breath and worse, not better. Huffing is a type of cough. It also involves taking a breath in and actively exhaling. It is more like "huffing" onto a mirror or window to steam it up. It is not as forceful as a cough but can work better and be less tiring.

Chest physical therapy (CPT or chest PT) or postural drainage and percussion (PD & P) is an ACT that often includes postural drainage and chest percussion. With postural drainage, the person gets in varied positions (postures) that drain mucus from different lung parts.

Gravity pulls mucus from small to large airways where it can be coughed up. With chest percussion the chest is clapped and vibrated to dislodge and move mucus. This is done in varied positions to drain all lung parts.

Oscillating positive expiratory pressure (oscillating PEP) is an ACT where the person blows all the way out many times through a device. Types of oscillating PEP devices include the Flutter®, Acapella®, Cornet®, and intrapulmonary percussive ventilation (IPV). Breathing with these devices vibrates the large and small airways. This vibration thins, dislodges, and moves mucus. After blowing through the device many times, the person coughs or huffs. This cycle is repeated many times.

High-frequency chest wall oscillation also is called the Vest or Oscillator. An inflatable vest is attached to a machine that vibrates it at high frequency. The vest vibrates the chest to loosen and thin mucus. Every five minutes the person stops the machine and coughs or huffs.

Positive expiratory pressure (PEP) therapy gets air into the lungs and behind the mucus using extra (collateral) airways. PEP holds airways open, keeping them from closing. A PEP system includes a mask or mouthpiece attached to a resistor set by your CF care team. The person breathes in normally and breathes out a little harder against the resistance.

Active cycle of breathing technique (ACBT) involves a set of breathing techniques. It can be changed to meet each person's needs. It gets air behind mucus, lowers airway spasm, and clears mucus. It includes:

- **Breathing control:** Normal, gentle breathing with the lower chest while relaxing the upper chest and shoulders.

- **Thoracic expansion exercises:** Deep breaths in. Some use a three-second breath-hold to get more air behind the mucus. This may be done with chest clapping or vibrating, followed by breathing control.

- **Forced expiration technique:** Huffs of varied lengths with breathing control.

Autogenic drainage (AD) means "self-drainage." It uses varied airflows to move mucus. It aims to reach very high airflows in different lung parts. This moves mucus from small to large airways. AD has three parts:

- Dislodging mucus
- Collecting mucus
- Clearing mucus

The person inhales to different levels and then adjusts how they breathe out to heighten airflow and move mucus. At first, AD takes hard work and practice. It is best for people over eight years old.

Conclusion

This is a brief overview of some of the ACTs used. ACTs can be varied based on your disease, your care center, or even your country! Your CF care team will help you choose what is best for you. If you have questions, please contact your local CF care center.

Section 14.4

Postural Drainage and Percussion

"An Introduction to Postural Drainage and Percussion,"
© 2005 Cystic Fibrosis Foundation. Reprinted with permission.

Postural drainage and percussion (PD & P), also known as chest physical therapy, is a widely accepted technique to help people with cystic fibrosis (CF) breathe with less difficulty and stay healthy. PD & P uses gravity and percussion to loosen the thick, sticky mucus in the lungs so it can be removed by coughing. Unclogging the airways is critical to reducing the severity of lung infections.

PD & P is easy to perform using the techniques you will learn here. For the child with CF, PD & P can be performed by physical therapists, respiratory therapists, nurses, parents, siblings and even friends.

PD & P is sometimes used along with other types of treatments, such as inhaled bronchodilators and antibiotics. If ordered, bronchodilators should be taken before PD & P to open the airways, and aerosolized antibiotics should be taken after PD & P to treat the opened airways. Your doctor or therapist will recommend a routine for you or your child.

Becoming Familiar with the Lungs

Learning more about the respiratory system and its relationship to internal organs can help you to understand why PD & P treatments are effective, and how each lung segment is drained.

Draining the Lung Segments

The goal of PD & P is to clear mucus from each of the five lobes of the lungs by draining mucus into the larger airways so that it can be coughed out. The right lung is composed of three lobes: the upper lobe, the middle lobe and the lower lobe. The left lung is made up of only two lobes: the upper lobe and the lower lobe.

The lobes are divided into smaller divisions called segments. The upper lobes on the left and right sides are each made up of three segments: apical, posterior, and anterior. The left upper lobe includes the lingula, which corresponds to the middle lobe on the right. The lower lobes each include four segments: superior, anterior, basal, lateral basal, and posterior basal.

Each segment of the lung contains a network of air tubes, air sacs, and blood vessels. These sacs allow for the exchange of oxygen and carbon dioxide between the blood and air. It is these segments that are being drained. Note the position of each lung segment in Figure 14.1.

Performing PD & P

The performance of PD & P involves a combination of techniques including: multiple bronchial drainage positions, percussion, vibration, deep breathing, and coughing.

Although individual PD & P techniques will be further detailed, a brief summary of the complete treatment follows. Once the person is in one of several prescribed bronchial drainage positions, the caregiver performs percussion on the chest wall. This treatment usually is given for a period of three to five minutes, sometimes followed by vibration over the same lung segment for approximately fifteen seconds (or during five exhalations). The person is then encouraged to cough or huff vigorously to get rid of mucus, clearing the lungs.

It is important to know that for some infants, toddlers, children, and adults, certain postural drainage positions may worsen heartburn

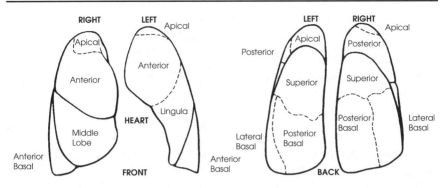

Figure 14.1. External Anatomy of the Lung

and cause vomiting. Specifically, when some people lay with their heads down (lower than the stomach), they can get reflux. This is stomach acid (heartburn) or food coming up from the stomach. It can cause discomfort, wheezing, or vomiting. Reflux may also lead to earlier lung infection or damage. If these things occur, tell your therapist and/or doctor. There are other positions or airway clearance techniques (ACTs) that might be better.

Description of PD & P Techniques

Postural drainage uses gravity to help move mucus from the lungs up to the throat. The person lies or sits in various positions so that the segment to be drained is uppermost on the patient's body. The segment is then drained using percussion, vibration, and gravity. For a complete description of these positions, see figures 14.4 through 14.15. Your CF care team may tailor these positions to your or your child's needs.

Percussion or clapping by the caregiver on the chest wall over the lung segment to be drained forces secretions into the larger airways. The hand is cupped as if to hold water but with the palm facing down as in Figure 2. The cupped hand conforms to the chest wall and traps a cushion of air to soften the clapping.

Percussion is done vigorously and rhythmically, but should not be painful or sting if the hand is cupped properly. Each percussion also should have a hollow sound. The majority of the movement is in the wrist with the arm relaxed, making percussion less tiring to perform.

Percussion should be done only over the ribs. Special attention must be taken to avoid percussing over the spine, breastbone, stomach and

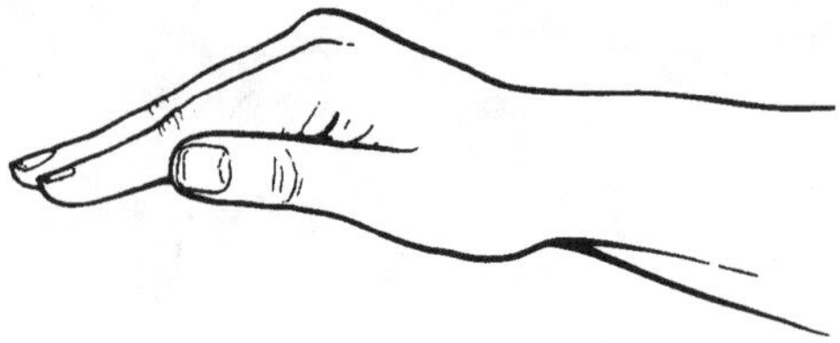

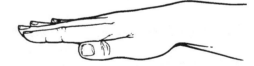

Figure 14.2. Cupped Hand

lower ribs, or back to prevent trauma to the spleen on the left, the liver on the right, and the kidneys in the lower back.

Various mechanical devices may be used in place of the traditional cupped palm method for percussion. Ask your doctor or therapist for advice.

Vibration gently shakes secretions into the larger airways. The caregiver places a hand firmly on the chest wall over the appropriate segment and tenses the muscles of the arm and shoulder to create a fine shaking motion. Then, the caregiver applies a light pressure over the area being vibrated. (The caregiver also may place one hand over the other, then press the top and bottom hand into each other to vibrate.) Vibration is done with the flattened hand, not the cupped hand, as in Figure 14.3. Exhalation should be as slow and as complete as possible.

Figure 14.3. Flat Hand

Deep breathing moves the loosened mucus and may stimulate coughing. Diaphragmatic breathing/belly breathing or lower chest breathing is used to encourage deep breathing to move air into the lower lungs. The belly moves outward when the person breathes in and sinks in when he or she breathes out.

Coughing is essential in clearing the airways. A forced but not strained exhalation, following a deep inhalation, may stimulate a productive cough. The mucus can then be coughed out. To increase the cough's effectiveness while decreasing the strain to the person, coughing may be assisted by supporting the sides of the lower chest with the hands or elbows.

Huffing

At the end of each drainage position, the person can take a deep breath, and then expel it quickly in a "huff." This "huff" forces the air and mucus out, making the cough more effective.

Timing of PD & P

Generally, each treatment session can last for twenty to forty minutes. PD & P is best done before meals or one and a half to two hours after eating to minimize the chance of vomiting. Early morning and bedtime sessions usually are recommended. The length of PD & P and the number of treatment sessions may need to be increased if the person is more congested. The recommended positions and durations of treatment are prescribed by the CF doctor or therapist.

Enhancing PD & P for the Person and Caregiver

Both the person and the caregiver should try to be comfortable during PD & P. Before beginning PD & P, the person should remove tight clothing, jewelry, buttons, and zippers around the neck, chest, and waist. Light, soft clothing, such as a T-shirt, may be worn and an extra towel or layer of clothing can be used to lessen any sting from percussion. Do not perform PD & P on bare skin. The therapist or caregiver should remove rings and other bulky jewelry such as watches or bracelets. An ample supply of tissues or a place to cough out the mucus should be provided.

Performing PD & P Comfortably and Carefully

If the head down position is recommended, the person's head should be well supported. The person can bend at the hips and knees to allow for both a stronger cough and a more comfortable position. The caregiver should not lean forward when treating the person, but should remain in an upright position to protect his or her back. To achieve this, the table on which the person lies should be positioned at a comfortable height for the caregiver.

Purchasing Equipment

Equipment such as drainage tables, electrical and nonelectrical palm percussors, and vibrators may be helpful and can be purchased from medical equipment stores. Older children and adults may find percussors useful when performing their own PD & P, but younger children may be frightened by the noise of a percussor.

Ask your doctor or therapist at your CF care center for recommendations on equipment.

Tips for Achieving the Proper Positions

To enable you to perform PD & P more frequently and effectively, select a method of achieving the proper bronchial drainage angles that is easy to set up. Some people use a firm padded board or table. These tilt boards, or drainage tables, can be elevated at one end by placing blocks on the floor. Tables that adjust to various angles or heights can be constructed or bought.

Pillows, sofa cushions, bundles of newspapers under pillows for support, cribs with adjustable mattress heights/tilts, foam wedges, and bean bag chairs work for many families. Infants can be positioned with or without pillows in the caregiver's lap.

Making PD & P More Enjoyable

An additional benefit of PD & P is that it promotes a special time together. On a regular basis, PD & P offers a specific time for you to enjoy each other's company.

To enhance the quality of the time you spend with your caregiver or child doing PD & P, do one of the following:

- Schedule PD & P around a favorite TV show.

- Play a favorite tape of songs or stories.

- Spend time playing, talking, or singing before, during, and after PD & P.

- For kids, encourage blowing or coughing games during PD & P, such as blowing pinwheels or coughing the deepest cough.

- Ask willing and capable relatives, friends, brothers, and sisters to perform PD & P occasionally. This can provide a welcome break from the daily routine.

- Minimize interruptions.

Identifying ways that make PD & P more enjoyable at all ages can help you keep a regular routine and get maximum health benefits.

Summary of Postural Drainage Positions

Lung segments are drained using gravity as the patient lies or sits in different positions. Percussion and vibration are performed on the front, back and sides of the person's chest and are followed by deep breathing and coughing.

Figure 14.4 summarizes all positions used for bronchial drainage. Details and explanations are provided for people of all ages in figures 14.5 through 14.15 of this chapter.

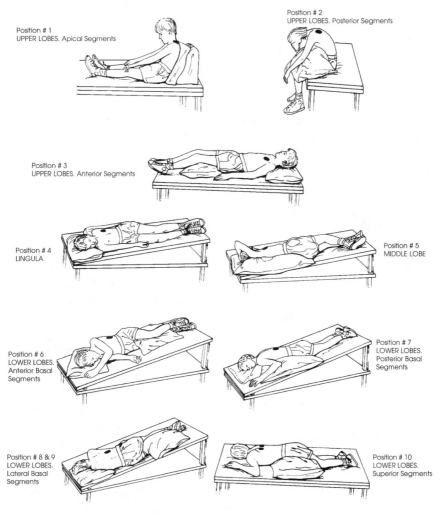

Position # 1
UPPER LOBES. Apical Segments

Position # 2
UPPER LOBES. Posterior Segments

Position # 3
UPPER LOBES. Anterior Segments

Position # 4
LINGULA

Position # 5
MIDDLE LOBE

Position # 6
LOWER LOBES.
Anterior Basal
Segments

Position # 7
LOWER LOBES.
Posterior Basal
Segments

Position # 8 & 9
LOWER LOBES.
Lateral Basal
Segments

Position # 10
LOWER LOBES.
Superior Segments

Figure 14.4. Summary of Postural Drainage Positions

Instructions for Postural Drainage Positions

The following diagrams describe the drainage positions necessary to drain each lung segment. In the diagrams, shaded areas on the chest indicate the location of the segment that is to be drained in each position.

The maneuvers vary slightly with the person's age. Here, the diagrams illustrate the first PD position for 1) an infant with the caregiver holding the infant on his or her lap, 2) an older child or adult who performs PD & P independently (assistance may be needed to treat some positions) and 3) a child or adult with the caregiver assisting with PD & P. The remaining diagrams illustrate a caregiver giving PD & P to a child, and can be adapted for infants and adults.

Instructions are shown using a drainage table, but alternatives are available. Pillows may be used for added comfort, but should not lessen the angle necessary for drainage. If the person tires easily, the sequence of positions can be varied, but all segments should be treated regularly.

Please remember to percuss and vibrate only over the ribs. Avoid percussing and vibrating over the spine, breastbone, stomach and lower ribs, or back to prevent trauma to the spleen on the left, the liver on the right, and the kidneys in the lower back. Do not percuss or vibrate on bare skin.

Position #1: Upper Lobes, Apical Segments (Infant)

Lean the infant back from a sitting position at a 30-degree angle on a pillow in your lap. Percuss and vibrate over the muscular area between the collarbone and the top of the shoulder blade. Percuss and vibrate on both the left and right sides. (Infant shown without T-shirt for illustration purposes only.)

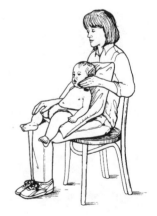

Figure 14.5. Position # 1: Upper Lobes, Apical Segments (Infant)

Position #1: Upper Lobes, Apical Segments (Adult)

Sit on a chair and lean backward on a pillow at a 30-degree angle. Percuss and vibrate over the muscular area between the collarbone and the top of the shoulder blade on both the left and right sides of the chest.

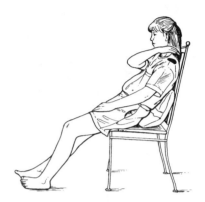

Figure 14.6. Position #1: Upper Lobes, Apical Segments (Adult)

Position #1: Upper Lobes, Apical Segments (Child)

The child sits on the flat drainage table and leans on a pillow at a 30 degree angle against the caregiver. Percuss and vibrate over the muscular area between the collarbone and the top of the shoulder blade on both the left and right sides. (Child shown without T-shirt for illustration purposes only.)

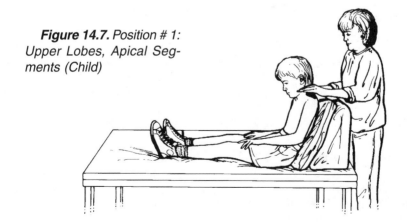

Figure 14.7. Position # 1: Upper Lobes, Apical Segments (Child)

Position #2: Upper Lobes, Posterior Segments (Child)

The child sits on the flat drainage table and leans forward over a folded pillow at a 30-degree angle. Stand behind the child and percuss and vibrate on the upper back on the left and right sides of the chest. (Child shown without T-shirt for illustration purposes only.)

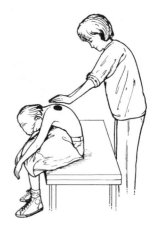

Figure 14.8. Position #2: Upper Lobes, Posterior Segments (Child)

Position #3: Upper Lobes, Anterior Segments (Child)

The child lies on his or her back on a flat drainage table. Percuss and vibrate between the collarbone and nipple on both the left and right sides of the chest. (Child shown without T-shirt for illustration purposes only.)

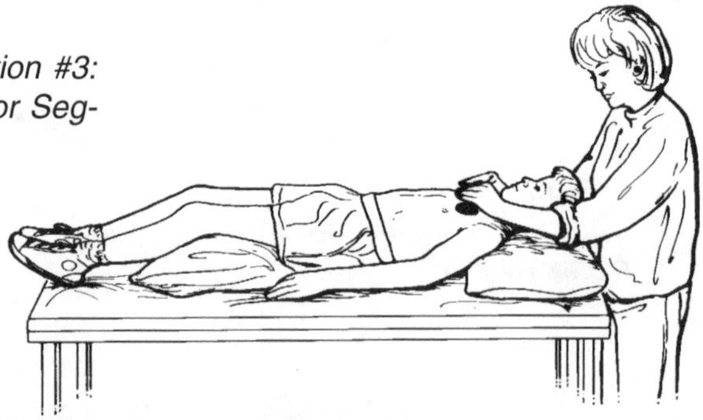

Figure 14.9. Position #3: Upper Lobes, Anterior Segments (Child)

Position #4: Lingula (Child)

Elevate the foot of the table fourteen inches (about 15 degrees). The child lies head down on the right side and rotates 1/4 turn backward.

A pillow may be placed behind the child (from shoulder to hip) and the child may flex his or her knees. Percuss and vibrate just outside the left nipple area. For females with tenderness around the breasts, percuss and vibrate with the heel of hand under the armpit and fingers extended forward beneath the breasts. (Child shown without T-shirt for illustration purposes only.)

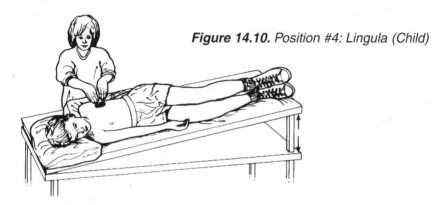

Figure 14.10. Position #4: Lingula (Child)

Position #5: Middle Lobe (Child)

Elevate the foot of the table fourteen inches (about 15 degrees). The child lies head down on the right side and rotates 1/4 turn backward. A pillow may be placed behind the child (from shoulder to hip) and the child may flex his or her knees. Percuss and vibrate just outside the right nipple area. For females with tenderness around the breasts, percuss and vibrate with the heel of hand under the armpit and fingers extended forward beneath the breasts. (Child shown without T-shirt for illustration purposes only.)

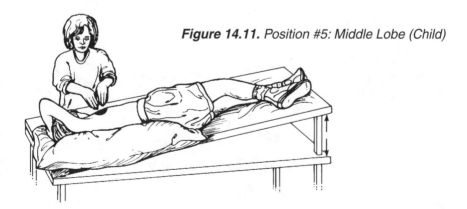

Figure 14.11. Position #5: Middle Lobe (Child)

Position #6: Lower Lobes, Anterior Basal Segments (Child)

Elevate the foot of the drainage table eighteen inches (about 30 degrees). The child lies on his or her right side with the head down and a pillow behind the back. Percuss and vibrate over the lower ribs on the left side of the chest, as shown in the diagram. To drain the right side of the chest, the child lies on his or her left side with the head down and a pillow behind the back. Percuss and vibrate over the lower ribs on the right side of the chest. (Child shown without T-shirt for illustration purposes only.)

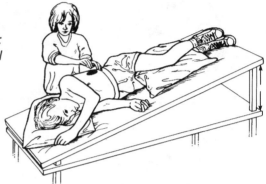

Figure 14.12. Position #6: Lower Lobes, Anterior Basal Segments (Child)

Position #7: Lower Lobes, Posterior Basal Segments (Child)

Elevate the foot of the drainage table eighteen inches (about 30 degrees). The child lies on his or her abdomen, head down, with a pillow under the hips. Percuss and vibrate on both the left and right sides of the spine. Do not percuss or vibrate over the spine or lower ribs. (Child shown without T-shirt for illustration purposes only.)

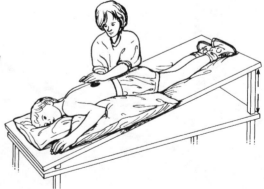

Figure 14.13. Position #7: Lower Lobes, Posterior Basal Segments (Child)

Positions #8 and #9: Lower Lobes, Lateral Basal Segments (Child)

Elevate the foot of the table eighteen inches (about 30 degrees). The child lies on his or her left side, head down, and leans 1/4 turn forward toward the table. The child can flex his or her upper leg over a pillow for support. Percuss and vibrate over the uppermost portion of the lower ribs to drain the right side, as shown in the diagram. To drain the left side, the child lies on his or her right side in the same position. Percuss and vibrate over the uppermost portion of the lower left ribs. (Child shown without T-shirt for illustration purposes only.)

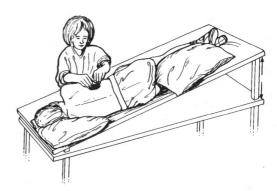

Figure 14.14. Positions #8 and #9: Lower Lobes, Lateral Basal Segments (Child)

Position #10: Lower Lobes, Superior Segments

The child lies on his or her abdomen on a flat drainage table with two pillows under the hips. Percuss and vibrate over the middle part of the back at the bottom of the shoulder blade on both the left and right side of the spine. Do not percuss or vibrate over the spine. (Child shown without T-shirt for illustration purposes only.)

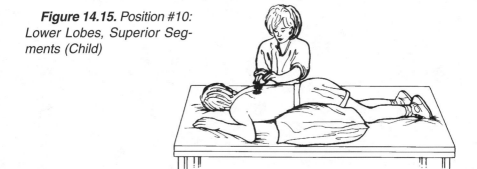

Figure 14.15. Position #10: Lower Lobes, Superior Segments (Child)

Chapter 15

Surgical Treatment of Respiratory Disorders

Chapter Contents

Section 15.1

Common Reasons for Lung Surgery

Excerpted from "A Patient's Guide to Lung Surgery,"
© 2008 University of Southern California Department of Cardiothoracic
Surgery. All rights reserved. Reprinted with permission.

Surgery is often done to get a closer look at the inside of the lungs and to help treat lung problems. If a mass is found in the lung, surgery can help determine its cause. If necessary, the mass may also be removed. Surgery may be done for other conditions, as well, such as collapsed lung or fluid around the lung.

A Lung Mass

If a mass has been found in the lung, a biopsy (sample) can be removed and examined to determine whether the growth is benign (not cancerous) or malignant (cancerous). In addition, the exact location and size of the mass can be measured, and other areas can be examined to check whether the mass has spread. If the mass needs to be removed, its size, location, and spread determine how much of the surrounding lung also needs to be removed. Removal of part or all of a lung is called lung resection.

A Collapsed Lung

If a portion of the lung wall is thin or ruptured, air may leak into the pleural space. When air collects in the pleural space, the lung may collapse. This is known as collapsed lung or pneumothorax. Tubes placed during surgery can drain air from the pleural space so the lung re-expands. During surgery, the wall of the lung can also be repaired so it won't collapse again.

Fluid around the Lungs

Fluid may collect in the area around the lungs. One common cause of fluid around the lungs is a lung infection, which may be a complication of certain types of surgery or an illness such as pneumonia. During surgery, tubes can be placed in the pleural space to drain fluid and help the lungs heal.

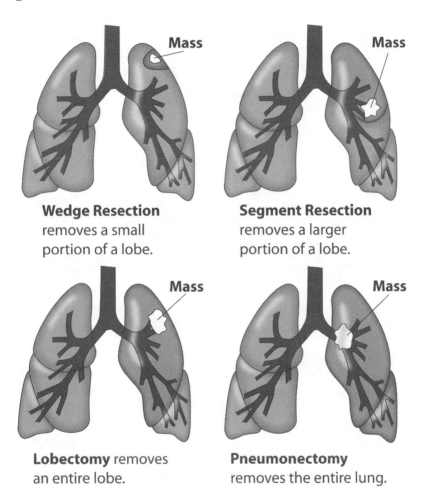

Wedge Resection removes a small portion of a lobe.

Segment Resection removes a larger portion of a lobe.

Lobectomy removes an entire lobe.

Pneumonectomy removes the entire lung.

Figure 15.1. Surgical Techniques for Treating a Lung Mass

Section 15.2

Lung Surgery for the Treatment of Cancer

Surgical Resection

Lung surgery for cancer includes the removal of the tumor, lymph nodes, and sections of the lung that contain the tumor. It is the treatment of choice in several types and stages of lung cancer, either alone or in combination with chemotherapy or radiation therapy. It is also used to remove cancerous tumors that have spread to the lungs from other parts of the body. The surgeon will recommend one of several approaches for removal of the tumor.

Surgical Approach

Thoracoscopy (also called VATS—Video Assisted Thoracic Surgery): A minimally invasive technique. Three small (approximately one-inch) incisions are made in your side. A video-scope is placed through one of the incisions. This scope allows the surgeon to see your lungs. A stapler and grasper are inserted in the other incisions. The tumor is removed through a plastic bag in order to prevent the spread of cancer. The incisions are closed by sutures, which will eventually dissolve. Thoracoscopy is used when the tumor is small and located on the outer edges of the lungs.

Thoracotomy: Thoracotomy is used when the tumor is not accessible with the thoracoscope. An incision is made in your side, between your ribs. The incision is approximately seven to nine inches long. Your ribs are separated and one may be cut. The tumor, lymph nodes, and surrounding lung are removed. Your muscle and skin are closed with sutures or staples.

Modified approach: Sometimes conventional approaches need to be modified in order for the tumor, lymph nodes, and affected lung to be adequately removed. Your surgeon will describe the specific approach to be used for you.

Results

No matter which approach is used, the surgeon will remove the tumor and send it to pathology for analysis. The pathologist will inspect the tissue for cancer cells. The final pathology report usually takes ten to fourteen days. The surgeon will notify you of your diagnosis as soon as he knows the results, or at your follow-up appointment, two weeks after discharge.

Risks and Potential Complications

The main risks of lung surgery for cancer are: prolonged air leak (see below), pneumonia or infection, bleeding, need for a blood transfusion, stroke, heart attack, and death. Preoperative chemotherapy and /or radiation therapy can increase the chance of these risks.

Prolonged Air Leak

No matter which approach is used, one or more chest tubes will be placed in your side during the operation. These tubes drain fluid and air from around the lungs. Most patients have an air leak after lung surgery. This happens when air from the lung tissue (usually at the internal suture line) leaks out into the chest cavity. If the volume of air inside the chest becomes too great, the pressure could cause the lung tissue to collapse. The chest tubes prevent this from happening. Most air leaks stop within three to five days after surgery. When they last longer, it is called a prolonged air leak. This is the most common complication of chest surgery. These leaks always heal, but it can mean you will need to stay in the hospital longer than expected.

Chest Tubes

During surgery, one or more chest tubes will be placed into your side. These chest tubes are used for drainage and to monitor air leakage. The tube is hooked up to an empty container, which will collect any fluid that drains out from your chest. The chest tube will remain in until the drainage stops and there is no air leakage.

Pain Control

Operations create pain. We make every effort to minimize your discomfort through oral medications, intravenous (IV) medications, and epidural catheters. You will be asked frequently about your pain. Please be honest. It is very important for the pain to be under control because taking deep breaths and moving are essential for quick recovery.

Patient-controlled analgesia (PCA): This is pain medicine that is given through your IV. You will be able to press a button connected to the pain medicine and dose yourself as needed. You do not need to worry about overdosing or becoming addicted. Limits will be programmed into the pump and you will not become dependent while you are having real pain.

Epidural catheter: This is a very small tube placed in your back at the time of surgery. Pain medication is infused through the catheter, which will bathe the spinal cord and prevent pain. You may have a PCA button for your epidural pain medicine (see above).

Oral medications: Oral medications are most often given on an "as needed" schedule. This means that you must ask the nurse to give you the medicine. Usually, there is a four-hour interval between doses. Please let your nurse know if you need your medicine more frequently or if it makes you too sleepy.

Deep Breathing, Coughing, and Incentive Spirometry

It is very important to cough and deep breathe after surgery. Your lungs need to be fully expanded to prevent infection and collapse. Please practice coughing and deep breathing before you come in for surgery.

Deep breathing: Fill your lungs up slowly over a count of five, hold for a count of five, exhale slowly over a count of five. Repeat ten times per hour while you are awake.

Coughing: Take two slow breaths filling your lungs up as much as possible. Begin your cough as you exhale the second time. Make sure you hold a pillow or towel over your incision (also called "splinting" your incision) during your cough. This will decrease the pain. Repeat ten times per hour while you are awake.

Incentive spirometry: Hold the spirometer securely in two hands and place your mouth on the mouthpiece. Exhale around the mouthpiece and make a tight seal on the mouthpiece. Inhale slowly to the count of five while you watch the disc move upward. Hold for a count of five, loosen the seal around the mouthpiece, and exhale. Repeat ten times per hour while you are awake.

Activity

Walking and moving frequently are very important components of your recovery. The more you push yourself to exercise and move, the quicker and less painful your recovery will be. You may not feel up to moving, *but you must*. You will be up in the chair the night of surgery and walking in your room the next morning.

Section 15.3

Thoracotomy

Excerpted from "A Patient's Guide to Lung Surgery,"
© 2008 University of Southern California Department of Cardiothoracic Surgery. All rights reserved. Reprinted with permission.

Thoracotomy: Preparing for Surgery

During thoracotomy, your surgeon directly views your lungs and the area around them. Surgical procedures may be done, such as removing part or all of a lung if a mass is present. Your surgeon will give you instructions on how to get ready for the procedure and explain what the surgery can do to help treat your condition:

- Have blood tests or other routine tests that your doctor recommends.

- Ask your doctor about donating your own blood in advance of surgery.

- If you smoke, stop immediately.

- Tell your doctor about any medications you're taking (including aspirin), and ask if you should stop them.

- Don't eat or drink anything after midnight the night before your surgery.

Risks and Complications

The risks associated with thoracotomy include the following:

- Risks of general anesthesia
- Wound infection
- Bleeding
- Inflammation of the lungs (pneumonia)
- Air leak through the lung wall, requiring a longer hospital stay
- Worsening of any existing heart problems
- Blockage of a blood vessel in the leg (deep vein thrombosis) with potential for blood clots in the lung (pulmonary embolism)

The Thoracotomy Procedure

Once you're asleep, you're positioned comfortably on your side and covered with sterile drapes. Your surgeon then makes an incision across your side. Your rib cage is separated to expose your lungs.

The lung to be operated on is deflated, while a breathing tube helps your other lung continue working. The deflated lung can then be examined and any necessary procedure performed, including removing part or all of the lung. In some cases, nearby lymph nodes may be removed, as well.

When the procedure is finished, one or more tubes are placed in the chest temporarily to drain fluid and air. Then the rib cage is repaired and the muscle and skin are closed with sutures or staples.

In the Recovery Area

After surgery, you'll be moved to a recovery area where you can be closely monitored. When you first wake up from the anesthesia, you may feel groggy, thirsty, or cold. If the breathing tube given to you during surgery remains in place, you won't be able to talk.

Flexible tubes in your chest drain air, blood, and fluid. Intravenous (IV) lines give you fluid and medications. Monitors record your heartbeat and the amount of oxygen in your blood. You may spend one or more days in this special monitoring unit before you're moved to a regular hospital room.

During your recovery, you'll be given pain medications to help make you more comfortable. You may also be taught exercises to improve your breathing and your range of motion while you heal. The hospital stay after a thoracotomy varies from patient to patient, but it's often a week or longer.

Section 15.4

Lung Volume Reduction Surgery

Excerpted from "Lung Volume Reduction Surgery for Severe Emphysema," © 2008 University of Southern California Department of Cardiothoracic Surgery. All rights reserved. Reprinted with permission.

Many people who suffer with emphysema have portions of the lung which are more affected than others. This finding led to the development of a surgical approach to treat emphysema. Lung volume reduction surgery (LVRS) is a procedure which removes approximately 20 to 35 percent of the poorly functioning, space-occupying lung tissue from each lung. By reducing the lung size, the remaining lung and surrounding muscles (intercostals and diaphragm) are able to work more efficiently. This makes breathing easier and helps patients achieve greater quality of life.

Good Candidates

It is very important that this operation is only offered to people who are likely to benefit from the procedure with the lowest risk of complications. A good candidate for LVRS is someone who has stopped smoking for at least four months and has disabling emphysema despite complete compliance with optimum medical therapy. The patient must be able to participate in a pulmonary rehabilitation program prior to and after surgery. Any other medical conditions that the candidate may have must be well controlled and must not present unacceptable risks for complications from the procedure. Most importantly, the patient must have a pattern of emphysema that is amenable to surgical management. This means that there are space-occupying, poorly functioning areas of the lung which can be removed to improve lung function. Imaging studies including chest x-ray, computed axial tomography (CAT) scan, and lung perfusion studies are done to determine this.

The National Emphysema Treatment Trial (NETT) was a prospective, randomized, multicenter trial which compared the results of LVRS to medical therapy which showed that there were three groups of patients that tend to benefit from LVRS. The following groups of patients are candidates for LVRS:

- **Group 1:** Patients with predominantly upper lobe emphysema and low exercise capacity. These patients have improved survival and functional outcomes after LVRS compared to medical therapy.

- **Group 2:** Patients with predominantly upper lobe emphysema and high exercise capacity. These patients have improved functional outcomes after LVRS but no difference in survival compared to medical therapy.

- **Group 3:** Patients with non–upper lobe emphysema and low exercise capacity. These patients have improved survival after LVRS but no difference in survival compared to medical therapy.

Poor Candidates

The NETT also identified patients who are unlikely to benefit from LVRS and have high risk for death after the procedure. The following groups of patients are not candidates for LVRS:

- Patients with non–upper lobe emphysema and high exercise capacity.

- Patients with extremely poor pulmonary function (forced expiratory volume in the first second (FEV1) 20 percent or less than predicted) and either homogenous distribution of emphysema on CT scan or extremely poor carbon monoxide diffusing capacity (DLCO 20 percent or less than predicted).

What to Expect

To optimize exercise capacity and improve early postoperative recovery, patients must participate in a six- to ten-week pulmonary rehabilitation program prior to surgery. The operation requires general anesthesia and can be done through either a breast bone incision or smaller chest incisions using video surgery. A special surgical stapler is used to remove the diseased lung tissue and seal the remaining lung from leaking blood and air. Immediately after the procedure patients are awakened from the general anesthetic and allowed to breath on their own. Pain medicine is given through an epidural catheter to help control postoperative discomfort. Drainage tubes are left in the chest to drain any excess air or fluid from the chest after surgery. These are removed once the air and fluid leakage stops. Physical therapy is reinstituted early during the recovery phase during the hospitalization. Patients are discharged from the hospital once the patient is mobile, tolerating a regular diet, and drainage tubes have been removed.

Anticipated Benefits

- Relief of shortness of breath
- Improved lung function
- Increased energy level and physical mobility
- Improved ability to function at normal daily activities
- May decrease need for supplemental oxygen

Potential Complications

There are significant risks associated with LVRS because of the poor baseline lung function. The major risks associated with this procedure are:

- Prolonged air leakage is the most common complication after LVRS.
- Approximately 40 percent of patients will have this problem. Some patients will actually go home with a chest drain in place for a few days to help manage this.
- Pneumonia (15 percent) can occur in emphysema patients, especially in patients who have a history of recurrent bouts.
- Bleeding (2 to 5 percent).
- Stroke (less than 1 percent).
- Heart attack (1 percent).
- Death: The chance of dying after LVRS is approximately 3 to 8 percent.

Section 15.5

Pneumonectomy

Pneumonectomy literally means "lung excision." The term refers to a number of different procedures, all of which involve the surgical removal of part or all of a lung. Pneumonectomy may be used for diagnosis or treatment of a variety of diseases, and the uses of pneumonectomy have greatly expanded over time.

Uses of Pneumonectomy:

The first modern pneumonectomies were performed in the latter half of the nineteenth century. At the time, most were done to treat severe tuberculosis infection of the lungs. For patients with rampant infection, pneumonectomy could be life saving.

With the development of effective anti-tuberculosis medicines in the mid-twentieth century, intractable tuberculosis became much less common. Surgical treatment of lung cancer had been attempted since the 1920s, but the decline of tuberculosis meant that cancer began to account for a much larger proportion of pneumonectomies. Today, cancer therapy remains one of the leading indications for pneumonectomy.

In the 1980s, lung transplantation techniques improved sufficiently to become an option for patients with incurable lung diseases. Both single and double lung transplants are now performed. Pneumonectomy is an essential part of any lung transplant, as it involves taking healthy lungs out of a donor, removing the recipient's diseased lungs, and implanting the new lungs.

In the 1990s, a new form of pneumonectomy called lung volume reduction surgery sparked considerable interest as a treatment for severe emphysema. Removing part of a lung from a patient who has trouble breathing may seem crazy, but it can be highly effective. The most severely damaged portions of the lungs are removed, which takes pressure off the healthier tissue, and allows the lungs to work more efficiently. Careful patient selection is key, as only certain emphysema patients can benefit from the surgery.

In addition to the above, pneumonectomy has been used for some time to perform lung biopsies. X-rays, computed tomography (CT) scans, sputum analysis, and other techniques frequently allow noninvasive diagnosis of medical problems. However, there are cases where a lung disease can only be accurately diagnosed by removing a portion of the lung for study. This continues to be a major use of pneumonectomy.

Extent of Pneumonectomy:

Pneumonectomy is called either partial or complete, depending upon how much lung tissue is removed.

Partial pneumonectomy is removal of a portion of a lung, rather than the entire organ. Often, this is done as a biopsy procedure, which may be necessary to diagnose certain infections, cancers, or other diseases. Usually, this requires removal of only a small part of the lung.

Sometimes, it is necessary to remove larger parts of the lung. For example, this may be used to treat lung cancer if the tumor is localized to one portion of the lung. Frequently, this involves removal of one or more of the three lobes of the right lung, or of the two lobes in the left lung. Removal of a lobe of the lung is known as lobectomy.

Lung volume reduction surgery for advanced emphysema also utilizes partial pneumonectomy. The upper portions of one or both lungs are removed to create more room for the less diseased lower parts.

Complete pneumonectomy is the removal of an entire lung. This may be performed for more extensive cancers in the lung, when partial pneumonectomy is not enough but there is still hope for a cure. Many lung transplant procedures involve double pneumonectomies, removing both diseased lungs to allow insertion of two healthy lungs from an organ donor.

Techniques of Pneumonectomy

There are two general methods of pneumonectomy, and many more specific techniques. Which is performed depends on multiple factors, including the goals of the surgery, the health of the patient, and the experience of the surgeon. In some cases, a surgery may begin with one technique and be completed with another. In others, different surgical approaches may be combined to give the best results.

Open pneumonectomy: This is the original pneumonectomy surgery, and it involves making a large opening in the chest wall to expose the lung. Depending upon the procedure, this may involve opening the chest from the front through the sternum, or from the side, between or through ribs. Opening the chest tends to give the surgeon the best access to the lung, and may be the only practical approach for some procedures such as lung transplantation. However, the surgery has the major disadvantage that it involves a very large incision over most of the chest, which makes recovery slower and more painful, and may increase the risk of bleeding or infection. This technique is still very much in use, but the trend in recent years has been toward less invasive approaches.

Video-assisted thoracoscopic surgery (VATS): This technique came into use during the 1990s, and has since become the preferred approach for many procedures. Rather than creating a large opening in the chest, several small slits or punctures are made between ribs. A thin, rod-like light and video camera known as a thoracoscope is inserted through one of the openings into the chest cavity, allowing the surgeon to see the inside of the chest on a monitor screen. Thin grasping and cutting tools with long handles are inserted through the other openings. The surgeon can then move the tools inside the chest to perform the surgery, watching the progress through the thoracoscope.

VATS has sometimes been described as performing surgery through a keyhole. In some cases, VATS may be performed with the assistance of surgical robots, which can move the instruments in more precise or complex ways than a surgeon's hands.

VATS has the obvious advantage that recovery is faster and less painful than with open pneumonectomy. It tends to be safer to medically fragile patients, as it puts less stress on the body. Some studies have found lower death and complication rates for VATS than with open surgical approaches.

Unfortunately, VATS cannot be used in all cases. Surgeries that involve removal of large amounts of lung tissue may be impossible. VATS may not allow the surgeon to see or reach key parts of the lung, and for some procedures, this reduces the odds of success. Similarly, extensive scar tissue or cancer in the chest may make a VATS approach very difficult. VATS tends to take longer to perform than open pneumonectomy, and prolonging surgery may negate the other medical advantages of the procedure.

Sometimes, pneumonectomy may be started via VATS, and converted to open pneumonectomy if there are unexpected complications. It is possible that the surgeon will not be able to tell what will work best until he or she sees inside the chest.

Risks and Complications of Pneumonectomy

Pneumonectomy is always a major surgery, and carries considerable risk. All of the blood in the body flows through the lungs, and any disruption of this can put a great deal of stress on the heart, kidneys, and other organs. Surgery inside the chest can lead to bleeding or infection, and this can be catastrophic in some cases. Pain in the chest wall after surgery can be quite severe, and can become permanent in some patients.

Because the lungs are air-filled, any surgery that cuts them can lead to persistent air leakage into the chest cavity. This complication, known as pneumothorax, can usually be treated with suction tubes into the chest until the leaks seal themselves, but occasionally the leaks can prove extremely difficult to stop.

Removal of any portion of the lung reduces the ability of the organ to bring oxygen into the blood and remove carbon dioxide. Young, healthy individuals may be able to tolerate loss of a considerable amount of lung tissue. However, older and sicker patients may not have enough reserve to lose very much. A careful assessment of baseline lung function is critical to determine if the patient will be able to survive the surgery.

Questions to Ask Your Doctor about Pneumonectomy

Pneumonectomy must never be undertaken lightly, and it is important that you have a good understanding of what is planned. Information elsewhere in this book can give you some background. Your doctor can also provide a great deal of information and education about pneumonectomy.

At a minimum, you should know the answers to the following questions before surgery:

- Why do I need a pneumonectomy? What will happen if I do not have the surgery?

- What kind of pneumonectomy is planned? How extensive will it be?

- Which technique of pneumonectomy will be used? Why is this the best choice for me?

- How risky will pneumonectomy be for me?

- What will my life be like after I recover from this surgery?

229

Section 15.6

Chest Tube Thoracostomy

Excerpted from "Chest Tube Insertion," © 2008 A.D.A.M., Inc.
Reprinted with permission. Updated May 3, 2007.

Chest tubes are inserted to drain blood, fluid, or air and to allow
the lungs to fully expand. The tube is placed between the ribs and into
the space between the inner lining and the outer lining of the lung
(pleural space).

The area where the tube will be inserted is numbed (local anesthesia). Sometimes sedation is also used. The chest tube is inserted
through an incision between the ribs into the chest and is connected
to a bottle or canister that contains sterile water. Suction is attached
to the system for drainage. A stitch (suture) and adhesive tape keep
the tube in place.

The chest tube usually stays in place until the x-rays show that
all the blood, fluid, or air has drained from the chest and the lung has
fully re-expanded. When the chest tube is no longer needed, it can be
easily removed. Most people don't need medications to sedate or numb
them while the chest tube is removed. Antibiotics may be used to prevent or treat infection.

In certain people, the chest tube may be inserted using a minimally
invasive technique guided by x-ray. Sometimes chest tubes are placed
during major lung or heart surgery while the person is under general
anesthesia.

Why the Procedure Is Performed

Chest tubes are used to treat conditions that can cause the lung
to collapse, such as:

- Air leaks from the lung into the chest (pneumothorax);
- Bleeding into the chest (hemothorax);
- After surgery or trauma in the chest (pneumothorax or he-
  mothorax);
- Lung abscesses or pus in the chest (empyema).

Risks

Risks for any anesthesia are:

- Reactions to medications;
- Problems breathing.

Risks for any surgery are:

- Bleeding;
- Infection.

Outlook (Prognosis)

Most people completely recover from the chest tube insertion and removal. There is only a small scar.

Recovery

You will stay in the hospital until the chest tube is removed. While the chest tube is in place, the nursing staff will carefully check for possible air leaks, breathing difficulties, and the need for additional oxygen. You'll need to breathe deeply and cough often to help re-expand the lung, assist with drainage, and prevent fluids from collecting in the lungs.

Chapter 16

Lung Transplantation

Why Are Lung Transplants Needed?

What Lungs Do When They Are Healthy

Every cell in your body requires oxygen to do its job. When a cell uses oxygen, it produces carbon dioxide, which then has to be quickly removed.

Your lungs have the all-important job of providing the oxygen your body needs and expelling the carbon dioxide. The lungs do their job when you breathe—oxygen *in*, carbon dioxide *out*. Your blood carries oxygen *from* the lungs to cells and carries carbon dioxide *to* the lungs for disposal when you exhale. Your heart is the pump that propels blood to and from the lungs.

When lungs are healthy, you are rarely aware of the automatic process of breathing. The only time you feel "short of breath" is when your lungs have to work harder to supply oxygen and get rid of carbon dioxide—for example, when you exercise hard or when oxygen is in short supply at high altitude.

What Happens When Your Lungs Are Not Healthy

When your lungs are not healthy, you may feel "short of breath" and fatigued almost all the time. Unhealthy or damaged lungs are not able to keep the flow and exchange of oxygen and carbon dioxide moving at the rate your cells need to function efficiently. The cells then send out a signal that tells you to work harder at breathing—much like your body cells send a thirsty-feeling signal that makes you want to drink more when there is a danger of dehydration.

This constant fatigue and struggle to breathe diminishes your quality of life. Your life may even be shortened if your body is unable to get enough oxygen and remove carbon dioxide. If your lungs become so damaged that even extra oxygen and other therapies are inadequate to improve your condition, you may be a candidate for lung transplantation.

Diseases and Conditions That Affect the Lungs

A number of diseases and conditions can cause the lungs to become so unhealthy that one or both lungs need to be replaced with a transplant. These diseases and conditions include:

- Chronic obstructive pulmonary disease (COPD) and/or emphysema due to tobacco smoking, alpha1-antitrypsin deficiency (an inherited condition), or other causes;
- Pulmonary fibrosis (scarring of the lung);
- Sarcoidosis;
- Cystic fibrosis;
- Bronchiectasis (chronic airway infection and damage);
- Primary pulmonary hypertension;
- Lymphangioleiomyomatosis (LAM);
- Langerhans cell histiocytosis of the lung (also known as eosinophilic granuloma or histiocytosis X);
- Congenital heart disease with Eisenmenger syndrome.

Other rare conditions may also be considered for transplantation.

What Kind of Transplants Can Be Considered?

Single-Lung or Double-Lung

The transplant team's assessment of your medical needs and the availability of donor lungs are considered in determining whether one or both lungs should be transplanted.

Heart-Lungs

Both lungs and the heart are replaced when both have irreversible damage, either due to one disease or a combination of diseases that affect both organs.

Pediatric Lung Transplantation

Lung transplantation in children is usually considered for:

- Cystic fibrosis with end-stage lung disease;
- Pulmonary hypertension;
- Pulmonary fibrosis.

Can You Be Considered for Lung Transplantation?

To be considered for lung transplantation, you must:

- Have a condition for which transplantation is considered an effective treatment;
- Have severe and progressive lung disease that no longer responds to medical treatment;
- Be willing to accept the risks of surgery and subsequent medical treatment;
- Be physically capable of undergoing surgery and subsequent medical treatment;
- Not be smoking or abusing alcohol or drugs.

Even if you otherwise qualify, the transplant team may determine that you are not a good candidate—for example, because of severe, coexisting medical conditions that may be worsened by a surgical procedure and follow-up treatments with powerful immunosuppressive (antirejection) drugs.

How Will Your Transplant Candidacy Be Evaluated?

While you may be referred to a transplant center by your physician, this does not mean that you are automatically accepted as a transplant candidate. You will be evaluated, physically and psychologically. You and members of your family will be interviewed by the transplant center team. You will undergo a number of testing procedures

235

that are used to assess your physical condition. These tests may include:

Heart

- Catheterization of the heart to examine blood supply and pressure (this test requires a catheter to be threaded through a large vein into your heart and dye injected into the heart through the catheter while an x-ray picture is taken);
- Nuclear cardiology studies to determine heart function and blood supply (these require injection of a radioactive substance to "tag" red blood cells);
- Electrocardiogram to determine heart electrical activity;
- Echocardiogram (ultrasound) to assess heart muscle and valve function and to estimate pulmonary pressures.

Lungs

- Ventilation-perfusion lung scan to determine blood and air supply to the lungs (this requires an injection of radioactive "tracer" into a vein);
- Pulmonary function tests to measure lung size and function (requires inhaling/exhaling into a machine);
- Chest CT scan to get a three-dimensional x-ray picture of your lungs.

Other

- Laboratory tests of blood to determine your blood type, help determine the risk of rejecting a transplanted lung or getting a serious infection, and look at the function of your other organs;
- Bone density test;
- Exercise capacity;
- Any other tests that physicians may believe are needed to complete a thorough evaluation.

All information from tests, interviews, and your medical history will be considered in determining whether you can be a candidate for lung transplantation. The team will also assess whether you have adequate financial resources and social support to meet the requirements of the program. Different transplant centers may have additional criteria for transplantation evaluation.

Benefits and Risks of Lung Transplantation

Benefits

Lung transplantation has the potential both to lengthen life expectancy and substantially improve quality of life. It is impossible to predict how long you may survive after transplantation. The most critical period for survival is the first year after transplantation; this is the period when surgical complications, rejection, and infection (see Risks below) are the greatest threat to survival. Patients who survive the first year are more likely to survive three years or longer after transplantation. There are patients alive today who had lung transplantation ten or even fifteen years ago.

Each lung transplant center has survival statistics for its transplantation programs. For American transplant programs, these statistics are available from the United Network for Organ Sharing (UNOS). You should discuss this information with your physician and the transplant team.

Risks

Rejection and infection are the two major complications of lung transplantation. You must cooperate completely with your physicians to try to keep these complications from developing or to keep them under control if they do occur.

Rejection: Because your transplanted lung(s) is "foreign" to your body, your body's immune system will try to destroy it—just as it tries to destroy "foreign" bacteria and viruses when they invade. Your immune system helps protect you from illness, but the process has to be "turned off" to keep your transplanted lung(s) from being destroyed.

Immunosuppressive (antirejection) medications prescribed by your doctors will help slow down and control the rejection process. Other medications may be necessary to control and treat rejection if your immune system breaks through the immunosuppressive blockade. Following your doctors' orders and taking all medications as prescribed help to prevent or control rejection. However, sometimes rejection can occur even despite your best efforts.

The most likely time for rejection to begin is during the first three months after transplantation surgery. Symptoms of rejection include fever, chills, flu-like aches, and shortness of breath. Your transplant team will instruct you regarding who to call to immediately report any such symptoms. Regular check-ups, x-rays, and breathing tests are also necessary to detect rejection that can occasionally occur without noticeable symptoms. Some programs take tiny biopsies of the lung through a device called a bronchoscope to screen for this "silent" rejection.

Immunosuppressive medications you will be taking in combination may include prednisone, cyclosporine or tacrolimus, azathioprine or mycophenolate, or other medications. The dosages of these drugs may be adjusted frequently by your physicians in response to drug levels, rejection, or side effects.

Infection: Because you will be taking immunosuppressive medications, your immune system will be less able to fight off invading bacteria and viruses. You will be much more susceptible to infections, which can become severe.

You have an important role in the prevention of infection—by following instructions to avoid exposure to infection, and immediately reporting any symptoms of infection.

Other complications: Many other complications are possible, including medication side effects, long-term problems with function of the transplanted lungs, and certain types of cancer. Your physicians and the transplant team will discuss these potential complications with you before transplantation and help you manage them after transplantation.

What Will Happen When You Are Accepted into a Lung Transplant Program?

Once you are accepted into a medical center's transplant program, you will be placed on the waiting list for a lung transplant. Each medical center has its own rules to follow, but, in general, you will:

- Be given regular tests while you are waiting;

- Be put on a regimen of "healthy living" that will get you into the best possible physical condition for surgery, with exercise, good nutrition, no smoking, and limited or no use of alcohol;

- Be put in touch with the medical center's social services to help you with problems, such as lodging and transportation, legal issues, and finances;

- Be counseled, along with members of your family, as to what to expect before, during, and after lung transplantation;

- Be told what to do when it is your time to receive a donor lung—for example, how to get to the medical center as quickly as possible if you live in a city or town other than the one where the medical center is located.

How Will You Get Your Donor Lung?

In the United States, all organs available for transplantation are listed on a national transplant waiting list maintained by the United Network for Organ Sharing (UNOS). The UNOS list matches donor organs to potential recipients, based on a number of criteria:

- Compatibility of donor and recipient (blood type, lung size)

- The severity of the recipient's lung disease, and the likelihood of a lung transplant improving his or her survival

Every medical center matches donors and recipients through UNOS, but each center has its own rules for accepting or declining transplant candidates.

Other countries may have other criteria for allocation of donor lungs, such as the amount of time the recipient has been on the waiting list.

Your donor lung(s) come from a person who has died and whose organs have been made available for transplantation. You will never know the name of your organ donor, because transplant centers respect donor confidentiality. Working through your transplant center, you can send an anonymous letter of appreciation to the donor's family.

What Is the Surgical Procedure?

A transplant operation will require many hours—about one hour to prepare you for anesthesia and to attach necessary monitoring lines, four to eight hours of surgery for a single-lung transplant, and six to twelve hours for a double-lung transplant. Additional time may be required if you have had prior chest surgery.

Single-lung transplants are usually done through an incision made on the right or left side, depending on which lung is being replaced. Double-lung transplants are generally done using an incision across the entire chest, just below the breast.

The operation begins when the donor lung arrives in the operating room. Your lung(s) is removed and the donor lung is placed in the

239

chest cavity. The surgeon connects the blood vessels to and from the lung (pulmonary artery and pulmonary vein) and the main airway (bronchus) of the donor lung to your airway. The same connections are made for the other lung if you are having a double-lung transplant.

For a heart-lung transplant, you are connected to a heart-lung machine that circulates your blood while the operation is in progress. After both lungs and the heart are removed, the donor lungs are attached as described in the paragraph above. The donor heart is attached to a "cuff" of the old heart's atrium that was left in place for just that purpose, and the main artery (aorta) is attached to the aorta of the donor heart.

After surgery is completed, you will be taken to an intensive care unit (ICU) for postsurgical recovery and monitoring. You will be in the ICU for at least several days. While you are in the ICU, you will have a breathing tube and mechanical ventilation for one or two days, a nasogastric tube to remove stomach contents that might be aspirated or make you nauseous, chest tubes to drain blood and postsurgical fluids from the chest cavity, a Foley catheter to drain urine, and intravenous (IV) catheters in your neck and arm for monitoring and for providing necessary fluids and medications. After leaving the ICU, you will go to a hospital room. The average stay in a hospital varies between transplant programs but is generally one to three weeks. However, since many complications can occur, some people are in the ICU and in the hospital for much longer—sometimes many weeks or even months.

What Happens after Discharge?

During the first ninety days after discharge from the hospital, you will make frequent trips to the medical center for blood tests, breathing tests, x-rays, and other monitoring of your condition. If you are doing well after ninety days, trips to the medical center may be less frequent.

You are also instructed to self-monitor your weight, blood pressure, pulse, temperature, lung function, and (if you are diabetic) blood sugar.

Of primary importance is the following: no smoking, limited use of alcohol, and good nutrition.

As soon as you are able, you will start a program of exercise rehabilitation. This may be conducted at the medical center or at a rehabilitation facility under professional supervision.

Commitment of You and Your Family

Lung transplantation requires full commitment from you and your family to:

- Maintain optimism during the months or years you may be on the waiting list for a donor lung;

- Cooperate with your physicians, especially in taking transplant medications;

- Maintain a healthy lifestyle to make the most of your second chance at life.

Questions You Should Ask Your Physician and Medical Center

Is transplantation my best option for treatment of my condition?

What are organ and patient survival rates at this institution for the type of transplant I will need?

How many transplants of this type are done every year at this institution? How many by my physicians and surgeons?

How long have they been doing this type of transplant surgery?

What costs of transplantation and rehabilitation are covered by my insurance? What out-of-pocket costs will I have to pay?

Part Three

Infectious and Inflammatory Diseases of the Respiratory System

Chapter 17

Bacterial Infections

Chapter Contents

Section 17.1

Hot Tub Lung

"Aqua Lung: Indoor Hot Tubs Found to Be Source of Lung Disease, National Jewish Physician Reports at American Thoracic Society Conference," © 2000 National Jewish Medical and Research Center. All rights reserved. For additional information, visit http://www .nationaljewish.org or call 1-800-222-LUNG. Reviewed by David A. Cooke, M.D., March 2008.

Microscopic organisms contained in aerosols generated by indoor hot tubs can cause lung disease in the people who regularly use them, a National Jewish Medical and Research Center physician reported in May 2000 at the American Thoracic Society (ATS) International Conference.

National Jewish physicians recently treated nine people, including four children, for a lung disease caused by nontuberculous mycobacteria (NTM). NTM—specifically *Mycobacteria avium* and *fortuitum*—were found in the hot tub water and/or in the air of the homes of the people diagnosed. The hot tubs are located inside of homes, near family and living rooms, and bedrooms.

"The jets from hot tubs aerosolize the bacteria, which is how this becomes a problem," said Cecile Rose, M.D., MPH, a National Jewish physician specializing in treating people with environment and occupational lung diseases, and reporting the research findings at ATS. "Bubbles—rich with the bacteria—rise up, burst, and disperse the bacteria throughout a room."

Unlike its bacterial cousin tuberculosis—transmitted by infected humans—NTM is not contagious. In nature, these organisms live in brackish ocean water, like tide pools. But indoor hot tubs, which generally produce a substantial mist, may be causing this lung disease to become more prevalent. The organisms enter the air when a mist, called aerosolization, is produced and the bacteria are suspended in water droplets.

People with NTM often suffer from fever, tiredness, night sweats, cough, and weight loss. "For people with mild cases of NTM, removing the hot tub from the home is the primary treatment," she said.

In more severe cases, and those reported on at the ATS conference, treatment involved corticosteroids and/or corticosteroids and anti-mycobacterial antibiotics. Sometimes three to four antibiotics must be given at once.

This respiratory problem is often misdiagnosed as sarcoidosis—characterized by inflamed, microscopic growths called granulomas most often found in the lungs—or tuberculosis. "This disease mimics other granulomatous lung diseases, but few people understand the link between hot tub exposure and the symptoms of disease," she said. In instances when the lung problems are misdiagnosed, and in three cases reported at the ATS conference they were, patients remained in the home, prolonging their exposure to NTM.

Nevertheless, Dr. Rose adds, "Because luxury items like hot tubs are becoming more common, I believe there will be an increasing recognition and understanding of the risk associated with their use among doctors and consumers."

Section 17.2

Legionellosis (Legionnaires Disease)

Reprinted from "Legionellosis: Legionnaires' Disease (LD) and Pontiac Fever," U.S. Centers for Disease Control and Prevention, October 12, 2005.

Legionellosis is an infection caused by the bacterium *Legionella pneumophila*. The disease has two distinct forms:

- Legionnaires disease, the more severe form of infection, which includes pneumonia, and

- Pontiac fever, a milder illness.

Legionnaires disease acquired its name in 1976 when an outbreak of pneumonia occurred among persons attending a convention of the American Legion in Philadelphia. Later, the bacterium causing the illness was named *Legionella*.

What is Legionnaires disease?

Legionnaires disease is caused by a type of bacteria called *Legionella.* The bacteria got its name in 1976, when many people who went to a Philadelphia convention of the American Legion suffered from an outbreak of this disease, a type of pneumonia (lung infection). Although this type of bacteria was around before 1976, more illness from Legionnaires disease is being detected now. This is because we are now looking for this disease whenever a patient has pneumonia.

Each year, between eight thousand and eighteen thousand people are hospitalized with Legionnaires disease in the United States. However, many infections are not diagnosed or reported, so this number may be higher. More illness is usually found in the summer and early fall, but it can happen any time of year.

What are the symptoms of Legionnaires disease?

Legionnaires disease can have symptoms like many other forms of pneumonia, so it can be hard to diagnose at first. Signs of the disease can include: a high fever, chills, and a cough. Some people may also suffer from muscle aches and headaches. Chest x-rays are needed to find the pneumonia caused by the bacteria, and other tests can be done on sputum (phlegm), as well as blood or urine to find evidence of the bacteria in the body.

These symptoms usually begin two to fourteen days after being exposed to the bacteria.

A milder infection caused by the same type of *Legionella* bacteria is called Pontiac fever. The symptoms of Pontiac fever usually last for two to five days and may also include fever, headaches, and muscle aches; however, there is no pneumonia. Symptoms go away on their own without treatment and without causing further problems.

Pontiac fever and Legionnaires disease may also be called "Legionellosis" separately or together.

How serious is it? What is the treatment?

Legionnaires disease can be very serious and can cause death in up to 5 to 30 percent of cases. Most cases can be treated successfully with antibiotics (drugs that kill bacteria in the body), and healthy people usually recover from infection.

Where do Legionella *bacteria come from?*

The *Legionella* bacteria are found naturally in the environment, usually in water. The bacteria grow best in warm water, like the kind found in hot tubs, cooling towers, hot water tanks, large plumbing systems, or parts of the air-conditioning systems of large buildings. They do not seem to grow in car or window air-conditioners.

How do people get Legionnaires disease?

People get Legionnaires disease when they breathe in a mist or vapor (small droplets of water in the air) that has been contaminated with the bacteria. One example might be from breathing in the steam from a whirlpool spa that has not been properly cleaned and disinfected.

The bacteria are *not* spread from one person to another person.

Outbreaks are when two or more people become ill in the same place at about the same time, such as patients in hospitals. Hospital buildings have complex water systems, and many people in hospitals already have illnesses that increase their risk for *Legionella* infection.

Other outbreaks have been linked to aerosol sources in the community, or with cruise ships and hotels, with the most likely sources being whirlpool spas, cooling towers (air-conditioning units from large buildings), and water used for drinking and bathing.

Who gets this disease?

People most at risk of getting sick from the bacteria are older people (usually sixty-five years of age or older), as well as people who are smokers, or those who have a chronic lung disease (like emphysema).

People who have weak immune systems from diseases like cancer, diabetes, or kidney failure are also more likely to get sick from *Legionella* bacteria. People who take drugs to suppress (weaken) the immune system (like after a transplant operation or chemotherapy) are also at higher risk.

What should I do if I think I was exposed to Legionella *bacteria?*

Most people exposed to the bacteria do not become ill. If you have reason to believe you were exposed to the bacteria, talk to your doctor or local health department. Be sure to mention if you have traveled in the last two weeks.

A person diagnosed with Legionnaires disease in the workplace is not a threat to others who share office space or other areas with him or her. However, if you believe that your workplace was the source of the person's illness, contact your local health department.

Section 17.3

Psittacosis

What is psittacosis?

Psittacosis is a disease caused by bacteria called *Chlamydia psittaci*. It is a disease of birds that can also affect people.

Who gets psittacosis?

Persons most likely to get psittacosis are those who handle infected household birds, usually imported psittacine birds (parrots, parakeets). Workers in turkey processing plants have also been infected.

Where are organisms found?

The organisms are found in droppings, secretions, and dust from feathers of parakeets, parrots, and lovebirds; less often in poultry, pigeons, canaries, and sea birds. Birds that appear to be healthy can be carriers and shed the bacteria, particularly when subjected to the stresses of crowding and shipping.

How is psittacosis spread?

Transmission occurs when the bacteria are inhaled from dried bird droppings, secretions, or dust from feathers.

What are the symptoms of psittacosis?

The most common symptoms in humans are fever, headache, feeling of weakness, loss of appetite, muscle aches, chills, sore throat, cough, and sensitivity to light. These symptoms can present as a mild flu-like illness or can be very severe, especially in older persons.

How soon after exposure do symptoms appear?

The symptoms generally appear about ten days after exposure, but can appear as early as one week or as long as four weeks after exposure.

Do infected people need to be excluded from work or school?

No, but persons who are coughing should be instructed to cough into paper tissues which are then discarded in a sanitary fashion.

What is the treatment for psittacosis?

Antibiotics of the tetracycline group are administered for ten to fourteen days after temperature returns to normal.

How can psittacosis be prevented?

Controlling the disease in the bird population helps reduce the risk for people. However, birds that seem healthy can shed the bacteria and new birds may reintroduce the bacteria, so prevention depends on properly designed and managed facilities that raise and sell birds and the use of protective clothing, including wearing masks or respirators, and gloves by those working with birds. Sick birds should be diagnosed and treated. If they are sold while they are being treated, the new owner should be informed and be sure that treatment is completed.

Bird cages should be cleaned regularly with disinfectants (alcohol, Lysol, or bleach solution) and the contents of the cage should be disposed of properly.

Section 17.4

Tuberculosis

Reprinted from "Tuberculosis: General Information,"
U.S. Centers for Disease Control and Prevention, July 2007.

What is tuberculosis (TB)?

Tuberculosis (TB) is a disease caused by germs that are spread from person to person through the air. TB usually affects the lungs, but it can also affect other parts of the body, such as the brain, the kidneys, or the spine. A person with TB can die if they do not get treatment.

What are the symptoms of TB?

The general symptoms of TB disease include feelings of sickness or weakness, weight loss, fever, and night sweats. The symptoms of TB disease of the lungs also include coughing, chest pain, and the coughing up of blood. Symptoms of TB disease in other parts of the body depend on the area affected.

How is TB spread?

TB germs are put into the air when a person with TB disease of the lungs or throat coughs, sneezes, speaks, or sings. These germs can stay in the air for several hours, depending on the environment. Persons who breathe in the air containing these TB germs can become infected; this is called latent TB infection.

What is the difference between latent TB infection and TB disease?

People with latent TB infection have TB germs in their bodies, but they are not sick because the germs are not active. These people do not have symptoms of TB disease, and they cannot spread the germs to others. However, they may develop TB disease in the future. They are often prescribed treatment to prevent them from developing TB disease.

People with TB disease are sick from TB germs that are active, meaning that they are multiplying and destroying tissue in their body. They usually have symptoms of TB disease. People with TB disease of the lungs or throat are capable of spreading germs to others. They are prescribed drugs that can treat TB disease.

What should I do if I have spent time with someone with latent TB infection?

A person with latent TB infection cannot spread germs to other people. You do not need to be tested if you have spent time with someone with latent TB infection. However, if you have spent time with someone with TB disease or someone with symptoms of TB, you should be tested.

What should I do if I have been exposed to someone with TB disease?

People with TB disease are most likely to spread the germs to people they spend time with every day, such as family members or coworkers. If you have been around someone who has TB disease, you should go to your doctor or your local health department for tests.

How do you get tested for TB?

There are two tests that can be used to help detect TB infection. The Mantoux tuberculin skin test is performed by injecting a small amount of fluid (called tuberculin) into the skin in the lower part of the arm. A person given the tuberculin skin test must return within forty-eight to seventy-two hours to have a trained health care worker look for a reaction on the arm. A second test is the QuantiFERON®-TB Gold test. The QuantiFERON®-TB Gold test is a blood test that measures how the patient's immune system reacts to the germs that cause TB.

What does a positive tuberculin skin test or QuantiFERON®-TB gold test mean?

A positive tuberculin skin test or QuantiFERON®-TB Gold test only tells that a person has been infected with TB germs. It does not tell whether or not the person has progressed to TB disease. Other tests, such as a chest x-ray and a sample of sputum, are needed to see whether the person has TB disease.

What is Bacille Calmette-Guérin (BCG)?

BCG is a vaccine for TB disease. BCG is used in many countries, but it is not generally recommended in the United States. BCG vaccination does not completely prevent people from getting TB. It may also cause a false positive tuberculin skin test. However, persons who have been vaccinated with BCG can be given a tuberculin skin test or QuantiFERON®-TB Gold test.

Why is latent TB infection treated?

If you have latent TB infection but not TB disease, your doctor may want you to take a drug to kill the TB germs and prevent you from developing TB disease. The decision about taking treatment for latent infection will be based on your chances of developing TB disease. Some people are more likely than others to develop TB disease once they have TB infection. This includes people with human immunodeficiency virus (HIV) infection, people who were recently exposed to someone with TB disease, and people with certain medical conditions.

How is TB disease treated?

TB disease can be treated by taking several drugs for six to twelve months. It is very important that people who have TB disease finish the medicine, and take the drugs exactly as prescribed. If they stop taking the drugs too soon, they can become sick again; if they do not take the drugs correctly, the germs that are still alive may become resistant to those drugs. TB that is resistant to drugs is harder and more expensive to treat. In some situations, staff of the local health department meet regularly with patients who have TB to watch them take their medications. This is called directly observed therapy (DOT). DOT helps the patient complete treatment in the least amount of time.

Chapter 18

Viral Infections

Chapter Contents

Section 18.1

Avian (Bird) Flu

You've probably heard news reports about a potentially dangerous avian flu. And like many people, you may be wondering how to react to the frightening headlines about people having died of the bird flu and the possibility of the flu someday spreading rapidly around the world, infecting humans.

While the bird flu can be serious, unless you have household chickens and live in a country where there's an outbreak now, the bird flu probably is not an immediate health threat for you or your family. Experts believe only 160 people have contracted the disease since it was identified as a threat eight years ago.

The avian flu that has affected birds and people in Asia, Europe, Africa, and the Middle East is different from the flu that many people get during the cold-weather months. Poultry—like chickens and turkeys—tend to get infected with the bird flu by migrating waterfowl (like ducks, geese, and swans), and spread it to other birds through their infected feces, saliva, or secretions. The people who have gotten sick or died from the bird flu in Asia have had direct contact with infected birds, or surfaces that have been contaminated by them. This strain of the bird flu—which is called H5N1—can't be spread from person to person.

Experts are concerned that this flu could mutate (undergo a genetic change) into a new form that can spread from person to person. Right now there's no vaccine for the bird flu, so they're worried that if it does mutate, it will be difficult to stop and will cause a pandemic, which is a global outbreak.

Health officials around the world are taking precautions to make sure that the bird flu doesn't spread, and to keep people safe from it if it does. Many countries—including the United States—aren't importing poultry from countries where there have been avian flu outbreaks.

Meanwhile, scientists are working on developing a vaccine to keep people from getting the avian flu.

In most places, there's no immediate threat from bird flu. All the same, the best thing you can do to safeguard your family from any contagious illness is to practice good hand-washing habits, teach your child to do the same, and take proper food safety precautions. (Never eat undercooked or uncooked poultry, and wash any kitchen surfaces where you have handled or worked with any uncooked meat.)

If you're traveling to a country where there has been a bird flu outbreak, it's best to talk with your doctor and look to agencies like the Centers for Disease Control and Prevention (CDC) and the World Health Organization (WHO).

Here are some more answers to questions about avian flu.

What is avian flu?

It is a form of the flu (influenza) virus that usually only infects birds and sometimes infects pigs. There are many different strains of the avian flu. Some of those strains only cause mild symptoms in birds, ruffling their feathers and reducing their egg production. Other strains, including some of the H5 strains, are more dangerous—they spread quickly, cause more severe symptoms, and are almost always fatal to the birds.

An estimated 160 people have contracted the H5N1 strain of the flu, and about half of them have died. In an effort to keep the flu from spreading, hundreds of birds in those countries have been destroyed. The WHO is estimating that it will take at least two years to contain this outbreak of the bird flu.

Where is the avian flu an urgent concern?

Over the past couple of years experts have recorded and confirmed outbreaks of H5N1 among birds in countries in Asia, Europe, Africa, and the Middle East.

Could avian flu become a concern in the United States?

The strain of flu virus that has spread in Asia, the Middle East, and Eastern Europe has not been found in birds—or humans—in the United States. There's a very low risk that people in the United States will get infected with the avian flu unless there's a global outbreak.

But this strain of the virus has been around since 1997. And the longer it lingers, spreading among birds in Asia, the more opportunities there are for the virus to infect people. The more people that are infected with the virus, the more opportunities the virus will have to mutate into a form that could spread from person to person. That could lead to a pandemic. As a precaution, the United States is not importing any birds from countries that have reported outbreaks of the bird flu.

How do birds spread the flu to other birds?

Researchers think that migrating birds, like ducks, geese, and swans can carry and spread the virus to other birds but generally don't get sick from it. Bird flu can sicken domesticated birds, like chickens and turkeys, and kill them.

A bird can get the bird flu from another bird by coming into close contact with its infected feces, secretions, or saliva, or surfaces, dirt, or cages that have been contaminated by them. That's why researchers think live bird markets, where birds are kept in close quarters, are places where the virus has rapidly spread.

The virus also can spread from farm to farm if birds' infected feces and saliva get on farming equipment, like tractor wheels, clothing, and cages.

How has avian flu spread to humans?

Experts think that the people who were infected by the bird flu had direct contact with infected poultry. They lived in rural areas where many families have small household poultry flocks, and slaughter, defeather, and butcher poultry themselves. Poultry also roam freely in some of those areas, and there are lots of opportunities to be exposed to their infected feces.

Can a person with avian flu spread it to other people?

It's unlikely that a person who gets infected with this strain of the avian flu would spread it to other people. All human cases of bird flu so far have happened because people came into close contact with infected birds.

What are the symptoms of avian flu in humans?

The symptoms of bird flu in people tend to be similar to the typical flu: fever, cough, sore throat, muscle aches. But this flu also can lead to eye infections, pneumonia, and severe coughing and breathing problems.

What are the signs of a pandemic?

If clusters of people start showing symptoms of the flu around the same time, in the same place, in a country where it's known that the virus is spreading, it would signal that the virus has mutated and is spreading from person to person. Doctors and public health officials would try to find out how the people got sick, and use that information to try to track and stop the disease from spreading.

What are public officials doing to prevent the spread of avian flu?

Officials in Japan, Korea, and Malaysia have announced that their local outbreaks have been controlled, and that there's no more of the virus there.

Even so, the WHO has started stockpiling antiviral medications and created an emergency plan in case there is a pandemic. The agency is providing guidance for all nations to do the same and is closely monitoring countries where there have been outbreaks, watching for further cases and any possible mutations.

U.S. president George Bush announced a plan that includes stockpiling medications to help reduce effects of the flu, producing more flu vaccine, and developing a vaccine for the avian flu.

Should I stop eating chicken and turkey?

It's safe to eat properly cooked chicken, turkey, and any other poultry in the United States. But do not eat raw (uncooked) or undercooked poultry or poultry products. When you're cooking, separate raw meat from cooked or ready-to-eat foods. Don't use the same cutting boards, knives, or utensils on uncooked meats and other foods. Heat can destroy flu viruses, so you should cook poultry until the temperature of the meat reaches at least 158 degrees Fahrenheit (70 degrees Celsius).

How can I protect my family from avian flu?

If you plan to travel to a country where there has been an outbreak, avoid any contact with chickens, ducks, geese, pigeons, turkeys, quail, or any wild birds. Stay away from live bird markets, local poultry farms, or any other settings where there might be infected poultry. Avoid touching surfaces that could have been contaminated by bird saliva, feces, or urine. Look to agencies like the CDC for travel advisories.

At this point, if you live in a country where there's not a bird flu outbreak, there aren't any special precautions you need to take. But in general, hand washing keeps viruses and other contagious illnesses from spreading. So no matter where you live or how healthy you are, be sure to frequently and thoroughly wash your hands with soap and water, particularly after going to the bathroom and before preparing meals and eating, and after taking care of a sick person. Encourage your child to develop healthy hand-washing habits.

Can the flu shot prevent avian flu?

No. There is no vaccine currently available for the avian flu, although there is one under development. However, experts stress that the strains of common flu virus that circle the globe each year are much more likely to pose a threat to human health during flu season. And in this case protection is available for that. So you may want to think about getting a flu shot for yourself and your family to help you stay well during the flu season, which runs from November to April, particularly if any of you are considered to be in a high-risk group. Pregnant women, babies from six to twenty-three months old, anyone who lives with or cares for infants under six months old, and people with certain chronic medical conditions are all considered high risk.

What's the treatment for avian flu?

Doctors hope that antiviral medications will help keep the flu from spreading if it mutates and becomes contagious to humans. These medications can't cure the bird flu, but they can make the symptoms less severe. Still, flu viruses can become resistant to these drugs, so they may not always work. More studies are underway to determine how effective these medications are.

Can my pet bird get infected with the avian flu?

Your pet bird could contract the avian flu if it is exposed to another bird that's carrying the virus. So it's important to keep your bird and its food and water inside, away from any place where it could be exposed to infected migrating or domestic birds. That way your pet won't be at risk for getting the bird flu.

In addition, there are many precautions you can take to guard against the bird flu virus and other illnesses:

- Don't allow your bird to drink or eat from ponds or other places that migrating birds may have flown over.

- Keep your pet bird's cage clean.

- Wash your hands after handling your pet bird, cleaning its cage, or after having any contact with your bird's secretions.

- If you have any questions about your bird's health, talk with your veterinarian.

Government officials from the United States and other countries have stopped importing live birds and bird products (like meat and eggs) from countries where there have been outbreaks of the bird flu. So if you buy a pet bird, it should not have been exposed to the virus.

That said, there is an illegal market for buying and selling exotic birds and other animals. So just to be safe, before you buy any animal to keep as a pet, find out where it was born and raised. If you have any questions, contact a veterinarian, officials with the U.S. Centers for Disease Control, or the World Health Organization.

Section 18.2

Bronchiolitis

Bronchiolitis is a common illness of the respiratory tract caused by an infection that affects the tiny airways, called the bronchioles, that lead to the lungs. As these airways become inflamed, they swell and fill with mucus, making breathing difficult.

Bronchiolitis:

- Most often affects infants and young children because their small airways can become blocked more easily than those of older kids or adults;

- Typically occurs during the first two years of life, with peak occurrence at about three to six months of age;

- Is more common in males, children who have not been breastfed, and those who live in crowded conditions.

Day-care attendance and exposure to cigarette smoke also can increase the likelihood that an infant will develop bronchiolitis.

Although it's often a mild illness, some infants are at risk for a more severe disease that requires hospitalization. Conditions that increase the risk of severe bronchiolitis include prematurity, prior chronic heart or lung disease, and a weakened immune system due to illness or medications.

Kids who have had bronchiolitis may be more likely to develop asthma later in life, but it's unclear whether the illness causes or triggers asthma, or whether children who eventually develop asthma were simply more prone to developing bronchiolitis as infants. Studies are being done to clarify the relationship between bronchiolitis and the later development of asthma.

Bronchiolitis is usually caused by a viral infection, most commonly respiratory syncytial virus (RSV). RSV infections are responsible for more than half of all cases of bronchiolitis and are most widespread in the winter and early spring. Other viruses associated with bronchiolitis include rhinovirus, influenza (flu), and human metapneumovirus.

Signs and Symptoms

The first symptoms of bronchiolitis are usually the same as those of a common cold:

- Stuffiness
- Runny nose
- Mild cough
- Mild fever

These symptoms last a day or two and are followed by worsening of the cough and the appearance of wheezes (high-pitched whistling noises when exhaling).

Sometimes more severe respiratory difficulties gradually develop, marked by:

- Rapid, shallow breathing;

- A rapid heartbeat;

- Drawing in of the neck and chest with each breath, known as retractions;

- Flaring of the nostrils;

- Irritability, with difficulty sleeping and signs of fatigue or lethargy.

The child may also have a poor appetite and may vomit after coughing. Less commonly, babies, especially those born prematurely, may have episodes where they briefly stop breathing (this is called apnea) before developing other symptoms.

In severe cases, symptoms may worsen quickly. A child with severe bronchiolitis may tire from the work of breathing and have poor air movement in and out of the lungs due to the clogging of the small airways. The skin can turn blue (called cyanosis), which is especially noticeable in the lips and fingernails. The child also can become dehydrated from working harder to breathe, vomiting, and taking in less during feedings.

Contagiousness

The infections that cause bronchiolitis are contagious. The germs can spread in tiny drops of fluid from an infected person's nose and mouth, which may become airborne via sneezes, coughs, or laughs, and also can end up on things the person has touched, such as used tissues or toys.

Infants in child-care centers have a higher risk of contracting an infection that may lead to bronchiolitis because they're in close contact with lots of other young children.

Prevention

The best way to prevent the spread of viruses that can cause bronchiolitis is frequent hand washing. It may help to keep infants away from others who have colds or coughs. Babies who are exposed to cigarette smoke are more likely to develop more severe bronchiolitis compared with those from smoke-free homes. Therefore, it's important to avoid exposing children to cigarette smoke.

Although a vaccine for bronchiolitis has not yet been developed, a medication can be given to lessen the severity of the disease. It contains antibodies to RSV and is injected monthly during peak RSV season. The medication is recommended only for infants at high risk of severe disease, such as those born very prematurely or those with chronic lung disease.

Incubation

The incubation period (the time between infection and the onset of symptoms) ranges from several days to a week, depending on the infection causing the bronchiolitis.

Duration

Cases of bronchiolitis typically last about twelve days, but kids with severe cases can cough for weeks. The illness generally peaks on about the second to third day after the child starts coughing and having difficulty breathing and then gradually resolves.

Professional Treatment

Fortunately, most cases of bronchiolitis are mild and require no specific professional treatment. Antibiotics aren't useful because bronchiolitis is caused by a viral infection, and antibiotics are only effective against bacterial infections. Medication may sometimes be given to help open a child's airways.

Infants who have trouble breathing, are dehydrated, or appear fatigued should always be evaluated by a doctor. Those who are moderately or severely ill may need to be hospitalized, watched closely, and given fluids and humidified oxygen. Rarely, in very severe cases, some babies are placed on respirators to help them breathe until they start to get better.

Home Treatment

The best treatment for most kids is time to recover and plenty of fluids. Making sure a child drinks enough fluids can be a tricky task, however, because infants with bronchiolitis may not feel like drinking. They should be offered fluids in small amounts at more frequent intervals than usual.

Indoor air, especially during winter, can dry out airways and make the mucus stickier. Some parents use a cool-mist vaporizer or humidifier in the child's room to help loosen mucus in the airway and relieve cough and congestion. If you use one, clean it daily with household bleach to prevent mold from building up. Avoid hot-water and steam humidifiers, which can be hazardous and can cause scalding.

To clear nasal congestion, try a bulb syringe and saline (saltwater) nose drops. This can be especially helpful just before feeding and sleeping. Sometimes, keeping the child in a slight upright position may help improve labored breathing. Give acetaminophen to reduce fever and make the child more comfortable.

When to Call the Doctor

Call your doctor if your child:

- Is breathing quickly, especially if this is accompanied by retractions or wheezing;
- Might be dehydrated due to poor appetite or vomiting;
- Is sleepier than usual;
- Has a high fever;
- Has a worsening cough;
- Appears fatigued or lethargic.

Seek immediate help if you feel your child is having difficulty breathing and the cough, retractions, or wheezing are getting worse, or if his or her lips or fingernails appear blue.

Section 18.3

Common Cold

Reprinted from the National Institute of Allergy and
Infectious Diseases, National Institutes of Health, August 16, 2007.

Overview

Sneezing, scratchy throat, runny nose—everyone knows the first signs of a cold, probably the most common illness known. Although the common cold is usually mild, with symptoms lasting one to two weeks, it is a leading cause of doctor visits and missed days from school and work. According to the Centers for Disease Control and Prevention, twenty-two million school days are lost annually in the United States due to the common cold.

In the course of a year, people in the United States suffer one billion colds, according to some estimates.

Children have about six to ten colds a year. One important reason why colds are so common in children is because they are often in close contact with each other in daycare centers and schools. In families with children in school, the number of colds per child can be as high as twelve a year. Adults average about two to four colds a year, although the range varies widely. Women, especially those aged twenty to thirty years, have more colds than men, possibly because of their closer contact with children. On average, people older than sixty have fewer than one cold a year.

In the United States, most colds occur during the fall and winter. Beginning in late August or early September, the rate of colds increases slowly for a few weeks and remains high until March or April, when it declines. The seasonal variation may relate to the opening of schools and to cold weather, which prompt people to spend more time indoors and increase the chances that viruses will spread to you from someone else.

Seasonal changes in relative humidity also may affect the prevalence of colds. The most common cold-causing viruses survive better when humidity is low—the colder months of the year. Cold weather also may make the inside lining of your nose drier and more vulnerable to viral infection.

Cause

The Viruses

More than two hundred different viruses are known to cause the symptoms of the common cold. Some, such as the rhinoviruses, seldom produce serious illnesses. Others, such as parainfluenza and respiratory syncytial virus, produce mild infections in adults but can precipitate severe lower respiratory infections in young children.

Rhinoviruses (from the Greek *rhin*, meaning "nose") cause an estimated 30 to 35 percent of all adult colds, and are most active in early fall, spring, and summer. More than 110 distinct rhinovirus types have been identified. These agents grow best at temperatures of about 91 degrees Fahrenheit, the temperature inside the human nose.

Scientists think coronaviruses cause a large percentage of all adult colds. They bring on colds primarily in the winter and early spring. Of the more than thirty kinds, three or four infect humans. The importance of coronaviruses as a cause of colds is hard to assess because, unlike rhinoviruses, they are difficult to grow in the laboratory.

Approximately 10 to 15 percent of adult colds are caused by viruses also responsible for other, more severe illnesses: adenoviruses, coxsackieviruses, echoviruses, orthomyxoviruses (including influenza A and B viruses, which cause flu), paramyxoviruses (including several parainfluenza viruses), respiratory syncytial virus, and enteroviruses.

The causes of 30 to 50 percent of adult colds, presumed to be viral, remain unidentified. The same viruses that produce colds in adults appear to cause colds in children. The relative importance of various viruses in pediatric colds, however, is unclear because it's difficult to isolate the precise cause of symptoms in studies of children with colds.

The Weather

There is no evidence that you can get a cold from exposure to cold weather or from getting chilled or overheated.

Other Factors

There is also no evidence that your chances of getting a cold are related to factors such as exercise, diet, or enlarged tonsils or adenoids. On the other hand, research suggests that psychological stress and allergic diseases affecting your nose or throat may have an impact on your chances of getting infected by cold viruses.

Transmission

You can get infected by cold viruses by either of these methods:

• Touching your skin or environmental surfaces, such as telephones and stair rails, that have cold germs on them and then touching your eyes or nose

• Inhaling drops of mucus full of cold germs from the air

Symptoms

Symptoms of the common cold usually begin two to three days after infection and often include the following:

• Mucus buildup in your nose

• Difficulty breathing through your nose

• Swelling of your sinuses

• Sneezing

• Sore throat

• Cough

• Headache

Fever is usually slight but can climb to 102 degrees Fahrenheit in infants and young children. Cold symptoms can last from two to fourteen days, but like most people, you'll probably recover in a week. If symptoms occur often or last much longer than two weeks, you might have an allergy rather than a cold.

Colds occasionally can lead to bacterial infections of your middle ear or sinuses, requiring treatment with antibiotics. High fever, significantly swollen glands, severe sinus pain, and a cough that produces mucus, may indicate a complication or more serious illness requiring a visit to your healthcare provider.

Treatment

There is no cure for the common cold, but you can get relief from your cold symptoms by doing the following:

• Resting in bed

• Drinking plenty of fluids

• Gargling with warm salt water or using throat sprays or lozenges for a scratchy or sore throat

- Using petroleum jelly for a raw nose
- Taking aspirin or acetaminophen, Tylenol, for example, for headache or fever

A word of caution: Several studies have linked aspirin use to the development of Reye syndrome in children recovering from flu or chickenpox. Reye syndrome is a rare but serious illness that usually occurs in children between the ages of three and twelve years. It can affect all organs of the body but most often the brain and liver. While most children who survive an episode of Reye syndrome do not suffer any lasting consequences, the illness can lead to permanent brain damage or death. The American Academy of Pediatrics recommends children and teenagers not be given aspirin or medicine containing aspirin when they have any viral illness such as the common cold.

Over-the-Counter Cold Medicines

Nonprescription cold remedies, including decongestants and cough suppressants, may relieve some of your cold symptoms but will not prevent or even shorten the length of your cold. Moreover, because most of these medicines have some side effects, such as drowsiness, dizziness, insomnia, or upset stomach, you should take them with care.

Over-the-Counter Antihistamines

Nonprescription antihistamines may give you some relief from symptoms such as runny nose and watery eyes which are commonly associated with colds.

Antibiotics

Never take antibiotics to treat a cold because antibiotics do not kill viruses. You should use these prescription medicines only if you have a rare bacterial complication, such as sinusitis or ear infections. In addition, you should not use antibiotics "just in case" because they will not prevent bacterial infections.

Steam

Although inhaling steam may temporarily relieve symptoms of congestion, health experts have found that this approach is not an effective treatment.

Prevention

There are several ways you can keep yourself from getting a cold or passing one on to others:

- Because cold germs on your hands can easily enter through your eyes and nose, keep your hands away from those areas of your body.
- If possible, avoid being close to people who have colds.
- If you have a cold, avoid being close to people.
- If you sneeze or cough, cover your nose or mouth.

Hand Washing

Hand washing with soap and water is the simplest and one of the most effective ways to keep from getting colds or giving them to others. During cold season, you should wash your hands often and teach your children to do the same.

When water isn't available, the Centers for Disease Control and Prevention (CDC) recommends using alcohol-based products made for washing hands.

Disinfecting

Rhinoviruses can live up to three hours on your skin. They also can survive up to three hours on objects such as telephones and stair railings. Cleaning environmental surfaces with a virus-killing disinfectant might help prevent spread of infection.

Unproven Prevention Methods

Echinacea

Echinacea is a dietary herbal supplement that some people use to treat their colds. Researchers, however, have found that while the herb may help treat your colds if taken in the early stages, it will not help prevent them.

One research study funded by the National Center for Complementary and Alternative Medicine, a part of the National Institutes of Health, found that echinacea is not effective at all in treating children aged two to eleven.

Vitamin C

Many people are convinced that taking large quantities of vitamin C will prevent colds or relieve symptoms. To test this theory, several large-scale, controlled studies involving children and adults have been conducted. To date, no conclusive data has shown that large doses of vitamin C prevent colds. The vitamin may reduce the severity or duration of symptoms, but there is no clear evidence.

Taking vitamin C over long periods of time in large amounts may be harmful. Too much vitamin C can cause severe diarrhea, a particular danger for elderly people and small children.

Complications

Colds occasionally can lead to bacterial infections of your middle ear or sinuses, requiring treatment with antibiotics. High fever, significantly swollen glands, severe sinus pain, and a cough that produces mucus may indicate a complication or more serious illness requiring a visit to your healthcare provider.

Research

Thanks to basic research, scientists know more about the rhinovirus than almost any other virus, and have powerful new tools for developing antiviral drugs. Although the common cold may never be uncommon, further investigations offer the hope of reducing the huge burden of this universal problem.

Research on Rhinovirus Transmission

Much of the research on the transmission of the common cold has been done with rhinoviruses, which are shed in the highest concentration in nasal secretions. Studies suggest a person is most likely to transmit rhinoviruses in the second to fourth day of infection, when the amount of virus in nasal secretions is highest.

Researchers also have shown that using aspirin to treat colds increases the amount of virus in nasal secretions, possibly making the cold sufferer more of a hazard to others.

Vaccine

Because so many different viruses can cause the common cold, the outlook for developing a vaccine that will prevent transmission of all of them is dim. Scientists, however, continue to search for a solution to this problem.

Section 18.4

Hantavirus Pulmonary Syndrome

Excerpted from "Hantavirus Pulmonary Syndrome: What You Need to Know," U.S. Centers for Disease Control and Prevention, October 26, 2006.

What is hantavirus pulmonary syndrome (HPS)?

Hantavirus pulmonary syndrome (HPS) is a deadly disease caused by hantaviruses. Rodents can transmit hantaviruses through urine, droppings, or saliva. Humans can contract the disease when they breathe in aerosolized virus.

Who is at risk of contracting HPS?

Anyone who comes into contact with rodents that carry hantavirus is at risk of HPS. Rodent infestation in and around the home remains the primary risk for hantavirus exposure. Even healthy individuals are at risk for HPS infection if exposed to the virus.

Which rodents are known to be carriers of hantavirus that cause HPS in humans?

In the United States, deer mice, cotton and rice rats (in the Southeast), and the white-footed mouse (in the Northeast), are the only known rodent carriers of hantaviruses causing HPS.

How is HPS transmitted?

Hantavirus is transmitted by infected rodents through urine, droppings, or saliva. Individuals become infected with HPS after breathing fresh aerosolized urine, droppings, saliva, or nesting materials. Transmission can also occur when these materials are directly introduced into broken skin, the nose or the mouth. If a rodent with the virus bites someone, the virus may be spread to that person, but this type of transmission is rare.

Can you contract HPS from another person?

HPS in the United States cannot be transmitted from one person to another. You cannot get the virus from touching or kissing a person who has HPS or from a health care worker who has treated someone with the disease. In addition, you cannot contract the virus from a blood transfusion in which you receive blood from a person who survived HPS.

Can you contract HPS from other animals?

Hantaviruses that cause HPS in the United States are only known to be transmitted by certain species of rodents. HPS in the United States is not known to be transmitted by farm animals, dogs, or cats, or from rodents purchased from a pet store.

How long can hantavirus remain infectious in the environment?

The length of time hantaviruses can remain infectious in the environment is variable and depends on environmental conditions, such as temperature and humidity, whether the virus is indoors or outdoors or exposed to the sun, and even on the rodent's diet (which would affect the chemistry of its urine). Viability for two or three days has been shown at normal room temperature. Exposure to sunlight will decrease the time of viability, and freezing temperatures will actually increase the time that the virus remains viable. Since the survival of infectious virus is measured in terms of hours or days, only active infestations of infected rodents result in conditions that are likely to lead to human hantavirus infection.

How do I prevent HPS?

Seal up, trap up, clean up: Seal up rodent entry holes or gaps with steel wool, lath metal, or caulk. Trap rats and mice by using an appropriate snap trap. Clean up rodent food sources and nesting sites and take precautions when cleaning rodent-infested areas.

What are the recommendations for cleaning a rodent-infested area?

- Put on rubber, latex, vinyl, or nitrile gloves.

- Do not stir up dust by vacuuming, sweeping, or any other means.

- Thoroughly wet contaminated areas with a bleach solution or household disinfectant. Hypochlorite (bleach) solution: Mix 1 ½ cups of household bleach in one gallon of water.

- Once everything is wet, take up contaminated materials with damp towel and then mop or sponge the area with bleach solution or household disinfectant.

- Spray dead rodents with disinfectant and then double-bag along with all cleaning materials. Bury, burn, or throw out rodent in appropriate waste disposal system. (Contact your local or state health department concerning other appropriate disposal methods.)

- Disinfect gloves with disinfectant or soap and water before taking them off.

- After taking off the clean gloves, thoroughly wash hands with soap and water (or use a waterless alcohol-based hand rub when soap is not available).

Can I use a vacuum with HEPA filter to clean up rodent-contaminated areas?

HEPA vacuums are not recommended since they blow air around and may create aerosols.

How do I clean papers, books, and delicate items?

Books, papers, and other items that cannot be cleaned with a liquid disinfectant or thrown away should be left outdoors in the sunlight for several hours or in an indoor area free of rodents for approximately one week before final cleaning. After that time, the virus should no longer be infectious. Wear rubber, latex, or vinyl gloves and wipe the items with a cloth moistened with disinfectant.

I do not want to bleach my clothes or stuffed animals; is there anything else I can do?

Wash clothing or stuffed animals in the washing machine using hot water and regular detergent. Laundry detergent can break down the virus's lipid envelope, rendering it harmless. Machine dry laundry on a high setting or hang it to air dry in the sun. The Centers for Disease

Control and Prevention (CDC) does not recommend simply running the clothing through the dryer without washing first.

How do I clean rugs, carpets, and upholstered furniture?

Disinfect carpets and upholstered furniture with a disinfectant or with a commercial-grade steam cleaner or shampoo.

What precautions should I take if I think I have been exposed to hantavirus?

If you have been exposed to rodents or rodent infestations and have symptoms of fever, deep muscle aches, and severe shortness of breath, see your doctor immediately. Inform your doctor of possible rodent exposure so that he or she is alerted to the possibility of rodent-borne diseases, such as HPS.

Section 18.5

Human Metapneumovirus

Human metapneumovirus (HMPV) is a newly identified virus that causes a spectrum of respiratory illness, ranging from mild upper respiratory tract infections to severe bronchiolitis and pneumonia. HMPV was first identified by researchers in the Netherlands in 2001 as a cause of respiratory tract disease in Dutch children. However, the virus has been thought to be infecting humans for at least fifty years.[1]

HMPV has been recently identified in children and adults with acute respiratory tract infections (ARTI) in various parts of the world. The first evidence of HMPV in the United States was found in New Haven, Connecticut, in the 2001–2002 fall/winter season.[2]

HMPV is associated with a rate of community acquired respiratory illness similar to that of the parainfluenza viruses and influenza virus but substantially less than that associated with respiratory syncytial virus (RSV).[3] RSV, in addition to parainfluenza virus, adenovirus, and influenza virus are common known causes of lower respiratory tract disease in infants and children.

However, HMPV may be responsible for a significant portion of the more than 150,000 bronchiolitis hospitalizations in infants and children younger than five years. Researchers estimate that the cause of 15 to 34 percent of bronchiolitis and pneumonia cases cannot be determined.[4]

Little is known about of the nature of the HMPV infection, but a recent study found that the severity of illness in HMPV-positive patients is similar to those illnesses in RSV-positive patients. Therefore, while the incidence of HMPV infection may not compare with that of RSV infection, the disease severity may be very similar.[5]

Clinical symptoms of HMPV infection also seem to be indistinguishable from RSV infections. Symptoms include high fever, severe cough, difficulty breathing, abnormally rapid breathing, wheezing, vomiting, and diarrhea.

Researchers suggest that HMPV may stimulate asthmatic episodes in children with asthma. One study found that asthma was the most frequently recorded hospital discharge diagnosis among HMPV-positive children.[6] Another found that 14 percent of HMPV cases had an exacerbation of asthma.[7]

The mean age of HMPV infection was 11.6 months, 78 percent of illnesses occurred between December and April, and the hospitalization rate was 2 percent. Males are more likely than females to have HMPV infection.[8]

HMPV also causes RSV-like disease in elderly adults; the at-risk population is elderly persons with COPD.[9]

For more information on human metapneumovirus, call your local American Lung Association at 800-LUNG-USA (800-586-4872).

Sources

1. Nissen MD, Sloots TP, Mackay I, Siebert D. Human metapneumovirus. *EMedicine* (serial online) 2004 Jun. Available from: http://www.emedicine.com/med/topic3564.htm.

2. Esper F, Boucher D, Weibel C, Martinello RA, Kahn JS. Human metapnuemovirus infection in the United States: Clinical manifestations associated with a newly emerging respiratory infection in children. *Pediatrics* 2003 Jun. Vol. 111(6): 1407–10.

3. Mullins JA, Erdman DD, Weinberg GA, Edwards K, Hall CB, Walker FJ, et al. Human metapneumovirus infection among children hospitalized with acute respiratory illness. *Emerging Infectious Disease* (serial online) 2004 Apr. Available from: http://www.cdc.gov/ncidod/EOD/vol10no4/03-0555.htm.

4. Esper F, Boucher D, Weibel C, Martinello RA, Kahn JS. Human metapnuemovirus infection in the United States: Clinical manifestations associated with a newly emerging respiratory infection in children. *Pediatrics* 2003 Jun. Vol. 111(6): 1407–10.

5. Mullins JA, Erdman DD, Weinberg GA, Edwards K, Hall CB, Walker FJ, et al. Human metapneumovirus infection among children hospitalized with acute respiratory illness. *Emerging Infectious Disease* (serial online) 2004 Apr. Available from: http://www.cdc.gov/ncidod/EOD/vol10no4/03-0555.htm.

6. Ibid.

7. Williams JV, Harris RA, Tollefson SJ, Halburnt-Rush LL, et al. Human metapneumovirus and lower respiratory tract disease in otherwise healthy infants and children. *New England Journal of Medicine* 2004 Jan. Vol. 350(5): 443–50.

8. Ibid.

9. Nissen MD, Sloots TP, Mackay I, Siebert D. Human metapneumovirus. *EMedicine* (serial online) 2004 Jun. Available from: http://www.emedicine.com/med/topic3564.htm.

Section 18.6

Influenza

"What Is Influenza (Also Called Flu)" is reprinted from "Key Facts about Seasonal Influenza (Flu)," U.S. Centers for Disease Control and Prevention, November 16, 2007. "Questions and Answers: Cold Versus Flu" is reprinted from U.S. Centers for Disease Control and Prevention, September 18, 2006.

What Is Influenza (Also Called Flu)?

The flu is a contagious respiratory illness caused by influenza viruses. It can cause mild to severe illness, and at times can lead to death. The best way to prevent the flu is by getting a flu vaccination each year.

Every year in the United States, on average:

- Between 5 and 20 percent of the population gets the flu;

- More than 200,000 people are hospitalized from flu complications; and

- About 36,000 people die from flu.

Some people, such as older people, young children, and people with certain health conditions (such as asthma, diabetes, or heart disease), are at high risk for serious flu complications.

Symptoms of Flu

Symptoms of flu include the following:

- fever (usually high)
- headache
- extreme tiredness
- dry cough
- sore throat
- runny or stuffy nose
- muscle aches

Stomach symptoms, such as nausea, vomiting, and diarrhea, also can occur but are more common in children than adults.

Complications of Flu

Complications of flu can include bacterial pneumonia, ear infections, sinus infections, dehydration, and worsening of chronic medical conditions, such as congestive heart failure, asthma, or diabetes.

How Flu Spreads

Flu viruses spread mainly from person to person through coughing or sneezing of people with influenza. Sometimes people may become infected by touching something with flu viruses on it and then touching their mouth or nose. Most healthy adults may be able to infect others beginning one day before symptoms develop and up to five days after becoming sick. That means that you may be able to pass on the flu to someone else before you know you are sick, as well as while you are sick.

Preventing Seasonal Flu: Get Vaccinated

The single best way to prevent the flu is to get a flu vaccination each year. There are two types of vaccines:

- **The "flu shot":** An inactivated vaccine (containing killed virus) that is given with a needle. The flu shot is approved for use in people six months of age and older, including healthy people and people with chronic medical conditions.

- **The nasal-spray flu vaccine:** A vaccine made with live, weakened flu viruses that do not cause the flu (sometimes called LAIV for "live attenuated influenza vaccine"). LAIV is approved for use in healthy people two to forty-nine years of age who are not pregnant.

About two weeks after vaccination, antibodies develop that protect against influenza virus infection. Flu vaccines will not protect against flu-like illnesses caused by non-influenza viruses.

When to Get Vaccinated

October or November is the best time to get vaccinated, but you can still get vaccinated in December and later. Flu season can begin as early as October and last as late as May.

Who Should Get Vaccinated?

In general, anyone who wants to reduce their chances of getting the flu can get vaccinated. However, certain people should get vaccinated each year either because they are at high risk of having serious flu-related complications or because they live with or care for high-risk persons. During flu seasons when vaccine supplies are limited or delayed, the Advisory Committee on Immunization Practices (ACIP) makes recommendations regarding priority groups for vaccination.

People who should get vaccinated each year are:

- People at high risk for complications from the flu, including:
  - Children aged six months until their fifth birthday;
  - Pregnant women;
  - People fifty years of age and older;
  - People of any age with certain chronic medical conditions; and
  - People who live in nursing homes and other long-term care facilities.

- People who live with or care for those at high risk for complications from flu, including:
  - Household contacts of persons at high risk for complications from the flu (see above);
  - Household contacts and out of home caregivers of children less than six months of age (these children are too young to be vaccinated);
  - Health care workers.

- Anyone who wants to decrease their risk of influenza.

Use of the Nasal Spray Flu Vaccine

Vaccination with the nasal-spray flu vaccine is an option for healthy people two to forty-nine years of age who are not pregnant, even healthy persons who live with or care for those in a high-risk group. The one exception is healthy persons who care for persons with severely weakened immune systems who require a protected environment; these healthy persons should get the inactivated vaccine.

Who Should Not Be Vaccinated

Some people should not be vaccinated without first consulting a physician. They include:

- People who have a severe allergy to chicken eggs.

- People who have had a severe reaction to an influenza vaccination in the past.

- People who developed Guillain-Barré syndrome (GBS) within six weeks of getting an influenza vaccine previously.

- Children less than six months of age (influenza vaccine is not approved for use in this age group).

- People who have a moderate or severe illness with a fever. These people should wait to get vaccinated until their symptoms lessen.

If you have questions about whether you should get a flu vaccine, consult your health-care provider.

Questions and Answers: Cold Versus Flu

What is the difference between a cold and the flu?

The flu and the common cold are both respiratory illnesses but they are caused by different viruses. Because these two types of illnesses have similar flu-like symptoms, it can be difficult to tell the difference between them based on symptoms alone. In general, the flu is worse than the common cold, and symptoms such as fever, body aches, extreme tiredness, and dry cough are more common and intense. Colds are usually milder than the flu. People with colds are more likely to have a runny or stuffy nose. Colds generally do not result in serious health problems, such as pneumonia, bacterial infections, or hospitalizations.

How can you tell the difference between a cold and the flu?

Because colds and flu share many symptoms, it can be difficult (or even impossible) to tell the difference between them based on symptoms alone. Special tests that usually must be done within the first few days of illness can be carried out, when needed, to tell if a person has the flu.

What are the symptoms of the flu versus the symptoms of a cold?

In general, the flu is worse than the common cold, and symptoms such as fever, body aches, extreme tiredness, and dry cough are more common and intense. Colds are usually milder than the flu. People with colds are more likely to have a runny or stuffy nose. Colds generally do not result in serious health problems, such as pneumonia, bacterial infections, or hospitalizations.

Section 18.7

Respiratory Syncytial Virus

What is respiratory syncytial virus (RSV)? What does RSV cause?

RSV is a lung infection caused by a virus. Although it can affect anyone, RSV is generally considered as the most frequent cause of lower respiratory tract infections in infants and young children. Each year about 125,000 infants are hospitalized with RSV in the United States.

What are the symptoms of an RSV infection?

Many persons with RSV infection show no symptoms. In adults and children older than three years, RSV symptoms are usually those of a simple upper respiratory tract illness. The illness typically begins with a low-grade fever, runny nose, cough, and, sometimes, wheezing. In children younger than age three, RSV can cause a lower respiratory tract illness, such as bronchiolitis or pneumonia, and more severe cases can result in respiratory failure. Symptoms may include a worsening croupy cough, unusually rapid breathing, difficulty breathing (the chest may suck in with each breath), and a bluish color of the lips or fingernails caused by low levels of oxygen in the blood. RSV has also been found to be a frequent cause of middle ear infections (otitis media) in preschool children.

How common is RSV?

RSV infections occur all over the world, most often in outbreaks that can last up to five months, from late fall through early spring. RSV epidemics spread easily in households, daycare centers, and schools.

Who is likely to get RSV?

Most children are infected at least once by age two and continue to be reinfected throughout life. RSV is the most common cause of bronchiolitis and pneumonia in infants and children under the age of one. The majority of children hospitalized for an RSV infection are under the age of six months. The elderly and premature babies or those with lung or heart problems or with weak immune systems have an especially high risk. Those who are exposed to tobacco smoke, attend daycare, live in crowded conditions, or have school-aged siblings could also be at higher risk.

How is RSV spread?

Typically a parent, or more likely an older sibling, comes down with what seems like a bad cold first. The virus is found in discharges from the nose and throat of an infected person. People can get RSV infection by breathing in droplets after an infected person has coughed; by hand-to-mouth contact after touching an infected person; and, by hand-to-mouth after touching a surface that an infected person has touched or coughed on. The time period from exposure to illness is usually about four days. After an infection, a person may be still contagious for a week.

How can you prevent RSV?

Exercise typical cold precautions during the peak of RSV season:

- Wash your hands often. Do not touch your eyes, nose, or mouth without washing your hands first. Soap and water and disinfectants easily inactivate the virus.

- If possible, avoid exposure to sick persons. Parents with high-risk young infants should avoid crowds.

- When RSV infects a daycare center, it is not unusual to see most, if not all of the children come down with an RSV infection. Make sure that all children and employees use good hand washing techniques and that all children and employees cover their faces when coughing or sneezing. Used tissues should be thrown away in a lined trashcan immediately after use.

- It is important that infants do not share toys, bottles, etc. Surfaces and toys shared by two or more children should be cleaned and disinfected regularly.

- Whenever a school-age child comes down with a cold, keep the child away from an infant brother or sister until the symptoms pass.

What do I do if I think anyone in my family has RSV?

Consult with your healthcare provider. Any breathing difficulties in an infant should be considered an emergency, so seek immediate help.

How are RSV infections diagnosed?

The diagnosis is usually made by the pattern of a child's symptoms (a clinical diagnosis), especially if he or she has a cold and is wheezing. RSV can be confirmed by checking for the virus in nasal washings or by growing the virus from nasal swabs.

How are RSV infections treated?

There is currently no vaccine to prevent RSV infection. Because RSV infection is often resolved on its own, treatment of mild symptoms is not necessary for most people. For babies and children who are at high risk of developing severe RSV, preventive medication is available. Parents of an infant who is premature, has a serious heart or lung disease, or has a weak immune system should contact their doctor or healthcare provider. Antibiotics are not useful in the treatment of RSV or any other viral disease.

Should I worry about RSV when I travel out of the country?

RSV is common worldwide, but no additional precautions are needed when traveling. The number of infections usually peaks in the late fall, winter, and early spring in the United States and Europe. In tropical climates, epidemics occur during the rainy season.

Section 18.8

Severe Acute Respiratory Syndrome (SARS)

Reprinted from "Frequently Asked Questions about SARS,"
U.S. Centers for Disease Control and Prevention, May 3, 2005.

The Disease

What is severe acute respiratory syndrome (SARS)?

Severe acute respiratory syndrome (SARS) is a viral respiratory illness that was recognized as a global threat in March 2003, after first appearing in southern China in November 2002.

What are the symptoms and signs of SARS?

The illness usually begins with a high fever (measured temperature greater than 100.4°F (>38.0°C). The fever is sometimes associated with chills or other symptoms, including headache, general feeling of discomfort, and body aches. Some people also experience mild respiratory symptoms at the outset. Diarrhea is seen in approximately 10 to 20 percent of patients. After two to seven days, SARS patients may develop a dry, nonproductive cough that might be accompanied by or progress to a condition in which the oxygen levels in the blood are low (hypoxia). In 10 to 20 percent of cases, patients require mechanical ventilation. Most patients develop pneumonia.

What is the cause of SARS?

SARS is caused by a previously unrecognized coronavirus, called SARS-associated coronavirus (SARS-CoV). It is possible that other infectious agents might have a role in some cases of SARS.

How is SARS spread?

The primary way that SARS appears to spread is by close person-to-person contact. SARS-CoV is thought to be transmitted most readily

285

by respiratory droplets (droplet spread) produced when an infected person coughs or sneezes. Droplet spread can happen when droplets from the cough or sneeze of an infected person are propelled a short distance (generally up to three feet) through the air and deposited on the mucous membranes of the mouth, nose, or eyes of persons who are nearby. The virus also can spread when a person touches a surface or object contaminated with infectious droplets and then touches his or her mouth, nose, or eye(s). In addition, it is possible that SARS-CoV might be spread more broadly through the air (airborne spread) or by other ways that are not now known.

What does "close contact" mean?

Close contact is defined as having cared for or lived with a person known to have SARS or having a high likelihood of direct contact with respiratory secretions and/or body fluids of a patient known to have SARS. Examples include kissing or embracing, sharing eating or drinking utensils, close conversation (within three feet), physical examination, and any other direct physical contact between people. Close contact does not include activities such as walking by a person or briefly sitting across a waiting room or office.

If I were exposed to SARS-CoV, how long would it take for me to become sick?

The time between exposure to SARS-CoV and the onset of symptoms is called the "incubation period." The incubation period for SARS is typically two to seven days, although in some cases it may be as long as ten days. In a very small proportion of cases, incubation periods of up to fourteen days have been reported.

How long is a person with SARS infectious to others?

Available information suggests that persons with SARS are most likely to be contagious only when they have symptoms, such as fever or cough. Patients are most contagious during the second week of illness. However, as a precaution against spreading the disease, the Centers for Disease Control and Prevention (CDC) recommends that persons with SARS limit their interactions outside the home (for example, by not going to work or to school) until ten days after their fever has gone away and their respiratory (breathing) symptoms have gotten better.

Is a person with SARS contagious before symptoms appear?

To date, no cases of SARS have been reported among persons who were exposed to a SARS patient before the onset of the patient's symptoms.

What medical treatment is recommended for patients with SARS?

CDC recommends that patients with SARS receive the same treatment that would be used for a patient with any serious community-acquired atypical pneumonia. SARS-CoV is being tested against various antiviral drugs to see if an effective treatment can be found.

If there is another outbreak of SARS, how can I protect myself?

If transmission of SARS-CoV recurs, there are some common-sense precautions that you can take that apply to many infectious diseases. The most important is frequent hand washing with soap and water or use of an alcohol-based hand rub. You should also avoid touching your eyes, nose, and mouth with unclean hands and encourage people around you to cover their nose and mouth with a tissue when coughing or sneezing.

Global SARS Outbreak, 2003

How many people contracted SARS worldwide during the 2003 outbreak? How many people died of SARS worldwide?

From November 2002 through July 2003, a total of 8,098 people worldwide became sick with severe acute respiratory syndrome that was accompanied by either pneumonia or respiratory distress syndrome (probable cases), according to the World Health Organization (WHO). Of these, 774 died. By late July 2003, no new cases were being reported, and WHO declared the global outbreak to be over.

How many people contracted SARS in the United States during the 2003 outbreak? How many people died of SARS in the United States?

In the United States, only eight persons were laboratory-confirmed as SARS cases. There were no SARS-related deaths in the United States.

All of the eight persons with laboratory-confirmed SARS had traveled to areas where SARS-CoV transmission was occurring.

SARS Situation, 2004

What is the current SARS situation in the world?

In April 2004, the Chinese Ministry of Health reported several new cases of possible SARS in Beijing and in Anhui Province, which is located in east-central China. As of April 26, 2004, the Ministry of Health had reported eight possible SARS cases: six in Beijing and two in Anhui Province. One of the patients in Anhui Province died. Nearly one thousand contacts of these patients with possible SARS were put under medical observation, including 640 in Beijing and 353 in Anhui.

In addition, health authorities reported that two doctors who treated one of one of the patients during her hospitalization in Anhui developed fever. A person in close contact with one of the doctors also developed fever.

To date, all diagnosed cases and cases under investigation have been linked to chains of transmission involving close personal contact with an identified case. There is no evidence of wider transmission in the community.

SARS-Associated Coronavirus

What are coronaviruses?

Coronaviruses are a group of viruses that have a halo or crown-like (corona) appearance when viewed under a microscope. These viruses are a common cause of mild to moderate upper-respiratory illness in humans and are associated with respiratory, gastrointestinal, liver, and neurologic disease in animals.

If coronaviruses usually cause mild illness in humans, how could this new coronavirus be responsible for a potentially life-threatening disease such as SARS?

There is not enough information about the new virus to determine the full range of illness that it might cause. Coronaviruses have occasionally been linked to pneumonia in humans, especially people with weakened immune systems. The viruses also can cause severe disease in animals, including cats, dogs, pigs, mice, and birds.

How long can SARS-CoV survive in the environment?

Preliminary studies in some research laboratories suggest that the virus may survive in the environment for several days. The length of time that the virus survives likely depends on a number of factors. These factors could include the type of material or body fluid containing the virus and various environmental conditions such as temperature or humidity. Researchers at CDC and other institutions are designing standardized experiments to measure how long SARS-CoV can survive in situations that simulate natural environmental conditions.

Laboratory Testing

Is there a laboratory test for SARS?

Yes, several laboratory tests can be used to detect SARS-CoV. A reverse transcription polymerase chain reaction (RT-PCR) test can detect SARS-CoV in clinical specimens such as blood, stool, and nasal secretions. Serologic testing also can be performed to detect SARS-CoV antibodies produced after infection. Finally, viral culture has been used to detect SARS-CoV.

What is a PCR test?

PCR (or polymerase chain reaction) is a laboratory method for detecting the genetic material of an infectious disease agent in specimens from patients. This type of testing has become an essential tool for detecting infectious disease agents.

What does serologic testing involve?

A serologic test is a laboratory method for detecting the presence and/or level of antibodies in an infectious agent in serum from a person. Antibodies are substances made by the body's immune system to fight a specific infection.

What does viral culture and isolation involve?

For a viral culture, a small sample of tissue or fluid that may be infected is placed in a container along with cells in which the virus can grow. If the virus grows in the culture, it will cause changes in the cells that can be seen under a microscope.

Chapter 19

Fungal Infections

Chapter Contents

Section 19.1

Aspergillosis

Definition

Aspergillosis is an infection, growth, or allergic response caused by the *Aspergillus* fungus.

Causes

Aspergillosis is caused by a fungus (*Aspergillus*), which is commonly found growing on dead leaves, stored grain, compost piles, or in other decaying vegetation.

There are several forms of aspergillosis:

- **Pulmonary aspergillosis–allergic bronchopulmonary type** is an allergic reaction to the fungus that develops with asthma.

- **Aspergilloma** is a growth (fungus ball) that develops in an area of previous lung disease such as tuberculosis or lung abscess.

- **Pulmonary aspergillosis–invasive type** is a serious infection with pneumonia that spreads to other parts of the body. This infection occurs almost exclusively in people with weakened immune systems due to cancer, acquired immunodeficiency syndrome (AIDS), leukemia, organ transplantation, chemotherapy, or other conditions or events that reduce the number of normal white blood cells.

Symptoms

Symptoms depend on the actual type of infection.
Symptoms of allergic aspergillosis may include:

- Fever;
- Malaise;
- Cough;
- Coughing up blood or brownish mucous plugs;
- Wheezing;
- Weight loss;
- Recurrent episodes of lung obstruction.

Additional symptoms seen in invasive aspergillosis:

- Chills;
- Headaches;
- Shortness of breath;
- Chest pain;
- Increased sputum production, which may be bloody;
- Bone pain;
- Blood in the urine;
- Decreased urine output;
- Meningitis;
- Vision problems;
- Sinusitis;
- Endocarditis.

Exams and Tests

Tests to diagnose aspergillosis infection may include:

- Chest x-ray;
- Computed tomography (CT) scan;
- Sputum stain and culture for *Aspergillus*;
- Tissue biopsy;
- *Aspergillus* antigen skin test;
- Aspergillosis precipitin antibody;
- Complete blood count.

293

Treatment

A fungus ball usually does not require treatment unless bleeding into the lung tissue is associated with the infection, then surgery is required.

Invasive aspergillosis is treated with several weeks of amphotericin B, an antifungal medication given by an intravenous line (IV). Itraconazole or voriconazole can also be used.

Endocarditis caused by *Aspergillus* is treated by surgically removing the infected heart valves. Long-term amphotericin B therapy is also needed.

Anti-fungal agents do not help people with allergic aspergillosis. Allergic aspergillosis is treated with prednisone taken by mouth.

Outlook (Prognosis)

Gradual improvement is seen in patients with allergic aspergillosis.

If invasive aspergillosis resists drug treatment, it eventually leads to death. The outlook for a person with invasive aspergillosis also depends on the underlying disease and immune system function.

Possible Complications

- Amphotericin B can cause kidney impairment and severely unpleasant side effects.

- Invasive lung disease can cause massive bleeding from the lung.

When to Contact a Medical Professional

Call the health care provider if symptoms of aspergillosis develop.

Prevention

Be careful when using medications that suppress the immune system. Prevention of AIDS prevents certain diseases, including aspergillosis, that are associated with a damaged or weakened immune system.

Section 19.2

Blastomycosis

What is blastomycosis?

Blastomycosis is an uncommon, but potentially serious fungal infection. It primarily affects the lungs and skin and is caused by the fungus *Blastomyces dermatitidis*. The illness that can result from exposure to this organism is extremely variable. Infected individuals may not develop any symptoms or may develop mild and rapidly improving respiratory symptoms; a progressive illness involving multiple organ systems can occur in untreated patients.

What are the signs and symptoms?

Some persons infected with *Blastomyces* fungus never develop symptoms. Evidence of their infection is only found by chance on a chest x-ray or blood test. Other individuals may develop an acute lung infection that begins with a fever and dry cough and may progress to weight loss, chest pain, and a persistent cough associated with the production of a thick sputum. Other symptoms may include muscle aches, night sweats, coughing up blood, shortness of breath, and chest tightness. The time from a person's exposure to the fungus to the time that symptoms develop can vary from three weeks to several months. Signs or symptoms and the infection may disappear spontaneously without treatment. However, in a small percentage of cases the infection may spread by blood to the skin, bone, or other organs. Blastomycosis of the skin appears as enlarging raised lesions with ulcerating centers. These usually occur on the exposed parts of the body, including the face, hands, wrists, feet, and ankles. In more severe cases, blood-borne fungal lesions may also occur in bones, the prostate gland, testes, and kidneys.

How is blastomycosis diagnosed?

Infected symptomatic individuals usually have abnormalities present on their chest x-rays. However, these abnormalities are not unique to blastomycosis and may occur with many other respiratory illnesses. The diagnosis of blastomycosis can be confirmed by the identification of the fungus *B. dermatitidis* in a culture of the sputum, skin, or biopsy specimen of infected tissue. Blood specimens may also be used to determine if an individual has had a previous blastomycosis infection; however, blood tests will not identify all cases and on occasion may be falsely positive. Similarly, skin tests are not accurate in diagnosing blastomycosis.

How does a person develop blastomycosis?

Blastomycosis develops when spores of the *B. dermatitidis* are breathed in and establish a primary infection in the lung. In nature, the fungus probably resides in the soil in decaying foliage and vegetation. Only under quite specific conditions of humidity, temperature, and nutrition can the fungus grow and produce the infecting particles, the spores. The spores become airborne when the soil in which the fungus is growing is disturbed. This aerosol is then inhaled by humans or other mammals. Thus, activities that involve disrupting the soil are likely to put a person at increased risk for acquiring blastomycosis.

Dogs may also develop blastomycosis because they also inhale the spores following disruption of the soil. Infected dogs cannot transmit the disease to humans, but do serve to indicate that an area may be infected with the fungus. Blastomycosis cannot be transmitted from person-to-person.

How is blastomycosis treated?

Once blastomycosis has been diagnosed, the disease can be treated with one of three anti-fungal drugs—itraconazole, amphotericin B, or fluconazole. For life-threatening blastomycosis or blastomycosis of the central nervous system, amphotericin B is the treatment of choice. Itraconazole or fluconazole are excellent for treatment of patients who are not critically ill or who have no central nervous system involvement.

How common is blastomycosis?

In spite of recent widespread publicity, blastomycosis is a relatively rare disease. From 1993 to 1997, an average of 117 cases of blastomycosis were reported to the Wisconsin Division of Public Health annually. It is likely that other persons are infected with the fungus but only develop minimal symptoms and are not diagnosed or reported to the Division of Health. Almost all cases of blastomycosis occur as isolated events and only rarely have outbreaks or clusters of cases been reported. Nationally, blastomycosis occurs along the Mississippi River Valley from Minnesota and Wisconsin to Arkansas, along the Ohio River Valley, and in the southeastern United States. Although cases of blastomycosis have been reported from all areas in Wisconsin, there appears to be an increase in the number of reported cases occurring in the northern and central counties. While *B. dermatitidis* is widely distributed geographically, the actual area infected with the fungus is likely to be small and may be limited to one rotting log or several square yards of infected soil. Depending upon environmental conditions, the area may be infected for only a brief time.

How can blastomycosis be prevented?

Currently, there is no way to identify areas where the organism exists. Therefore, until more is known about the existence of *B. dermatitidis* in nature, it cannot be successfully controlled in the environment. More effective skin and blood tests are needed to diagnose blastomycosis and to survey individuals in areas where blastomycosis is suspected to be prevalent. Through such surveys, high-risk areas in the environment could be identified and hopefully the necessary environmental conditions for the growth of *B. dermatitidis* characterized. Control efforts may then be possible.

Section 19.3

Coccidioidomycosis

Reprinted from "Valley Fever (Coccidioidomycosis)," State of California, Health and Human Services Agency. The text of this document is available online at http://www.cdph.ca.gov/healthinfo/discond/Documents/Valley%20fever.pdf; accessed October 2007.

What is valley fever and how common is it?

Valley fever can be a serious and sometimes deadly fungus infection. The valley fever fungus lives in soil and is spread, via spores, through the air. Spores are hardy forms of the fungus that can live for a long time in harsh environmental conditions such as heat, cold, and drought. Valley fever usually affects the lungs. When it affects other parts of the body, it is called disseminated valley fever.

An estimated 50,000 to 100,000 persons develop symptoms of valley fever each year in the United States, with an estimated 35,000 new infections per year in California alone.

Where is valley fever found?

It is found in limited areas of the southwestern U.S., Mexico, and parts of Central and South America that meet certain soil and climatic conditions.

How do people get valley fever?

Valley fever is spread through the air. The fungus spores get into the air when construction, natural disasters, or wind disturbs soil contaminated with the valley fever fungus. People breathe in the spores and then can get valley fever.

What are the signs and symptoms of valley fever?

About 60 percent of infected persons have no symptoms from infection by this fungus. The rest develop flu-like symptoms that can last a month. A small percentage of infected persons (less than 1 percent) develop disease that spreads outside the lungs to the brain, bone, and skin. Without proper treatment, valley fever can lead to severe pneumonia, meningitis, and death.

How is valley fever diagnosed?

Valley fever is diagnosed by an antibody blood test or culture.

Who is at risk for valley fever?

At highest risk for valley fever are farmers, construction workers, military personnel, archaeologists, and others who engage in activities that disturb the soil in areas where valley fever is common. People with weak immune systems, the elderly, African-Americans, Asians, and women in the third trimester of pregnancy are at increased risk for disseminated disease and can become seriously ill when infected. Anyone can get valley fever, but people who engage in activities that disturb the soil contaminated by the fungus are at increased risk. The disease is not spread from person to person.

Recent natural disasters have also triggered a rise in valley fever cases. The Central Valley of Southern California had a four-year epidemic of valley fever in the early 1990s after a severe drought. Cases of valley fever also increased in persons exposed to billowing dust released by the January 1994 earthquake in Northridge, California.

What is the treatment for valley fever?

Valley fever is treatable with a variety of oral and injectable antifungal agents.

How can valley fever be prevented?

There is no vaccine against valley fever. Persons at risk for valley fever should avoid exposure to dust and dry soil in areas where valley fever is common.

Section 19.4

Cryptococcosis

Cryptococcosis is a fungal infection caused by inhaling the fungus *Cryptococcus neoformans*, which is primarily found in soils enriched with pigeon droppings. In moist or desiccated pigeon dropping, *Cryptococcus neoformans* may remain viable for two years or longer.

Two varieties of *Cryptococcus neoformans* exist—*neoformans* and *gattii*. *Cryptococcus neoformans* var *neoformans* is the most common variety and mainly affects immunosuppressed patients such as those with human immunodeficiency virus (HIV) and acquired immunodeficiency syndrome (AIDS). *Cryptococcus neoformans* var *gattii* is much less common but affects mainly immunocompetent (normal immune function) individuals. This variety is restricted to subtropical and tropical areas and the fungus found on eucalyptus trees and the surrounding air.

Causes and Risk Factors

The most common cryptococcosis infections (*Cryptococcus neoformans* var *neoformans*) affect people with weakened immune systems, e.g. patients on high doses of corticosteroids, cancer chemotherapy patients, organ transplantation patients, and patients with acquired immune deficiency (AIDS) and human immunodeficiency virus infection (HIV). With the global emergence of AIDS, cryptococcosis is now one of the most common life-threatening fungal infections in these patients.

Infection is primarily through inhalation of Cryptococcus spores released from soil and bird droppings. It occurs in both humans and animals, but animal-to-human and human-to-human transmission via respiratory droplets has not been documented. Transmission via organ transplantation has been reported when infected donor organs were used. Infection via cuts through the skin is not common but may occur.

Clinical Features

The signs and symptoms of the disease are dependent on the site of infection. There are several main sites of infection.

Pulmonary (lung):

- In immunocompetent patients no signs or symptoms may be present. Often these patients will recover spontaneously without any medication.

- Immunosuppressed patients may present with mild-to-moderate symptoms, including fever, malaise, dry cough, chest pain.

- Severe infection may lead to pneumonia or adult respiratory distress syndrome.

Central nervous system (CNS):

- Meningitis is the most common presentation.

- Signs and symptoms include headache, altered mental status, confusion, lethargy, nausea and vomiting, blurred vision or double vision, seizures, and coma.

- This form of infection is fatal without appropriate therapy. Death may occur from two weeks to several years after the onset of symptoms.

Disseminated (widespread, involving other organs):

- In severe infections pulmonary and CNS disease is often associated with disseminated disease.

- Organs most commonly affected include the skin, prostate, and medullary cavity of the bones.

Cryptococcal skin infection:

- Skin infection occurs in 10 to 15 percent of patients infected with *Cryptococcus neoformans*.

- In immunocompetent patients, skin may be the only site of infection.

- In immunosuppressed patients, especially those with HIV infection or AIDS, skin infection is usually a sign of disseminated disease.

- Skin infection presents as:

- Papules (small bumps), pustules, nodules (larger lumps), and ulcers (sores);

- Bleeding into the skin, presenting as pinpoint red spots (petechiae) or bruising (ecchymoses).

Diagnosis

The following laboratory and radiology tests are performed to assist in the diagnosis of cryptococcal disease:

- Sputum culture and stain
- Lung biopsy
- Bronchoscopy
- Cerebrospinal fluid (CSF) culture and stain
- Chest x-ray
- Skin biopsy

Treatment

Treatment of cryptococcal disease depends on the patient's immunological status and the site of infection. It is based on the following categories of infection:

1. Pulmonary cryptococcosis in an immunocompetent patient

2. Pulmonary cryptococcosis in an immunosuppressed patient

3. CNS cryptococcosis

4. Disseminated nonpulmonary, non-CNS cryptococcosis

Immunocompetent patients with asymptomatic pulmonary disease do not usually require any treatment. If the disease does not resolve spontaneously then the anti-fungal fluconazole may be given for three to six months.

Treatment goals for categories 2, 3, and 4 differ on whether or not the patient also has HIV/AIDS. The goal in infected patients with HIV/AIDS is to first control the infection, followed by lifelong treatment to suppress *Cryptococcus neoformans*. For patients with cryptococcal disease not complicated by HIV/AIDS the treatment goal is to eradicate the fungi and achieve a permanent cure.

Several anti-fungal medications are used:

- Intravenous Amphotericin B is the drug of choice for the initial therapy of disseminated, pulmonary, and CNS cryptococcosis.

- Flucytosine should be used in conjunction with amphotericin B.

- Oral fluconazole can be used in less severe infections and is used for lifelong treatment to prevent relapses.

Section 19.5

Histoplasmosis

"Histoplasmosis," © 2007 Virginia Department of Health.
Reprinted with permission.

What is histoplasmosis?

Histoplasmosis is an infection caused by the fungus *Histoplasma capsulatum*. The symptoms vary greatly but it primarily affects the lungs. It rarely invades other parts of the body.

Who gets histoplasmosis?

Anyone can get histoplasmosis. Positive histoplasmosis skin tests are seen in as many as 80 percent of people living in some areas of the eastern and central United States, although most of these people never show any symptoms. It is often called the "cave sickness," as it is sometimes seen in persons who explore caves for a hobby. The more severe forms of this disease are seen more frequently in persons who have problems with their immune systems, such as persons with acquired immunodeficiency syndrome (AIDS). Bats, dogs, cats, rats, skunks, opossum, foxes, and other animals can get histoplasmosis and may play a role in spreading the disease.

How is this fungus spread?

The fungus grows in soil enriched with bat or bird (especially chicken) droppings that have gathered for three or more years. The fungus produces spores that get into the air if the contaminated soil is disturbed. Breathing in these spores causes infection. You cannot get histoplasmosis from another person.

What are the symptoms of histoplasmosis?

Most people with histoplasmosis have no symptoms. For those who do get sick, illness can vary from very mild respiratory disease to a serious illness involving the whole body. Most people have the mild respiratory form of illness with fever, chest pains, weakness, and sometimes a cough. The most serious forms of the disease can lead to death if they are not treated.

How soon after exposure do symptoms appear?

If symptoms appear, it is usually within five to eighteen days after exposure, with an average of ten days.

Where is the fungus that causes histoplasmosis found?

Histoplasma capsulatum is found throughout the world and is common in many areas of the United States, including parts of central and western Virginia. The fungus grows in soils that are mixed with lots of bird or bat droppings, e.g., around old chicken houses, roosts of starlings and blackbirds, in decaying trees, and in caves and other areas where bats live.

What is the treatment for histoplasmosis?

Treatment is not usually recommended for histoplasmosis; most people will get better without treatment. Specific antibiotics are used to treat severe cases of histoplasmosis. Persons who have had histoplasmosis usually do not get it again.

What can be done to prevent the spread of histoplasmosis?

It is not practical to test or decontaminate all possible places where the fungus may be found but the following steps can be taken to minimize exposure: avoid areas where the fungus might grow (such as those listed above); minimize exposure to dust by gently spraying possibly contaminated areas with water before disturbing the soil. Workers should wear disposable clothing and a National Institute for Occupational Safety and Health (NIOSH)/ Mine Safety and Health Administration (MSHA)–approved dust/mist respirator capable of filtering out particles larger than 1 micron in diameter.

Chapter 20

Chronic Inflammatory Lung Diseases

Chapter Contents

Section 20.1

Asthma

Reprinted from National Heart Lung and Blood Institute,
National Institutes of Health, May 2006.

What Is Asthma?

Asthma is a chronic disease that affects your airways. The airways are the tubes that carry air in and out of your lungs. If you have asthma, the inside walls of your airways are inflamed (swollen). The inflammation makes the airways very sensitive, and they tend to react strongly to things that you are allergic to or find irritating. When the airways react, they get narrower, and less air flows through to your lung tissue. This causes symptoms like wheezing (a whistling sound when you breathe), coughing, chest tightness, and trouble breathing, especially at night and in the early morning.

Asthma cannot be cured, but most people with asthma can control it so that they have few and infrequent symptoms and can live active lives.

When your asthma symptoms become worse than usual, it is called an asthma episode or attack. During an asthma attack, muscles around the airways tighten up, making the airways narrower so less air flows through. Inflammation increases, and the airways become more swollen and even narrower. Cells in the airways may also make more mucus than usual. This extra mucus also narrows the airways. These changes make it harder to breathe.

Asthma attacks are not all the same—some are worse than others. In a severe asthma attack, the airways can close so much that not enough oxygen gets to vital organs. This condition is a medical emergency. People can die from severe asthma attacks.

So, if you have asthma, you should see your doctor regularly. You will need to learn what things cause your asthma symptoms and how to avoid them. Your doctor will also prescribe medicines to keep your asthma under control.

Taking care of your asthma is an important part of your life. Controlling it means working closely with your doctor to learn what to do, staying away from things that bother your airways, taking medicines as directed by your doctor, and monitoring your asthma so that you can respond quickly to signs of an attack. By controlling your asthma every day, you can prevent serious symptoms and take part in all activities.

If your asthma is not well controlled, you are likely to have symptoms that can make you miss school or work and keep you from doing things you enjoy. Asthma is one of the leading causes of children missing school.

What Causes Asthma?

It is not clear exactly what makes the airways of people with asthma inflamed in the first place. Your inflamed airways may be due to a combination of things. We know that if other people in your family have asthma, you are more likely to develop it. New research suggests that being exposed to things like tobacco smoke, infections, and some allergens early in your life may increase your chances of developing asthma.

What Causes Asthma Symptoms and Attacks?

There are things in the environment that bring on your asthma symptoms and lead to asthma attacks. Some of the more common things include exercise, allergens, irritants, and viral infections. Some people have asthma only when they exercise or have a viral infection.

The list below gives some examples of things that can bring on asthma symptoms.

Allergens:

- Animal dander (from the skin, hair, or feathers of animals);
- Dust mites (contained in house dust);
- Cockroaches;
- Pollen from trees and grass;
- Mold (indoor and outdoor).

Irritants:

- Cigarette smoke;
- Air pollution;
- Cold air or changes in weather;
- Strong odors from painting or cooking;

- Scented products;
- Strong emotional expression (including crying or laughing hard) and stress.

Others:

- Medicines such as aspirin and beta-blockers;
- Sulfites in food (dried fruit) or beverages (wine);
- A condition called gastroesophageal reflux disease that causes heartburn and can worsen asthma symptoms, especially at night;
- Irritants or allergens that you may be exposed to at your work, such as special chemicals or dusts;
- Infections.

This is not a complete list of all the things that can bring on asthma symptoms. People can have trouble with one or more of these. It is important for you to learn which ones are problems for you. Your doctor can help you identify which things affect your asthma and ways to avoid them.

Who Is At Risk for Asthma?

In the United States, about twenty million people have been diagnosed with asthma; nearly nine million of them are children.

Asthma is closely linked to allergies. Most, but not all, people with asthma have allergies. Children with a family history of allergy and asthma are more likely to have asthma.

Although asthma affects people of all ages, it most often starts in childhood. More boys have asthma than girls, but in adulthood, more women have asthma than men.

Although asthma affects people of all races, African Americans are more likely than Caucasians to be hospitalized for asthma attacks and to die from asthma.

What Are the Signs and Symptoms of Asthma?

Common asthma symptoms include the following:

- **Coughing:** Coughing from asthma is often worse at night or early in the morning, making it hard to sleep.

- **Wheezing:** Wheezing is a whistling or squeaky sound when you breathe.

- **Chest tightness:** This can feel like something is squeezing or sitting on your chest.

- **Shortness of breath:** Some people say they can't catch their breath, or they feel breathless or out of breath. You may feel like you can't get enough air in or out of your lungs.

- **Faster breathing or noisy breathing.**

Not all people have these symptoms, and symptoms may vary from one asthma attack to another. Symptoms can differ in how severe they are: Sometimes symptoms can be mildly annoying, other times they can be serious enough to make you stop what you are doing, and sometimes symptoms can be so serious that they are life threatening.

Symptoms also differ in how often they occur. Some people with asthma have symptoms only once every few months, others have symptoms every week, and still other people have symptoms every day. With proper treatment, however, most people with asthma can expect to have few or no symptoms.

How Is Asthma Diagnosed?

Some things your doctor will ask about include the following:

- Periods of coughing, wheezing, shortness of breath, or chest tightness that come on suddenly, occur often, or seem to happen during certain times of the year or season

- Colds that seem to "go to the chest" or take more than ten days to get over

- Medicines you may have used to help your breathing

- Your family history of asthma and allergies

- Things that seem to cause your symptoms or make them worse

Your doctor will listen to your breathing and look for signs of asthma or allergies.

Your doctor will probably use a device called a spirometer to check how your lungs are working. This test is called spirometry. The test measures how much air you can blow out of your lungs after taking a deep breath, and how fast you can do it. The results will be lower than normal if your airways are inflamed and narrowed, or if the muscles around your airways have tightened up.

As part of the test, your doctor may give you a medicine that helps open narrowed airways to see if the medicine changes or improves your test results.

Spirometry is also used to check your asthma over time to see how you are doing.

Spirometry usually cannot be used in children younger than five years. If your child is younger than five years, the doctor may decide to try medicine for a while to see if the child's symptoms get better.

If your spirometry results are normal but you have asthma symptoms, your doctor will probably want you to have other tests to see what else could be causing your symptoms.

These include the following:

- Allergy testing to find out if and what allergens affect you.

- A test in which you use a peak flow meter every day for one to two weeks to check your breathing. A peak flow meter is a hand-held device that helps you monitor how well you are breathing.

- A test to see how your airways react to exercise.

- Tests to see if you have gastroesophageal reflux disease.

- A test to see if you have sinus disease.

Other tests, such as a chest x-ray or an electrocardiogram, may be needed to find out if a foreign object or other lung diseases or heart disease could be causing your symptoms. A correct diagnosis is important because asthma is treated differently from other diseases with similar symptoms.

Depending on the results of your physical exam, medical history, and lung function tests, your doctor can determine how severe your asthma is. This is important because the severity of your asthma will determine how your asthma should be treated. One way for doctors to classify asthma severity is by considering how often you have symptoms when you are not taking any medicine or when your asthma is not well controlled.

Based on symptoms, the four levels of asthma severity are as follows:

- **Mild intermittent (comes and goes):** You have episodes of asthma symptoms twice a week or less, and you are bothered by symptoms at night twice a month or less; between episodes, however, you have no symptoms and your lung function is normal.

- **Mild persistent asthma:** You have asthma symptoms more than twice a week, but no more than once in a single day. You are bothered by symptoms at night more than twice a month. You may have asthma attacks that affect your activity.

- **Moderate persistent asthma:** You have asthma symptoms every day, and you are bothered by nighttime symptoms more than once a week. Asthma attacks may affect your activity.

- **Severe persistent asthma:** You have symptoms throughout the day on most days, and you are bothered by nighttime symptoms often. In severe asthma, your physical activity is likely to be limited.

Anyone with asthma can have a severe attack—even people who have intermittent or mild persistent asthma.

How Is Asthma Treated?

Your doctor can work with you to decide about your treatment goals and what you need to do to control your asthma to achieve these goals. Asthma treatment includes the following:

- Working closely with your doctor to decide what your treatment goals are and learning how to meet those goals.

- Avoiding things that bring on your asthma symptoms or make your symptoms worse. Doing so can reduce the amount of medicine you need to control your asthma.

- Using asthma medicines. Allergy medicine and shots may also help control asthma in some people.

- Monitoring your asthma so that you can recognize when your symptoms are getting worse and respond quickly to prevent or stop an asthma attack.

With proper treatment, you should ideally have these results:

- Your asthma should be controlled.
- You should be free of asthma symptoms.
- You should have fewer attacks.
- You should need to use quick-relief medicines less often.
- You should be able to do normal activities without having symptoms.

311

Your doctor will work with you to develop an asthma self-management plan for controlling your asthma on a daily basis and an emergency action plan for stopping asthma attacks. These plans will tell you what medicines you should take and other things you should do to keep your asthma under control.

Medicines for Asthma

There are two main types of medicines for asthma:

- **Quick-relief medicines:** Taken at the first signs of asthma symptoms for immediate relief of these symptoms. You will feel the effects of these medicines within minutes.

- **Long-term control medicines:** Taken every day, usually over long periods of time, to prevent symptoms and asthma episodes or attacks. You will feel the full effects of these medicines after taking them for a few weeks. People with persistent asthma need long-term control medicines.

Quick-Relief Medicines

Everyone with asthma needs a quick-relief or "rescue" medicine to stop asthma symptoms before they get worse. Short-acting inhaled beta-agonists are the preferred quick-relief medicine. These medicines are bronchodilators. They act quickly to relax tightened muscles around your airways so that the airways can open up and allow more air to flow through.

You should take your quick-relief medicine when you first begin to feel asthma symptoms, such as coughing, wheezing, chest tightness, or shortness of breath. You should carry your quick-relief inhaler with you at all times in case of an asthma attack.

Your doctor may recommend that you take your quick-relief medicines at other times as well—for example, before exercise.

Long-Term Control Medicines

The most effective, long-term control medicine for asthma is an inhaled corticosteroid because this medicine reduces the airway swelling that makes asthma attacks more likely.

Inhaled corticosteroids (or steroids for short) are the preferred medicine for controlling mild, moderate, and severe persistent asthma. They are generally safe when taken as directed by your doctor.

312

In some cases, steroid tablets or liquid are used for short periods of time to bring asthma under control. The tablet or liquid form may also be used to control severe asthma.

Other long-term control medicines include the following:

- **Inhaled long-acting beta-agonists:** These medicines are bronchodilators, or muscle relaxers, not anti-inflammatory drugs. They are used to help control moderate and severe asthma and to prevent nighttime symptoms. Long-acting beta-agonists are usually taken together with inhaled corticosteroid medicines.

- **Leukotriene modifiers (montelukast, zafirlukast, and zileuton):** These are used either alone to treat mild persistent asthma or together with inhaled corticosteroids to treat moderate or severe asthma.

- **Cromolyn and nedocromil:** These are used to treat mild persistent asthma.

- **Theophylline:** This is used either alone to treat mild persistent asthma or together with inhaled corticosteroids to treat moderate persistent asthma. People who take theophylline should have their blood levels checked to be sure the dose is appropriate.

If you stop taking long-term control medicines, your asthma will likely worsen again.

Many people with asthma need both a short-acting bronchodilator to use when symptoms worsen and long-term daily asthma control medicines to treat the ongoing inflammation.

Over time, your doctor may need to make changes in your asthma medicine. You may need to increase your dose, lower your dose, or try a combination of medicines. Be sure to work with your doctor to find the best treatment for your asthma. The goal is to use the least amount of medicine necessary to control your asthma.

Most asthma medicines are inhaled. They go directly into your lungs, where they are needed. There are many kinds of inhalers, and many require different techniques. It is important to know how to use your inhaler correctly.

Use a Peak Flow Meter

As part of your daily asthma self-management plan, your doctor may recommend that you use a hand-held device called a peak flow meter at home to monitor how well your lungs are working.

313

You use the peak flow meter by taking a deep breath in and then blowing the air out hard into the peak flow meter. The peak flow meter then gives you a peak flow number that tells you how fast you moved the air out.

You will need to find out your "personal best" peak flow number. You do this by recording your peak flow number every day for a few weeks until your asthma is under control. The highest number you get during that time is your personal best peak flow. Then you can compare future peak flow measurements to your personal best peak flow, and that will show if your asthma is staying under control.

Your doctor will tell you how and when to use your peak flow meter and how to use your medicines based on the results. You may be advised to use your peak flow meter each morning to keep track of how well you are breathing.

Your peak flow meter can help warn you of a possible asthma attack even before you notice symptoms. If your peak flow meter shows that your breathing is getting worse, you should follow your emergency asthma action plan. Take your quick-relief or other medicines as your doctor directed. Then you can use the peak flow meter to see how your airways are responding to the medicine.

Ask your doctor about how you can take care of your asthma. You should know all of the following:

- What things tend to make your asthma worse and how to avoid them

- Early signs to watch for that mean your asthma is starting to get worse (like a drop in your peak flow number or an increase in symptoms)

- How and when to use your peak flow meter

- What medicines to take, how much to take, when to take them, and how to take them correctly

- When to call or see your doctor

- When you should get emergency treatment

Treating Asthma in Children

Children with asthma, like adults with asthma, should see a doctor for treatment of their asthma. Treatment may include allergy testing, finding ways to limit contact with things that bring on asthma attacks, and taking medicine.

314

Young children will need help from their parents and other care-givers to keep their asthma under control. Older children can learn to care for themselves and follow their asthma self-management plan with less supervision.

Asthma medicines for children are like those adults use, but doses are smaller. Children with asthma may need both a quick-relief (or "rescue") inhaler for attacks and daily medicine to control their asthma. Children with moderate or severe asthma should learn to use a peak flow meter to help keep their asthma under control. Using a peak flow meter can be very helpful because children often have a hard time describing their symptoms.

Parents should be alert for possible signs of asthma in children, such as coughing at night, frequent colds, wheezing, or other signs of breathing problems. If you suspect that your child has asthma or that your child's asthma is not well controlled, take your child to a doctor for an exam and testing.

Your doctor will choose medicines for your child based on the child's symptoms and test results. If your child has asthma, you will need to go to the doctor for regular follow-up visits and to make sure that your child uses the medicines properly.

Treating Asthma in Older Adults

Older adults may need to adjust their asthma treatment because of other diseases or conditions that they have. Some medicines (like beta blockers used for treating high blood pressure and glaucoma; aspirin; and nonsteroidal anti-inflammatory drugs) can interfere with asthma medicines or even cause asthma attacks. Be sure to tell your doctor about all medicines that you take, including over-the-counter ones.

Using steroids may affect bone density in adults, so ask your doctor about taking calcium and vitamin D supplements and other ways to help keep your bones strong.

Treating Asthma in Pregnancy

If you are pregnant, it is very important to both you and your baby to control your asthma. Uncontrolled asthma can lower the oxygen level in your blood, which means that your baby gets less oxygen too.

Most asthma medicines are generally safe to take during pregnancy. Doctors recommend that it is safer to take asthma medicines during pregnancy than to take the chance that you will have an attack.

If you are pregnant or thinking about becoming pregnant, talk to your doctor about your asthma and how to have a healthy pregnancy.

Treating Exercise-Induced Asthma

Regular physical activity is important for good health. If exercise brings on your asthma symptoms, talk to your doctor about the best ways to control your asthma when you are active. Some people with asthma use inhaled, quick-relief medicines before exercising to keep symptoms under control.

If you use your asthma medicines as directed, you should be able to take part in any physical activity or sport you choose. Many Olympic athletes have asthma.

Can Asthma Be Prevented?

We don't yet know how to prevent asthma, but there are some things that can lower your chances of having an asthma attack.

To prevent asthma symptoms, do the following things:

- Learn about your asthma and how to control it.

- Use medicines as directed by your doctor to prevent or stop attacks.

- Avoid things that make your asthma worse as much as possible.

- Get regular checkups from your doctor.

- Follow your asthma self-management plan.

Scientists do not yet know how to prevent the inflammation of the airways that leads to asthma. Scientists are exploring some theories:

- Babies exposed to tobacco smoke are more likely to get asthma. If a woman is exposed to tobacco smoke during pregnancy, her baby may also be more likely to get asthma.

- Obesity may be linked to asthma, as well as other health problems.

Living with Asthma

If you have asthma, it is important to learn how to take care of yourself. Work with your doctor on a daily asthma self-management plan that you are both happy with:

- Tell your doctor about all other medications you are taking, in case one of them affects your asthma.

- Follow your asthma self-management plan and have regular checkups.

- Learn to use your medication correctly. Ask your doctor to teach you how to use your inhaler. This is very important. If you do not use your inhalers correctly, less medication will get into your airways.

- If you are having problems taking your asthma medicine, let your doctor know right away.

You need to know what things bring on your asthma symptoms. Then do what you can to avoid or limit contact with these things:

- If animal dander is a problem for you, keep your pet out of the house or at least out of your bedroom, or find it a new home.

- Do not smoke or allow smoking in your home.

- If pollen is a problem for you, stay indoors with the air conditioner on, if possible, when the pollen count is high.

- To control dust mites, wash your sheets, blankets, pillows, and stuffed toys once a week in hot water. You can get special dust proof covers for your mattress and pillows.

- If cold air bothers you, wear a scarf over your mouth and nose in the winter.

- If you have symptoms when you exercise or do routine physical activities like climbing stairs, work with your doctor to find ways to be active without having asthma symptoms. Physical activity is important.

- If you are allergic to sulfites, avoid foods (like dried fruit) or beverages (like wine) that contain them.

Be alert for warning signs of an asthma attack:

- Watch for symptoms (for example, coughing, wheezing, chest tightness, and difficulty breathing) and use your quick-relief medicine as directed by your doctor.

- Use your peak flow meter as directed to monitor your asthma.

If your asthma is not under control, there will be signs that you should not ignore. The following are some signs that your asthma is getting worse:

- You have asthma symptoms more often than usual.

- Your asthma symptoms are worse than they used to be.

- Your asthma symptoms are bothering you a lot at night and making you lose sleep.

- You are missing school or work because of your asthma.

- Your peak flow number is low or varies a lot from day to day.

- Your asthma medicines do not seem to be working very well anymore.

- You have to use your short-acting quick-relief, or "rescue," inhaler more often. (Using quick-relief medicine every day or using more than one inhaler a month is too much.)

- You have to go to the emergency room or doctor because of an asthma attack. You end up in the hospital because of your asthma.

If your asthma seems to be getting worse, see your doctor. You may need to change your medicines or do other things to get your asthma under control.

Helping Your Child Live with Asthma

Children with asthma need the help of parents, other caregivers, teachers, and health care professionals to keep their asthma under control.

You can help your child with asthma keep it under control. For example, you can do the following:

- Take your child to the doctor for regular checkups and treatment.

- Make sure your child has an asthma self-management plan and that you know how to follow it.

- Help your child learn about asthma and how to control it.

- Help your child learn what things cause his or her asthma symptoms and how to avoid them, if possible.

- Protect your child from tobacco smoke by not smoking and not allowing people to smoke in your home.

- Find ways to reduce your child's exposure to allergens that bring on asthma attacks, like pollen, dust mites, cockroaches, or animal dander.

- Make sure your child knows how to take asthma medicines correctly (if your child is old enough to use an inhaler without your help).

- Make sure that your child uses a peak flow meter to help monitor and control asthma.

- Encourage your child to take part in physical activity. Work together to keep his or her asthma under control. Your child can be active.

- Talk to your child's other caregivers, teachers, or coaches about his or her asthma; give them copies of your child's asthma self-management plan.

Section 20.2

Exercise-Induced Asthma

Everyone needs to exercise, even people with asthma! A strong healthy body is one of your best defenses against disease. But some people with asthma have "exercise-induced asthma" (EIA). But with proper medical prevention and management you should be able to walk, climb stairs, run, and participate in activities, sports, and exercise without experiencing symptoms. You don't have to let EIA keep you from leading an active life or from achieving your athletic dreams.

What Is Exercise-Induced Asthma?

Exercise is a common cause of asthma symptoms. This is usually called exercise-induced asthma (EIA) or exercise-induced broncho-spasm (EIB). It is estimated that 80 to 90 percent of all individuals who have allergic asthma will experience symptoms of EIA with vigorous exercise or activity. For teenagers and young adults this is often the most common cause of asthma symptoms. Fortunately with better medications, monitoring, and management you can participate in physical activity and sports and achieve your highest performance level.

What Are the Symptoms of EIA?

Symptoms of exercised-induced asthma include coughing, wheezing, chest tightness, and shortness of breath. Coughing is the most common symptom of EIA and may be the only symptom you have. The symptoms of EIA may begin during exercise and will usually be worse five to ten minutes after stopping exercise. Symptoms most often resolve in another twenty to thirty minutes and can range from mild to severe. Occasionally some individuals will experience "late phase" symptoms four to twelve hours after stopping exercise. Late-phase symptoms are frequently less severe and can take up to twenty-four hours to go away.

What Causes EIA?

When you exercise you breathe faster due to the increased oxygen demands of your body. Usually during exercise you inhale through your mouth, causing the air to be dryer and cooler than when you breathe through your nasal passages. The decreases in warmth and humidity are both causes of bronchospasm. Exercise that exposes you to cold air such as skiing or ice hockey is therefore more likely to cause symptoms than exercise involving warm and humid air such as swimming. Pollution levels, high pollen counts, and exposure to other irritants such as smoke and strong fumes can also make EIA symptoms worse. A recent cold or asthma episode can cause you to have more difficulty exercising.

How Is EIA Diagnosed?

It is important to know the difference between being out of condition and having exercise-induced asthma. A well-conditioned person will usually only experience the symptoms of EIA with vigorous activity or exercise. To make a diagnosis, your doctor will take a thorough history and may perform a series of tests. During these tests, which may include running or a treadmill test, your doctor will measure your lung functions using a spirometer before, during, and after exercise. Monitoring your peak flows before, during, and after exercise can also help you and your doctor detect narrowing of your airways. Then, using guidelines established by your doctor, you can help prevent asthma symptoms, participate in and enjoy physical activity. Your doctor will also tell you what to do should a full-blown episode occur.

Treatment and Management of EIA

With proper treatment and management people with EIA can participate safely and achieve their full potential. Proper management requires that you take steps to prevent symptoms and carefully monitor your respiratory status before, during, and after exercise. Taking medication prior to exercising is important in preventing EIA. Proper warm up for six to ten minutes before periods of exercise or vigorous activity will usually help. Individuals who can tolerate continuous exercise with minimal symptoms may find that proper warm up may prevent the need for repeated medications.

What Types of Medications Treat/Prevent EIA?

There are three types of medications to prevent or treat the symptoms of EIA. Your healthcare provider can help you determine the best treatment program for you based on your asthma condition and the type of activity or exercise.

The first medication is a short-acting beta$_2$-agonist, also called a bronchodilator. This medication can prevent symptoms and should be taken ten to fifteen minutes before exercise. It will help prevent symptoms for up to four hours. This same medication can also be used to treat and reverse the symptoms of EIA should they occur.

The second medication is a long-acting bronchodilator. It needs to be taken thirty to sixty minutes prior to activity and only once within a twelve-hour period. Salmeterol can help prevent EIA symptoms for ten to twelve hours. This medication should only be used to prevent symptoms and should never be used to relieve symptoms once they occur because it does not offer any quick relief.

The third type of medication is cromolyn or nedocromil. They also need to be taken fifteen to twenty minutes prior to exercise. There is also some evidence that taking these medications will also help to prevent the late-phase reaction of EIA that is experienced by some individuals. These medications also should only be used as a preventative measure because they do not relieve symptoms once they begin. Some individuals use one of these medications in combination with a short-acting bronchodilator.

If you have frequent symptoms with usual activity or exercise, talk to your doctor. An increase in your long-term control medications may help. Long term anti-inflammatory medications such as inhaled steroids can reduce the frequency and severity of EIA.

Teachers and coaches should be informed if a child has exercise-induced asthma. They should be told that the child should be able to participate in activities, but that they may require medication prior to activity. Athletes should also disclose their medications and adhere to standards set by the U.S. Olympic Committee. Approved and prohibited medications can be obtained from the committee hotline (800-233-0393).

What Types of Sports are Best for People with EIA?

Activities that involve only short bursts of exercise or intermittent periods of activity are usually better tolerated. Such sports include walking, volleyball, basketball, and gymnastics or baseball. Swimming that involves breathing warm and moist air is often well tolerated. Aerobic sports such as distance running, soccer, or basketball are more likely to cause symptoms. In addition, cold air sports such as ice hockey or ice-skating may not be tolerated as well.

It is important to consult with your healthcare provider prior to beginning any exercise program and to pace yourself. With effective management people with EIA can perform and excel in a variety of sports. Many Olympic athletes and professional athletes with exercise-induced asthma have excelled in their sports, many winning Olympic gold medals.

Remember, with proper medical management you should be able to walk, climb stairs, run, and participate in activities, sports, and exercise without experiencing symptoms. Do not let EIA keep you from leading an active life or from achieving your athletic dreams.

Section 20.3

Bronchiectasis

Reprinted from National Heart Lung and Blood Institute,
National Institutes of Health, January 2006.

What Is Bronchiectasis?

Bronchiectasis is a lung disease that usually results from an infection or other condition that injures the walls of the airways in your lungs. The airways are the tubes that carry air in and out of your lungs.

This injury is the beginning of a cycle in which your airways slowly lose their ability to clear out mucus. The mucus builds up and creates an environment in which bacteria can grow. This leads to repeated serious lung infections. Each infection causes more damage to your airways.

Over time, your airways become stretched out, flabby, and scarred. They can no longer move air in and out.

This can affect how much oxygen reaches your body organs. If your lungs cannot move enough oxygen into your body, bronchiectasis can lead to serious illness, including heart failure.

Bronchiectasis can affect just one section of one of your lungs or many sections of both lungs.

Bronchiectasis usually begins in childhood, but symptoms may not appear until months or even years after you have started having repeated lung infections.

There are two types of bronchiectasis:

- Congenital bronchiectasis usually affects infants and children. It results from a problem in the development of the lungs in the fetus.

- Acquired bronchiectasis occurs in adults and older children. It is more common.

Bronchiectasis cannot be cured, but with proper care, most people who have it can enjoy a good quality of life.

What Causes Bronchiectasis?

Bronchiectasis is caused by injury to the lower airways. This injury may be caused by another disease, including any of the following:

- Cystic fibrosis, which leads to almost half of the cases of bronchiectasis in the United States.

- Severe pneumonia.

- Whooping cough (uncommon because most people are now vaccinated against it).

- Tuberculosis (TB) and other similar infections.

- Immunodeficiency disorders, such as human immunodeficiency virus (HIV) infection and acquired immunodeficiency syndrome (AIDS).

- Allergic bronchopulmonary aspergillosis, an allergic reaction to a fungus called *Aspergillus* that causes swelling in the airways.

- Kartagener syndrome, a rare inherited disease that involves the cilia. These are small hairlike structures that line your airways and normally clear out mucus.

- Other disorders that affect the function of the cilia.

Other conditions that can injure the lower airways and lead to bronchiectasis include the following:

- Blockage of your airways by a growth or a noncancerous tumor

- Blockage of your airways by something you inhaled—for example, a piece of a toy or a peanut that you inhaled when you were a child

- Fungal infections

What Are the Signs and Symptoms of Bronchiectasis?

The most common signs and symptoms are as follows:

- Daily cough, over months or years
- Daily production of large amounts of mucus, or phlegm
- Repeated lung infections
- Shortness of breath

- Wheezing
- Chest pain (pleurisy)

Over time, you may have more serious symptoms, including coughing up blood or bloody mucus, weight loss, fatigue, or sinus drainage.

Bronchiectasis can also lead to other serious health conditions, including collapsed lung, heart failure (if the disease advances to affect all parts of your airways), or brain abscess.

How Is Bronchiectasis Diagnosed?

There is no one specific test for bronchiectasis. Even in its later stages, the signs of the disease are similar to those of other conditions, so those conditions must be ruled out before a diagnosis can be made.

Your doctor may suspect bronchiectasis if you have a daily cough that produces large amounts of mucus.

Your doctor will determine if you have bronchiectasis by conducting a series of tests to identify any underlying causes that need to be treated, rule out other causes of your symptoms, and determine the amount of damage to your lungs.

The most commonly used tests to diagnose bronchiectasis are as follows:

- **Chest x-ray:** A chest x-ray takes a picture of your heart and lungs. It can show infection and scarring of your airway walls.

- **Computed tomography (CT) scan:** This test provides a computer-generated image of your airways and other tissue in your lungs. It has more detail than a regular chest x-ray. A CT scan is the defining test for bronchiectasis. It can show how much damage has been done to the airways and where the damage is.

Other tests your doctor may conduct include the following:

- **Blood tests:** These tests can show if you have a disease or condition that can lead to bronchiectasis. They can also show if you have an infection or low levels of certain infection-fighting blood cells.

- **Sputum culture:** Sputum contains mucus and often pus, blood, or bacteria. Laboratory tests of a sample of your sputum can show if you have bacteria, fungi, or tuberculosis.

- **Lung function tests:** These tests measure how well your lungs move air in and out. These tests show how much lung damage you have.

- **Sweat test or other tests for cystic fibrosis:** This is a patch test on your arm that measures the amount of salt (sodium chloride) in your sweat.

If your condition does not respond to treatment, your doctor may request a fiberoptic bronchoscopy. In this procedure, your doctor inserts a long, narrow, flexible tube with a light on the end through your nose or mouth into your airways. This tube is called a bronchoscope. It provides a video image of the airways and allows your doctor to collect samples of mucus. This test can show if something is blocking your lungs. You most likely would have this procedure as an outpatient in a hospital, under local anesthesia.

How Is Bronchiectasis Treated?

The goals of treatment are to treat any underlying conditions and respiratory infections, help remove mucus from your lungs, and prevent complications.

Early diagnosis and treatment of bronchiectasis are important. The sooner your doctor can start treating any underlying conditions that may be causing the bronchiectasis, the better the chances of preventing further damage to your lungs.

The mainstays of treatment for bronchiectasis are medications, especially antibiotics and chest physical therapy (CPT).

Medications

The main medicines used to treat bronchiectasis are as follows:

- Antibiotics are the main treatment for the repeated respiratory infections that bronchiectasis causes. Doctors usually prescribe oral antibiotics to treat these infections. For hard-to-treat infections, you may be given antibiotics through a tube into a vein in your arm. Your doctor may be able to help you arrange for a home care provider to give you intravenous antibiotics at home.

- Bronchodilators open your airways by relaxing the muscles around them. Inhaled bronchodilators can be breathed in as a fine mist from a metered-dose inhaler (puffer) or a nebulizer.

These medicines work quickly because the drug goes directly into your lungs. Doctors usually recommend that you use a broncho-dilator right before you do your chest physical therapy.

- Corticosteroids help reduce inflammation in your lungs. They work best when you take them with an inhaler.

- Mucus thinners, such as acetylcysteine, loosen the mucus.

- Expectorants help loosen the mucus in your lungs. They often come in combination with decongestants, which may provide additional relief. You do not need a prescription for them.

- Saline nasal washes help control sinusitis.

Chest Physical Therapy

CPT is also called chest clapping or percussion. It involves pounding your chest and back over and over with your hands or a device to loosen the mucus from your lungs so that you can cough it up. You should do CPT for bronchiectasis three or four times each day.

CPT is often called postural drainage. This means that you sit or lie on your stomach with your head down while you do CPT. This lets gravity and force help drain the mucus from your lungs.

Some people find CPT difficult or uncomfortable to do. Several devices have been developed that may help with CPT. The devices include the following:

- An electric chest clapper, known as a mechanical percussor.

- A removable inflatable therapy vest that uses high-frequency air waves to force the mucus that is deep in your lungs toward the upper airways so you can cough it up.

- A "flutter" device, a small handheld device that you breathe out through. It causes vibrations that dislodge the mucus.

- A positive expiratory pressure mask that creates vibrations that help break the mucus loose from the airway walls.

Several breathing techniques may also help loosen some of the mucus so you can cough it up:

- **Forced expiration technique (FET):** Forcing out a couple of breaths or huffs and then doing relaxed breathing

- **Active cycle breathing (ACB):** FET with deep breathing exercises that can loosen the mucus in your lungs

Depending on how serious your condition is, your doctor may also recommend oxygen therapy or surgery to remove a section of your lung.

Doctors usually do surgery only if other treatments have not helped and only one part of your lung is affected. If you have major bleeding, your doctor may recommend either surgery to remove the bleeding part of your lung or a procedure to control the bleeding.

Living with Bronchiectasis

If you have bronchiectasis, you should work closely with your doctor to develop self-management skills that can improve your quality of life. This means that you need to learn as much as you can about bronchiectasis and any underlying conditions that you have.

Avoiding respiratory infections should be a top priority. To do this:

- Have annual flu vaccinations;
- Have pneumonia vaccinations as directed by your doctor;
- Get regular aerobic exercise (walking and swimming, for example) to help loosen the mucus so it can be coughed up;
- Eat a healthy diet;
- Drink lots of fluids;
- Wash your hands often;
- Maintain a healthy weight.

Other things you can do to improve your condition include the following:

- Do not smoke.
- Avoid exposure to tobacco smoke.
- Avoid fumes and dust that can irritate your lungs.

Section 20.4

Chronic Bronchitis

What Is Chronic Bronchitis?

Chronic bronchitis is a disease of the lung. The lungs consist of a series of folded membranes (the alveoli), which are located at the ends of very fine branching air passages (bronchioles).

Chronic bronchitis is a persisting infection and inflammation of the larger airways of the lungs—the bronchi. There are two main bronchi in the lungs (the right and left), which divide from the trachea. Chronic bronchitis occurs as part of the disease complex known as chronic obstructive pulmonary disease (COPD), which also includes emphysema and small airways disease. Chronic bronchitis specifically refers to chronic cough and daily mucus production for at least three months of two or more consecutive years. Other causes of chronic cough must be excluded before making the diagnosis.

Predisposing Factors

Chronic bronchitis can affect both males and females of all ages but it tends to be most common in middle-aged males. The following predisposing factors have been identified:

- **Cigarette smoke:** This is by far the most important factor in the development of chronic bronchitis. The disease is four to ten times more common in heavy smokers regardless of age, sex, occupation, and place of dwelling. There is a direct relationship between intensity of smoking and reductions in lung function and mortality from disease. Those who smoke thirty cigarettes per day are twenty times more likely to die from chronic bronchitis and COPD than nonsmokers.

- **Pollution:** Nonsmokers exposed to heavy atmospheric pollution may occasionally develop chronic bronchitis. This results due to irritation of the airways from inhalation of toxins and fumes.

- **Family history:** There is some role of family history in the development of COPD and chronic bronchitis.

- **Airway infections:** Although infection is not considered responsible for the initiation of chronic bronchitis, it is important factor in maintaining disease and causing exacerbations.

Progression

Early on in chronic bronchitis you usually will have symptoms of cough productive of significant amounts of sputum without any significant breathlessness. The excess mucus production is caused by enlargement of mucous glands and increased numbers of mucus-secreting goblet cells in the airways. The small airways themselves then become inflamed but at this stage the disease is considered largely reversible. Cessation of smoking will resolve the airway inflammation.

As the disease progresses there is progressive abnormal cell growth (called squamous metaplasia) and fibrosis (hardening) of the bronchial walls. This causes airflow limitation and symptoms of shortness of breath. Symptoms of breathlessness are usually present on exertion. You may develop other signs of COPD, such as cyanosis (bluish discoloration of the lips and skin). Emphysema may also be present at this stage, causing more severe shortness of breath and chest tightness.

If your chronic bronchitis remains severe some other complications can develop, including:

- **Secondary polycythemia:** This is an increase in the number of red blood cells in the blood to try to compensate for reduced oxygen levels. The blood subsequently becomes "thicker" with sluggish flow, which can lead to clotting.

- **Right heart failure.**

- **Pneumothorax (punctured lung).**

- **Respiratory failure:** This is often caused by acute infective exacerbations. Death can sometimes occur from severe declines in respiratory function.

Probable Outcomes

Chronic bronchitis itself does not cause an increase in mortality unless there is an associated decline in lung function. Your overall prognosis therefore depends on:

- Whether you continue to smoke: stopping smoking will improve symptoms in 90 percent of patients. Even if you have severe disease, studies have shown that stopping smoking increases survival.

- Your current lung function.

- Presence of other complications such as heart failure and respiratory failure.

- Frequency of exacerbations.

Chronic bronchitis with severe breathlessness carries a poor prognosis with approximately 50 percent of patients dying by five years. Death is usually caused by a decline in lung function from infective exacerbations.

How Will It Affect Me?

Chronic bronchitis is defined clinically as cough productive of sputum for at least three months a year over two consecutive years. If airway limitation is also present you may experience symptoms of wheezing, chest tightness, and breathlessness. Your doctor will ask you lots of questions about your symptoms including when they started, their duration, and any triggering factors. Symptoms may be worsened by factors such as cold, foggy weather and atmospheric pollution. In addition your doctor will take a detailed medical history and family history to exclude other causes of cough and sputum production. Smoking history is essential as this is the major cause of chronic bronchitis.

It can be difficult to distinguish symptoms of chronic bronchitis from emphysema and both conditions commonly occur together. Therefore if you have cough and breathlessness your doctor may diagnose COPD, rather than chronic bronchitis alone.

Clinical Examination

Your doctor will perform a detailed examination of your respiratory system. This will include undressing your top, inspecting your chest, measuring your chest expansion, and listening to your breath sounds. Important signs your doctor will be looking for include:

- Productive cough.
- Cyanosis (bluish discoloration).
- Tachypnea: An increased respiratory rate.
- Use of accessory muscles.
- Hyper-expansion of the chest: In advanced disease the chest wall can become barrel shaped.
- Reduced chest expansion.
- Reduced breath sounds, wheeze, and crackles.
- Signs of heart failure such as peripheral edema (swelling) may be present in advanced disease.

Patients with chronic bronchitis are classically described as "blue bloaters" due to the presence of cyanosis and edema. They have reduced levels of ventilation and are not very breathless. There are low levels of oxygen in the blood and high levels of carbon dioxide, which can cause other signs such as bounding pulse, asterixis (flapping of the hands), and in severe cases, confusion and progressive drowsiness. Patients with predominantly emphysema on the other hand are described as "pink puffers," as they are very breathless and hyperventilating (with pursed lips) but have near normal levels of oxygen and carbon dioxide in the blood. However, these clinical signs aren't always reliable and do not always correlate with pathology.

How Is It Diagnosed?

Your doctor may perform a number of tests to confirm the diagnosis of chronic bronchitis and to detect the associated airway limitation. Tests may include:

- **Blood tests:** Specifically looking at the concentration of red blood cells which may be increased due to the chronic lack of oxygen in the body.
- **Chest x-ray:** This helps to show hyper-expansion of the lungs associated with chronic bronchitis and COPD. The lung fields will look enlarged and empty and may flatten out the diaphragm.
- **Electrocardiogram (ECG):** This can detect signs of right heart failure (a complication of chronic bronchitis and COPD).

- **Pulmonary/lung function tests:** Spirometry is the best test to detect airflow limitation and obstruction. Unlike asthma, the airflow limitation is not reversible.

- **Blood gases:** These may also be normal but in the later stages of disease you may have low oxygen and high carbon dioxide levels.

- **High-resolution computerized tomography (CT) scan:** This is sometimes used in patients with COPD. It is best for detecting emphysema and bullae (big dilated air spaces).

How Is It Treated?

Chronic bronchitis should be treated if airway limitation is present. Treatment follows the same general principles as treatment of COPD. The majority of treatments only control and improve symptoms. Only smoking cessation and oxygen therapy (in those with advanced disease) actually alter the course of disease. Stopping smoking is the best thing you can do, as quitting smoking, regardless of the stage and severity of disease, will slow down the rate of progression and prolong life. Other treatments are outlined below.

Drug Therapy

Drugs can be used for long-term suppression of symptoms or for treatment of acute exacerbations. Bronchodilators (such as Ventolin®, Seretide®, and Atrovent® via puffer or nebulizer) and corticosteroids are used for symptom control. Your doctor will usually give you a trial of oral steroids to see if you respond before using long-term inhaled steroids. Antibiotics are taken for short-term exacerbations of disease. Your doctor may also prescribe agents to reduce the thickness of your sputum (called mucolytics, for example acetylcysteine). Studies have shown these agents may reduce the frequency of exacerbations.

Pulmonary Rehabilitation

Chest physiotherapy has been shown to help remove secretions in the airways. Various techniques are available which assist sputum removal and improve your ventilation for patients. Your doctor will also enter you into exercise or pulmonary rehabilitation programs, which have been shown to increase exercise tolerance, relieve symptoms, and improve quality of life.

Oxygen Therapy

If you have severe airflow limitation you may require home oxygen therapy, sometimes for up to nineteen hours per day. Oxygen can be administered via nasal prongs or mask. This treatment has been shown to prolong life in patients with severe COPD who have stopped smoking.

Other

Vaccinations: It is important that you have your yearly influenza vaccination, and pneumococcal vaccine. This will help reduce effective exacerbations from these agents.

Diuretics: If your chronic bronchitis is complicated by right heart failure, you may be treated with tablets to remove the excess fluid.

For more health information on chronic bronchitis and appropriate treatment for yourself, please consult your local doctor.

Section 20.5

Chronic Obstructive Pulmonary Disease

Reprinted from "COPD," National Heart Lung and Blood Institute, National Institutes of Health, July 2007.

What Is Chronic Obstructive Pulmonary Disease?

Chronic obstructive pulmonary disease (COPD) is a lung disease in which the lungs are damaged, making it hard to breathe. In COPD, the airways—the tubes that carry air in and out of your lungs—are partly obstructed, making it difficult to get air in and out.

Cigarette smoking is the most common cause of COPD. Most people with COPD are smokers or former smokers. Breathing in other kinds of lung irritants, like pollution, dust, or chemicals, over a long period of time may also cause or contribute to COPD.

The airways branch out like an upside-down tree, and at the end of each branch are many small, balloon-like air sacs called alveoli. In healthy people, each airway is clear and open. The air sacs are small and dainty, and both the airways and air sacs are elastic and springy. When you breathe in, each air sac fills up with air like a small balloon; when you breathe out, the balloon deflates and the air goes out. In COPD, the airways and air sacs lose their shape and become floppy. Less air gets in and less air goes out because:

- The airways and air sacs lose their elasticity (like an old rubber band);
- The walls between many of the air sacs are destroyed;
- The walls of the airways become thick and inflamed (swollen);
- Cells in the airways make more mucus (sputum) than usual, which tends to clog the airways.

COPD develops slowly, and it may be many years before you notice symptoms like feeling short of breath. Most of the time, COPD is diagnosed in middle-aged or older people.

COPD is a major cause of death and illness, and it is the fourth-leading cause of death in the United States and throughout the world.

There is no cure for COPD. The damage to your airways and lungs cannot be reversed, but there are things you can do to feel better and slow the damage.

COPD is not contagious—you cannot catch it from someone else.

How the Lungs Work

The lungs provide a very large surface area (the size of a football field) for the exchange of oxygen and carbon dioxide between the body and the environment.

A slice of normal lung looks like a pink sponge filled with tiny bubbles or holes. These bubbles, surrounded by a fine network of tiny blood vessels, give the lungs a large surface to exchange oxygen (into the blood, where it is carried throughout the body) and carbon dioxide (out of the blood). This process is called gas exchange. Healthy lungs do this very well.

Here is how normal breathing works:

- You breathe in air through your nose and mouth. The air travels down through your windpipe (trachea) then through large and small tubes in your lungs called bronchial tubes. The larger tubes are bronchi, and the smaller tubes are bronchioles. Sometimes the word "airways" is used to refer to the various tubes or passages that air must travel through from the nose and mouth into the lungs. The airways in your lungs look something like an upside-down tree with many branches.

• At the ends of the small bronchial tubes, there are groups of tiny air sacs called alveoli. The air sacs have very thin walls, and small blood vessels called capillaries run in the walls. Oxygen passes from the air sacs into the blood in these small blood vessels. At the same time, carbon dioxide passes from the blood into the air sacs. Carbon dioxide, a normal byproduct of the body's metabolism, must be removed.

The airways and air sacs in the lung are normally elastic—that is, they try to spring back to their original shape after being stretched or filled with air, just the way a new rubber band or balloon would. This elastic quality helps retain the normal structure of the lung and helps to move the air quickly in and out. In COPD, much of the elastic quality is gone, and the airways and air sacs no longer bounce back to their original shape. This means that the airways collapse, like a floppy hose, and the air sacs tend to stay inflated. The floppy airways obstruct the airflow out of the lungs, leading to an abnormal increase in the lungs' size. In addition, the airways may become inflamed and thickened, and mucus-producing cells produce more mucus, further contributing to the difficulty of getting air out of the lungs.

Other Names for COPD

COPD has two alternative names: chronic obstructive airway disease and chronic obstructive lung disease.

In the United States, chronic obstructive pulmonary disease (COPD) includes emphysema and chronic bronchitis.

In the emphysema type of COPD, the walls between many of the air sacs are destroyed, leading to a few large air sacs instead of many tiny ones. Consequently, the lung looks like a sponge with many large bubbles or holes in it, instead of a sponge with very tiny holes. The large air sacs have less surface area for the exchange of oxygen and carbon dioxide than healthy air sacs. Poor exchange of the oxygen and carbon dioxide causes shortness of breath.

In chronic bronchitis, the airways have become inflamed and thickened, and there is an increase in the number and size of mucus-producing cells. This results in excessive mucus production, which in turn contributes to cough and difficulty getting air in and out of the lungs.

Most people with COPD have both chronic bronchitis and emphysema.

What Causes COPD?

Most cases of chronic obstructive pulmonary disease (COPD) develop after repeatedly breathing in fumes and other things that irritate and damage the lungs and airways. Cigarette smoking is the most common irritant that causes COPD. Pipe, cigar, and other types of tobacco smoke can also cause COPD, especially if the smoke is inhaled. Breathing in other fumes and dusts over a long period of time may also cause COPD. The lungs and airways are highly sensitive to these irritants. They cause the airways to become inflamed and narrowed, and they destroy the elastic fibers that allow the lung to stretch and then return to its resting shape. This makes breathing air in and out of the lungs more difficult.

Other things that may irritate the lungs and contribute to COPD include the following:

- Working around certain kinds of chemicals and breathing in the fumes for many years

- Working in a dusty area over many years

- Heavy exposure to air pollution

Being around secondhand smoke (smoke in the air from other people smoking cigarettes) also plays a role in an individual developing COPD.

Genes—tiny bits of information in your body cells passed on by your parents—may play a role in developing COPD. In rare cases, COPD is caused by a gene-related disorder called alpha 1 antitrypsin deficiency. Alpha 1 antitrypsin is a protein in your blood that inactivates destructive proteins. People with antitrypsin deficiency have low levels of alpha 1 antitrypsin; the imbalance of proteins leads to the destruction of the lungs and COPD. If people with this condition smoke, the disease progresses more rapidly.

Who Is at Risk for COPD?

Most people with chronic obstructive pulmonary disease (COPD) are smokers or were smokers in the past. People with a family history of COPD are more likely to get the disease if they smoke. The chance of developing COPD is also greater in people who have spent many years in contact with lung irritants, such as air pollution or chemical fumes, vapors, and dusts usually linked to certain jobs.

A person who has had frequent and severe lung infections, especially during childhood, may have a greater chance of developing lung damage that can lead to COPD. Fortunately, this is much less common today with antibiotic treatments.

Most people with COPD are at least forty years old or around middle age when symptoms start. It is unusual, but possible, for people younger than forty years of age to have COPD.

What Are the Signs and Symptoms of COPD?

The signs and symptoms of chronic obstructive pulmonary disease (COPD) include the following:

• Cough

• Sputum (mucus) production

• Shortness of breath, especially with exercise

• Wheezing (a whistling or squeaky sound when you breathe)

• Chest tightness

A cough that doesn't go away and coughing up lots of mucus are common signs of COPD. These often occur years before the flow of air in and out of the lungs is reduced. However, not everyone with a cough and sputum production goes on to develop COPD, and not everyone with COPD has a cough.

The severity of the symptoms depends on how much of the lung has been destroyed. If you continue to smoke, the lung destruction is faster than if you stop smoking.

How Is COPD Diagnosed?

Doctors consider a diagnosis of chronic obstructive pulmonary disease (COPD) if you have the typical symptoms and a history of exposure to lung irritants, especially cigarette smoking. A medical history, physical exam, and breathing tests are the most important tests to determine if you have COPD.

Your doctor will examine you and listen to your lungs. Your doctor will also ask you questions about your family and medical history and what lung irritants you may have been around for long periods of time.

Breathing Tests

Your doctor will use a breathing test called spirometry to confirm a diagnosis of COPD. This test is easy and painless and shows how well your lungs work. You breathe hard into a large hose connected to a machine called a spirometer. When you breathe out, the spirometer measures how much air your lungs can hold and how fast you can blow air out of your lungs after taking a deep breath.

Spirometry is the most sensitive and commonly used test of lung functions. It can detect COPD long before you have significant symptoms.

Based on this test, your doctor can determine if you have COPD and how severe it is. Doctors use the following classifications to describe the severity of COPD:

- **At risk (for developing COPD):** Breathing test is normal. Mild signs that include a chronic cough and sputum production.

- **Mild COPD:** Breathing test shows mild airflow limitation. Signs may include a chronic cough and sputum production. At this stage, you may not be aware that airflow in your lungs is reduced.

- **Moderate COPD:** Breathing test shows a worsening airflow limitation. Usually the signs have increased. Shortness of breath usually develops when working hard, walking fast, or doing other brisk activities. At this stage, a person usually seeks medical attention.

- **Severe COPD:** Breathing test shows severe airflow limitation. A person is short of breath after just a little activity. In very severe COPD, complications like respiratory failure or signs of heart failure may develop. At this stage, the quality of life is greatly impaired and the worsening symptoms may be life threatening.

Your doctor may also recommend tests to rule out other causes of your signs and symptoms. These tests include the following:

- **Bronchodilator reversibility testing:** This test uses the spirometer and medicines called bronchodilators. Bronchodilators work by relaxing tightened muscles around the airways and opening up airways quickly to ease breathing. Your doctor will use the results of this test to see if your lung problems are being caused by another lung condition such as asthma. However, since airways in COPD may also be constricted, your doctor can use the results of this test to help set your treatment goals.

- **Other pulmonary function testing:** For instance, your doctor could test diffusion capacity.

- **Chest x-ray:** A chest x-ray is a picture of your lungs. A chest x-ray may be done to see if another disease, like heart failure, may be causing your symptoms.

- **Arterial blood gas:** This is a blood test that shows the oxygen level in your blood. It is measured in people with severe COPD to see if oxygen treatment is recommended.

How Is COPD Treated?

Quitting smoking is the single most important thing you can do to reduce your risk of developing chronic obstructive pulmonary disease (COPD) and slow the progress of the disease.

Your doctor will recommend treatments that help relieve your symptoms and help you breathe easier. However, COPD cannot be cured.

The goals of COPD treatment are as follows:

- To relieve your symptoms with no or minimal side effects of treatment

- To slow the progress of the disease

- To improve exercise tolerance (your ability to stay active)

- To prevent and treat complications and sudden onset of problems

- To improve your overall health

The treatment for COPD is different for each person. Your family doctor may recommend that you see a lung specialist called a pulmonologist.

Treatment is based on whether your symptoms are mild, moderate, or severe.

Medicines and pulmonary rehabilitation (rehab) are often used to help relieve your symptoms and to help you breathe more easily and stay active.

COPD Medicines

Bronchodilators: Your doctor may recommend medicines called bronchodilators that work by relaxing the muscles around your airways. This type of medicine helps to open your airways quickly and make breathing easier. Bronchodilators can be either short acting or long acting:

- Short-acting bronchodilators last about four to six hours and are used only when needed.

- Long-acting bronchodilators last about twelve hours or more and are used every day.

Most bronchodilator medicines are inhaled, so they go directly into your lungs, where they are needed. There are many kinds of inhalers, and it is important to know how to use your inhaler correctly.

If you have mild COPD, your doctor may recommend that you use a short-acting bronchodilator. You then will use the inhaler only when needed.

If you have moderate or severe COPD, your doctor may recommend regular treatment with one or more inhaled bronchodilators. You may be told to use one long-acting bronchodilator. Some people may need to use a long-acting bronchodilator and a short-acting bronchodilator. This is called combination therapy.

Inhaled glucocorticosteroids (steroids): Inhaled steroids are used for some people with moderate or severe COPD. Inhaled steroids work to reduce airway inflammation. Your doctor may recommend that you try inhaled steroids for a trial period of six weeks to three months to see if the medicine is helping with your breathing problems.

Flu shots: The flu (influenza) can cause serious problems in people with COPD. Flu shots can reduce the chance of getting the flu. You should get a flu shot every year.

Pneumococcal vaccine: This vaccine should be administered to those with COPD to prevent a common cause of pneumonia. Revaccination may be necessary after five years in those older than sixty-five years of age.

Pulmonary Rehabilitation

Pulmonary rehabilitation (rehab) is a coordinated program of exercise, disease management training, and counseling that can help you stay more active and carry out your day-to-day activities. What is included in your pulmonary rehab program will depend on what you and your doctor think you need. It may include exercise training, nutrition advice, education about your disease and how to manage it, and counseling. The different parts of the rehab program are managed by different types of health care professionals (doctors, nurses, physical therapists, respiratory therapists, exercise specialists, dietitians) who work together to develop a program just for you. Pulmonary rehab programs can include some or all of the following aspects.

Medical evaluation and management: To decide what you need in your pulmonary rehab program, a medical evaluation will be done. This may include getting information on your health history and what medicines you take, doing a physical exam, and learning about your symptoms. A spirometry measurement may also be done before and after you take a bronchodilator medicine.

Setting goals: You will work with your pulmonary rehab team to set goals for your program. These goals will look at the types of activities that you want to do. For example, you may want to take walks every day, do chores around the house, and visit with friends. These things will be worked on in your pulmonary rehab program.

Exercise training: Your program may include exercise training. This training includes showing you exercises to help your arms and legs get stronger. You may also learn breathing exercises that strengthen the muscles needed for breathing.

Education: Many pulmonary rehab programs have an educational component that helps you learn about your disease and symptoms, commonly used treatments, different techniques used to manage symptoms, and what you should expect from the program. The education may include meeting with (1) a dietitian to learn about your diet and healthy eating; (2) an occupational therapist to learn ways that are easier on your breathing to carry out your everyday activities; or (3) a respiratory therapist to learn about breathing techniques and how to do respiratory treatments.

Program results (outcomes): You will talk with your pulmonary rehab team at different times during your program to go over the goals that you set and see if you are meeting them. For example, if your goal is to walk every day for thirty minutes, you will talk to members of your pulmonary team and tell them how often you are walking and for how long. The team is interested in helping you reach your goals.

Oxygen Treatment

If you have severe COPD and low levels of oxygen in your blood, you are not getting enough oxygen on your own. Your doctor may recommend oxygen therapy to help with your shortness of breath. You may need extra oxygen all the time or some of the time. For some people with severe COPD, using extra oxygen for more than fifteen hours a day can help them:

• Do tasks or activities with less shortness of breath;

• Protect the heart and other organs from damage;

• Sleep more during the night and improve alertness during the day;

• Live longer.

Surgery

For some people with severe COPD, surgery may be recommended. Surgery is usually done for people who have:

• Severe symptoms;

• Not had improvement from taking medicines;

• A very hard time breathing most of the time.

The two types of surgeries considered in the treatment of severe COPD are as follows:

• **Bullectomy:** In this procedure, doctors remove one or more very large bullae from the lungs of people who have emphysema. Bullae are air spaces that are formed when the walls of the air sacs break. The air spaces can become so large that they interfere with breathing.

• **Lung volume reduction surgery (LVRS):** In this procedure, surgeons remove sections of damaged tissue from the lungs of patients with emphysema. A major National Heart Lung and Blood Institute study of LVRS recently showed that patients whose emphysema was mostly in the upper lobes of the lung and who had this surgery, along with medical treatment and pulmonary rehabilitation, were more likely to function better after two years than patients who received medical therapy only. They also did not have a greater chance of dying than the other patients. A small group of these patients who also had low exercise capacity after pulmonary rehabilitation but before surgery were also more likely to function better after LVRS than similar patients who received medical treatment only.

A lung transplant may be done for some people with very severe COPD. A transplant involves removing the lung of a person with COPD and replacing it with a healthy lung from a donor.

How Can COPD Be Prevented from Progressing?

If you smoke, the most important thing you can do to stop more damage to your lungs is to quit smoking. For information on how to quit smoking, visit the website of the U.S. Office of the Surgeon General. Many hospitals have smoking cessation programs or can refer you to one.

It is also important to stay away from people who are smoking and places where you know there will be smokers.

Staying away from other lung irritants such as pollution, dust, and certain cooking or heating fumes is also important. For example, you should stay in your house when the outside air quality is poor.

Managing Complications and Preventing Sudden Onset of Problems

People with chronic obstructive pulmonary disease (COPD) often have symptoms that suddenly get worse. When this happens, you have a much harder time catching your breath. You may also have chest tightness, more coughing, change in your sputum, and a fever. It is important to call your doctor if you have any of these signs or symptoms.

Your doctor will look at things that might be causing these signs and symptoms to suddenly worsen. Sometimes the signs and symptoms are caused by a lung infection. Your doctor may want you to take an antibiotic medicine that helps fight off the infection.

Your doctor may also recommend additional medicines to help with your breathing. These medicines include bronchodilators and glucocorticosteroids.

Your doctor may recommend that you spend time in the hospital if any of the following are true:

- You have a lot of difficulty catching your breath.
- You have a hard time talking.
- Your lips or fingernails turn blue or gray.

- You are not mentally alert.
- Your heartbeat is very fast.
- Home treatment of worsening symptoms doesn't help.

Living with COPD

Although there is no cure for chronic obstructive pulmonary disease (COPD), your symptoms can be managed, and damage to your lungs can be slowed. If you smoke, quitting is the most important thing you can do to help your lungs. Information is available on ways to help you quit smoking. You also need to try to stay away from people who are smoking or places where there is smoking.

It is important to keep the air in your home clean. Here are some things that may help you in your home:

- Keep smoke, fumes, and strong smells out of your home.
- If your home is painted or sprayed for insects, have it done when you can stay away from your home.
- Cook near an open door or window.
- If you heat with wood or kerosene, keep a door or window open.
- Keep your windows closed and stay at home when there is a lot of pollution or dust outside.

If you are taking medicines, take them as ordered and make sure you refill them so you do not run out.

See your doctor at least two times a year, even if you are feeling fine. Make sure you bring a list of medicines you are taking to your doctor visit.

Ask your doctor or nurse about getting a flu shot and pneumonia vaccination.

Keep your body strong by learning breathing exercises and walking and exercising regularly.

Eat healthy foods. Ask your family to help you buy and fix healthy foods. Eat lots of fruits and vegetables. Eat protein food like meat, fish, eggs, milk, and soy.

If your doctor has told you that you have severe COPD, there are some things that you can do to get the most out of each breath. Make your life as easy as possible at home by doing the following:

- Asking your friends and family for help.

- Doing things slowly.
- Doing things sitting down.
- Putting things you need in one place that is easy to reach.
- Finding very simple ways to cook, clean, and do other chores. Some people use a small table or cart with wheels to move things around. Using a pole or tongs with long handles can help you reach things.
- Keeping your clothes loose.
- Wearing clothes and shoes that are easy to put on and take off.
- Asking for help moving your things around in your house so that you will not need to climb stairs as often.
- Picking a place to sit that you can enjoy and visit with others.

If you are finding that it is becoming more difficult to catch your breath, your coughing has gotten worse, you are coughing up more mucus, or you have signs of infection (such as a fever and feeling poorly), you need to call your doctor right away. Your doctor may do a spirometry test, blood work, and a chest x-ray. Your doctor may also:

- Order antibiotics, which are medicines that help fight off infection;
- Change the type and dosage of the bronchodilator and glucocorticosteroid medicines you have been taking;
- Order oxygen or increase the amount of oxygen you are currently using.

It is helpful to have certain information on hand in case you need to go to the hospital or doctor right away. You should plan now to make sure you have the following:

- The phone numbers for the doctor, hospital, and people who can take you to the hospital or doctor
- Directions to the hospital and doctor's office
- A list of the medicines you are taking

When to Get Emergency Help

You should get emergency help if any of the following are true:

346

- You find that is hard to talk or walk.

- Your heart is beating very fast or irregularly.

- Your lips or fingernails are gray or blue.

- Your breathing is fast and hard, even when you are using your medicines.

Section 20.6

Cystic Fibrosis

Cystic fibrosis (CF) is a genetic disorder that particularly affects the lungs and digestive system and makes kids who have it more vulnerable to repeated lung infections. Now, thanks to high-tech medical advances in drug therapy and genetics, children born with CF can look forward to longer and more comfortable lives. In the last ten years, research into all aspects of CF has helped doctors to understand the illness better and to develop new therapies. Ongoing research may someday lead to a cure.

What Is Cystic Fibrosis?

Currently affecting more than thirty thousand children and young adults in the United States, cystic fibrosis makes kids sick by disrupting the normal function of epithelial cells—cells that make up the sweat glands in the skin and that also line passageways inside the lungs, liver, pancreas, and digestive and reproductive systems.

The inherited CF gene directs the body's epithelial cells to produce a defective form of a protein called CFTR (or cystic fibrosis transmembrane conductance regulator) found in cells that line the lungs, digestive tract, sweat glands, and genitourinary system. When the CFTR protein is defective, epithelial cells can't regulate the way chloride (part of the salt called sodium chloride) passes across cell membranes. This disrupts the essential balance of salt and water needed to maintain a normal thin coating of fluid and mucus inside the lungs, pancreas, and passageways in other organs. The mucus becomes thick, sticky, and hard to move.

Normally, mucus in the lungs traps germs, which are then cleared out of the lungs. But in CF, the thick, sticky mucus and the germs it has trapped remain in the lungs, which become infected.

In the pancreas, thick mucus blocks the channels that would normally carry important enzymes to the intestines to digest foods. When this happens, the body can't process or absorb nutrients properly, especially fats. Kids with CF have problems gaining weight, even with a normal diet and a good appetite.

A Family's Risk for CF

Humans have twenty-three pairs of chromosomes made of the inherited genetic chemical deoxyribonucleic acid (DNA). The CF gene is found on chromosome number 7. It takes two copies of a CF gene—one inherited from each parent—for a child to show symptoms of CF. People born with only one CF gene (inherited from only one parent) and one normal gene are CF carriers. CF carriers do not show CF symptoms themselves, but can pass the problem CF gene to their children. Scientists estimate that about twelve million Americans are currently CF carriers. If two CF carriers have a child, there is a one in four chance that the child will have CF.

Almost 1,400 different mutations of the CF gene can lead to cystic fibrosis (some mutations cause milder symptoms than others). About 70 percent of people with CF have the disease because they inherited the mutant gene Delta F508 from both of their parents. This can be detected by genetic testing, which can be done in kids both before and after birth and in adults thinking about starting or enlarging their families.

Of all ethnic groups, Caucasians have the highest inherited risk for CF, and Asian Americans have the lowest. In the United States today, about 1 of every 3,600 Caucasian children is born with CF. This compares with 1 of every 17,000 African Americans and only 1 of every 90,000 Asian Americans. Although the chances of inherited risk may vary, CF has been described in every geographic area of the world among every ethnic population.

Scientists don't know exactly why the CF gene evolved in humans, but they have some evidence to show that it helped to protect earlier generations from the bacteria that cause cholera, a severe intestinal infection.

How CF Affects Kids

The diagnosis of CF is being made earlier and earlier, usually in infancy. However, about 15 percent of those with CF are diagnosed later in life (even adulthood). Symptoms usually center around the lungs and digestive organs and can be more or less severe.

A few kids with CF begin having symptoms at birth. Some are born with a condition called meconium ileus. Although all newborns have meconium—the thick, dark, putty-like substance that usually passes from the rectum in the first few days of life—in CF, the meconium can be too thick and sticky to pass and can completely block the intestines.

More commonly, though, babies born with CF don't gain weight as expected. They fail to thrive in spite of a normal diet and a good appetite. In these children, mucus blocks the passageways of the pancreas and prevents pancreatic digestive juices from entering the intestines. Without these digestive juices, the intestines can't absorb fats and proteins completely, so nutrients pass out of the body unused rather than helping the body grow. Poor fat absorption makes the stools appear oily and bulky and increases the child's risk for deficiencies of the fat-soluble vitamins (vitamins A, D, E, and K). Unabsorbed fats may also cause excessive intestinal gas, an abnormally swollen belly, and abdominal pain or discomfort.

Because CF also affects epithelial cells in the skin's sweat glands, kids with CF may have a salty "frosting" on their skin or taste "salty" when their parents kiss them. They may also lose abnormally large amounts of body salt when they sweat on hot days.

Cystic fibrosis is the most common cause of pancreatic insufficiency in children, but a condition called Shwachman-Diamond syndrome (SDS) is the second most common cause. SDS is a genetic condition that causes a reduced ability to digest food because digestive enzymes don't work properly. Some of the symptoms of SDS are similar to those of CF, so it may be confused with cystic fibrosis. However, in children with SDS, the sweat test is normal.

Because CF produces thick mucus within the respiratory tract, a child with CF may suffer from nasal congestion, sinus problems, wheezing, and asthma-like symptoms. As CF symptoms progress, the child may develop a chronic cough that produces globs of thick, heavy, discolored mucus. They may also suffer from repeated lung infections.

As chronic infections reduce lung function, the ability to breathe often decreases. A person with CF may eventually begin to feel short of breath, even when resting. Despite aggressive medical therapy, lung disease develops in nearly all patients with CF and is a common cause of disability and shortened life span.

Identifying a Child with CF

By performing genetic tests during pregnancy, parents can now learn whether their unborn children may have CF. But even when genetic tests confirm CF, there's still no way to predict beforehand whether a specific child's CF symptoms will be severe or mild. Genetic testing can also be done on a child after birth, and can be performed on parents, siblings, and other relatives who are considering having a family.

After birth, the standard diagnostic test for CF is called the sweat test—an accurate, safe, and painless way to diagnose CF. In the sweat test, a small electric current is used to carry the chemical pilocarpine into the skin of the forearm. This stimulates sweat glands in the area to produce sweat. Over a period of thirty to sixty minutes, sweat is collected on filter paper or gauze and tested for chloride.

To diagnose CF, two sweat tests are generally performed in a lab accredited by the Cystic Fibrosis Foundation. A child must have a sweat chloride result of greater than 60 on two separate sweat tests to make the diagnosis of CF. Sweat test normal values for infants are lower.

Several other tests are standard parts of the routine care used to monitor a child's CF:

- Chest x-rays

- Blood tests to evaluate nutritional status

- Bacterial studies that confirm the growth of *Pseudomonas aeruginosa*, *Staphylococcus aureus*, or *Haemophilus influenza* bacteria in the lungs (these bacteria are common in CF but may not affect healthy people exposed to CF)

- Pulmonary function tests (PFTs) to measure the effects of CF on breathing (PFTs are done as soon as the child is old enough to be able to cooperate in the testing procedure; infant PFTs are currently being studied)

Treating Kids with CF

When kids are first diagnosed with CF, they may or may not have to spend some time in the hospital, depending on their condition. If they do, they'll have diagnostic tests, especially baseline measurements of their breathing (lung function) and a nutritional assessment. Before they leave, their doctors will make sure that their lungs are clear and that they've started a diet with digestive enzymes and vitamins that will help them to gain weight normally. Afterward, they'll probably see their doctor for follow-up visits at least once every one to three months.

The basic daily care program varies from child to child, but usually includes pulmonary therapy (treatments to maintain lung function) and nutritional therapy (a high-calorie, high-fat diet with vitamin supplements). Kids with CF can also take oral doses of pancreatic enzymes to help them digest food better. They may also occasionally need oral or inhaled antibiotics to treat lung infections and mucolytic medication (a mucus-thinning drug) to keep mucus fluid and flowing.

A new treatment for CF, which is still being researched, is an inhaled spray containing normal copies of the CF gene. These normal genes deliver the correct copy of the CF gene into the lungs of CF patients. Since 1993, more than one hundred CF patients have been treated with CF gene therapy, and test trials are underway in at least nine different U.S. medical centers and other centers around the world. Another new therapy, called protein repair therapy, aims at repairing the defective CFTR protein. Numerous medications, including a spice called curcumin, are also being tested.

Caring for a child with CF can be tough at times, but parents need not feel alone. Doctors can usually refer them to a local support group linked to the Cystic Fibrosis Foundation.

Section 20.7

Emphysema

What Is Emphysema?

Emphysema is a condition in which the walls between the alveoli or air sacs within the lung lose their ability to stretch and recoil. The air sacs become weakened and break. Elasticity of the lung tissue is lost, causing air to be trapped in the air sacs and impairing the exchange of oxygen and carbon dioxide. Also, the support of the airways is lost, allowing for airflow obstruction.

Symptoms of emphysema include shortness of breath, cough, and a limited exercise tolerance. Emphysema and chronic bronchitis frequently co-exist together to comprise chronic obstructive pulmonary disease (COPD). COPD does not include other obstructive lung diseases such as asthma.

What Causes Emphysema?

Cigarette smoking is by far the most common cause of emphysema. Smoking is responsible for approximately 80 to 90 percent of deaths due to COPD.[1]

In addition, it is estimated that one hundred thousand Americans living today were born with a deficiency of a "lung protector" protein known as alpha 1-antitrypsin (AAT). Another twenty-five million Americans carry a single deficient gene that could be passed on to their children.[2]

In the absence of AAT, an inherited form of emphysema called alpha 1-antitrypsin deficiency–related emphysema is almost inevitable. Symptoms of AAT deficiency emphysema usually begin between thirty-two and forty-one years of age. Smoking significantly increases the severity of emphysema in AAT-deficient individuals.

How Serious Is Emphysema?

Over 3.1 million Americans have been diagnosed with emphysema, of which 91 percent were forty-five years of age or older. Emphysema rarely occurs in those under forty-five.[3] Men tend to have higher rates of emphysema. In 2002 the emphysema prevalence rate was 52 percent higher in males compared to females.

Together with chronic bronchitis and other chronic lower respiratory diseases, excluding asthma, chronic obstructive pulmonary disease (COPD) is the fourth leading cause of death in the United States, claiming the lives of more than 120,000 Americans.[4]

How Does Emphysema Develop?

Emphysema begins with the destruction of air sacs (alveoli) in the lungs where oxygen from the air is exchanged for carbon dioxide in the blood. The walls of the air sacs are thin and fragile. Damage to the air sacs is irreversible and results in permanent "holes" in the tissues of the lower lungs.

As air sacs are destroyed, the lungs are able to transfer less and less oxygen to the bloodstream, causing shortness of breath. The lungs also lose their elasticity, which is important to keep airways open. The patient experiences great difficulty exhaling.

Emphysema doesn't develop suddenly. It comes on very gradually. Years of exposure to the irritation of cigarette smoke usually precede the development of emphysema.

A person may initially visit the doctor because he or she has begun to feel short of breath during activity or exercise. As the disease progresses, a brief walk can be enough to bring on difficulty in breathing. Some people may have had chronic bronchitis before developing emphysema.

Treatment for Emphysema

Doctors can help persons with emphysema live more comfortably with their disease. The goal of treatment is to provide relief of symptoms and prevent progression of the disease with a minimum of side effects. The doctor's advice and treatment may include:

- **Quitting smoking:** The single most important factor for maintaining healthy lungs.

- **Bronchodilator drugs (prescription drugs that relax and open air passages in the lungs):** May be prescribed to treat emphysema if there is a tendency toward airway constriction or tightening. These drugs may be inhaled as aerosol sprays or taken orally.

- **Antibiotics:** If you have a bacterial infection, such as pneumococcal pneumonia.

- **Steroids:** These may be used for relapses or "acute exacerbations."

- **Exercise:** Including breathing exercises to strengthen the muscles used in breathing as part of a pulmonary rehabilitation program to condition the rest of the body. (The term "pulmonary" refers to the lungs.)

- **Alpha 1-proteinase inhibitor (A1PI):** Only if a person has AAT deficiency-related emphysema. A1PI is not recommended for those who develop emphysema as a result of cigarette smoking or other environmental factors.

- **Lung transplantation:** A major procedure, which can be effective.

- **Lung volume reduction surgery:** A surgical procedure in which the most severely diseased portions of the lung are removed to allow the remaining lung and breathing muscles to work better. The short-term results are promising but those with severe forms are at higher risk of death. Recently, the Centers for Medicare and Medicaid Services (CMS) announced that they intend to cover LVRS for people with non-high-risk severe emphysema, who meet the criteria stated in the National Emphysema Treatment Trial (NETT). In addition, CMS has decided that LVRS is "reasonable and necessary" only for qualified patients that undergo therapy before and after the surgery. CMS is currently composing accreditation standards for LVRS facilities and will use these standards to determine where the surgery will be covered.[5]

Prevention of Emphysema

Continuing research is being done to find answers for many questions about emphysema, especially about the best ways to prevent the disease.

Researchers know that quitting smoking can prevent the occurrence and decrease the progression of emphysema. Other environmental controls can also help prevent the disease.

If an individual has emphysema, the doctor will work hard to prevent the disease from getting worse by keeping the patient healthy and clear of any infection. The patient can participate in this prevention effort by following these general health guidelines:

- Emphysema is a serious disease. It damages your lungs, and it can damage your heart. See your doctor at the first sign of symptoms.

- Don't smoke. The majority of those who get emphysema are smokers. Continued smoking makes emphysema worse, especially for those who have AAT deficiency, the inherited form of emphysema.

- Maintain overall good health habits, which include proper nutrition, adequate sleep, and regular exercise to build up your stamina and resistance to infections.

- Reduce your exposure to air pollution, which may aggravate symptoms of emphysema. Refer to radio or television weather reports or your local newspaper for information about air quality. On days when the ozone (smog) level is unhealthy, restrict your activity to early morning or evening. When pollution levels are dangerous, remain indoors and stay as comfortable as possible.

- Consult your doctor at the start of any cold or respiratory infection because infection can make your emphysema symptoms worse. Ask about getting vaccinated against influenza and pneumococcal pneumonia.

For more information on emphysema, please review the Chronic Bronchitis and Emphysema Morbidity and Mortality Trend Report in the Data and Statistics section of the American Lung Association website or call the American Lung Association at 800-LUNG-USA (800-586-4872).

Sources:

1. U.S. Department of Health and Human Services. *The Health Consequences of Smoking*. A Report of the Surgeon General, 2004.

2. Alpha1 Network. What is Alpha-1? www.alphaone.org

3. National Center for Health Statistics, *National Health Interview Survey*, 1997–2002. Information cited in: American Lung

Association, Epidemiology and Statistics Unit, *Trends in Chronic Bronchitis and Emphysema: Morbidity and Mortality,* April 2004.

4. National Vital Statistics System. Deaths: Final Data for 2002. October 2004.

5. Centers for Medicare and Medicaid Services. Decision Memo for Lung Volume Reduction Surgery (CAG00115R) www.cms .hhs.gov/mcd/viewdecisionmemo.asp?id=96.

Section 20.8

Interstitial Lung Disease and Pulmonary Fibrosis

What Is Interstitial Lung Disease?

Interstitial Lung Disease (ILD) is a general term that includes a variety of chronic lung disorders. When a person has ILD, the lung is affected in three ways. First, the lung tissue is damaged in some known or unknown way. Second, the walls of the air sacs in the lung become inflamed. Finally, scarring (or fibrosis) begins in the interstitium (or tissue between the air sacs), and the lung becomes stiff.

Breathlessness during exercise can be one of the first symptoms of these diseases. A dry cough also may be present. These are common symptoms that many people ignore. Someone with these symptoms may wait until they feel quite ill before going to the doctor.

People with different types of ILD may have the same kind of symptoms but their symptoms may vary in severity. Their chest x-rays may look alike. Further testing is usually recommended to identify the specific type of ILD a person has. Some ILDs have known causes and some (idiopathic) have unknown causes.

Why is It Called Interstitial Lung Disease?

The tissue between the air sacs of the lungs is called the interstitium. Interstitial lung disease is named after this tissue because this is the tissue affected by fibrosis (scarring). Interstitial lung disease is sometimes also known as "interstitial pulmonary fibrosis." The terms interstitial lung disease, pulmonary fibrosis, and interstitial pulmonary fibrosis are often used to describe the same condition.

Interstitial Lung Diseases Are Puzzling

The course of these diseases is unpredictable. If they progress, the lung tissue thickens and becomes stiff. The work of breathing then becomes more difficult and demanding. Some of the diseases improve with medication if treated when inflammation occurs. Some people may need oxygen therapy as part of their treatment.

The diseases may run a gradual course or a rapid course. People with ILD may notice variations in symptoms—from very mild to moderate to very severe. Their condition may remain the same for long periods of time or it may change quickly. It's important to stay in touch with your doctor and report any changes in symptoms. You and your doctor can work together to manage ILD.

Common Link in Interstitial Lung Disease

While the progress and symptoms of these diseases may vary from person to person, there is one common link between the many forms of ILD. They all begin with an inflammation. The inflammation may affect different parts of the lung, as explained below:

- **The walls of the bronchioles (small airways):** When inflammation involves the bronchioles, it is called bronchiolitis.

- **The walls and air spaces of the alveoli (air sacs):** When inflammation involves the alveoli, it is called alveolitis.

- **The small blood vessels (capillaries) of the lungs:** When inflammation involves the small blood vessels, it is called vasculitis.

Inflammation of these parts of the lung may heal or may lead to permanent scarring of the lung tissue. When scarring of the lung tissue takes place, the condition is called pulmonary fibrosis.

Fibrosis, or scarring of the lung tissue, results in permanent loss of that tissue's ability to transport oxygen. The level of disability that a person experiences depends on the amount of scarring of the tissue. This is because the air sacs, as well as the lung tissue between and surrounding the air sacs, and the lung capillaries, are destroyed by the formation of scar tissue. If this happens, your doctor may prescribe oxygen to help you breathe easier.

Known Causes of Pulmonary Fibrosis

Several causes of pulmonary fibrosis are known. They include:

- **Occupational and environmental exposures:** Many jobs—particularly those that involve mining or that expose workers to asbestos or metal dusts—can cause pulmonary fibrosis. Workers doing these kinds of jobs may inhale small particles (like silica dusts or asbestos fibers) that can damage the lungs, especially the small airways and air sacs, and cause scarring (fibrosis). Agricultural workers also can be affected. Some organic substances, such as moldy hay, cause an allergic reaction in the lung. This reaction is called farmer's lung and can cause pulmonary fibrosis. Other fumes found on farms are directly toxic to the lungs.

- **Sarcoidosis:** A disease characterized by the formation of granulomas (areas of inflammatory cells), which can attack any area of the body but most frequently affects the lungs.

- **Drugs:** Certain medicines may have the undesirable side effect of causing pulmonary fibrosis. Check with your doctor about the medicines you are taking and ask about any possible side effects.

- **Radiation:** Treatment for breast cancer.

- **Connective tissue or collagen diseases:** Such as rheumatoid arthritis and systemic sclerosis.

- **Genetic or familial:** This is not as common as the other causes listed.

Idiopathic Pulmonary Fibrosis (IPF)

When all known causes of interstitial lung disease have been ruled out, the condition is called "idiopathic" (of unknown origin) pulmonary fibrosis (IPF).

There are several theories as to what may cause IPF, including viral illness and allergic or environmental exposure (including tobacco smoke). These theories are still being researched. Bacteria and other microorganisms are not thought to be the cause of IPF.

There is also a familial form of the disease, known as familial idiopathic pulmonary fibrosis. Additional research is being done to determine whether there is a genetic tendency to develop the disease, as well as to determine other causes of IPF.

What Are the Symptoms of IPF?

Shortness of breath is the main symptom of idiopathic pulmonary fibrosis. Since this is a symptom of many types of lung disease, making the correct diagnosis may be difficult. The shortness of breath may first appear during exercise. The condition then may progress to the point where any exertion is impossible. If the disease progresses, the person with IPF eventually may be short of breath even at rest.

Other symptoms may include a dry cough (without sputum). When the disease is severe and prolonged, heart failure with swelling of the legs may occur.

How Is IPF Diagnosed?

A very careful patient history is an important tool for diagnosis. The history will include environmental and occupational factors, hobbies, legal and illegal drug use, arthritis, and risk factors for diseases that affect the immune system. A physical examination, chest x-ray, pulmonary function tests, and blood tests are important. These tests will help your doctor rule out other lung diseases and determine the extent of disease.

Bronchoalveolar lavage (BAL)—a test which permits removal and examination of cells from the lower respiratory tract—may be used to diagnose IPF: this test helps a doctor identify inflammation in lung tissue, and also helps exclude infections and malignancies (cancer) as a cause of a patient's symptoms. The test is done during bronchoscopy, a special examination of the lung.

Lung biopsy—either done during bronchoscopy or as a surgical procedure that removes a sample of lung tissue for your doctor to study—this procedure is usually required for diagnosis of IPF.

Diagnostic Tests That May Be Used to Identify Pulmonary Fibrosis or Interstitial Lung Disease

1. Blood tests

2. Pulmonary function tests

3. Chest x-ray

4. Computed tomography (CT) scan

5. Bronchoscopy

6. Bronchoalveolar lavage

7. Lung biopsy

What Is the Treatment for IPF?

Corticosteroids may be administered to treat the inflammation present in some people with IPF. The success of this treatment for many forms of pulmonary fibrosis is variable and is still being researched. Other drugs are occasionally added when it is clear that the steroids are not effective in reversing the disease.

Some doctors may use corticosteroids in combination with other drugs when the diagnosis is first established. Which drug treatment plan is effective, and how long to use the drugs, is the focus of current research.

Oxygen therapy may be prescribed for some people with IPF. The need for oxygen will be determined by your doctor and may depend on the severity of disease, as well as your activity level. Talk with you doctor if you think you may need oxygen or if you have concerns about oxygen.

Influenza vaccine and pneumococcal pneumonia vaccine are both recommended for people with IPF or any lung disease. These two shots may help prevent infection and keep you healthy.

Lung transplantation may offer hope for selected people with severe IPF and other lung diseases. Speak with your doctor about eligibility criteria for lung transplant recipients.

Rehabilitation and education programs may help some people with IPF. Local support groups have been of benefit for people with IPF and their family members and friends.

Research supported by the American Lung Association has contributed significantly to scientific progress in understanding and treating respiratory disorders.

Section 20.9

Sarcoidosis

Reprinted from National Heart Lung and Blood Institute,
National Institutes of Health, June 2007.

What Is Sarcoidosis?

Sarcoidosis involves inflammation that produces tiny lumps of cells in various organs in your body. The lumps are called granulomas because they look like grains of sugar or sand. They are very small and can be seen only with a microscope.

These tiny granulomas can grow and clump together, making many large and small groups of lumps. If many granulomas form in an organ, they can affect how the organ works. This can cause symptoms of sarcoidosis.

Sarcoidosis can occur in almost any part of your body, although it usually affects some organs more than others. It usually starts in one of two places: lungs or lymph nodes, especially the lymph nodes in your chest cavity.

Sarcoidosis also often affects your skin, eyes, and liver.

Less often, sarcoidosis affects your spleen, brain, nerves, heart, tear glands, salivary glands, bones, and joints.

Rarely, sarcoidosis affects other organs, including your thyroid gland, breasts, kidneys, and reproductive organs.

Sarcoidosis almost always occurs in more than one organ at a time.

Sarcoidosis has an active and a nonactive phase. In the active phase, the granulomas form and grow. In this phase, symptoms can develop, and scar tissue can form in the organs where the granulomas occur. In the nonactive phase, the inflammation goes down, and the granulomas stay the same size or shrink. But the scars may remain and cause symptoms.

The course of the disease varies greatly among people.

- In many people, sarcoidosis is mild. The inflammation that causes the granulomas may get better on its own. The granulomas may stop growing or shrink. Symptoms may go away within a few years.

- In some people, the inflammation remains but doesn't get worse. You may also have symptoms or flare-ups and need treatment every now and then.

- In other people, sarcoidosis slowly gets worse over the years and can cause permanent organ damage. Although treatment can help, sarcoidosis may leave scar tissue in the lungs, skin, eyes, or other organs. The scar tissue can affect how the organs work. Treatment usually does not affect scar tissue.

Changes in sarcoidosis usually occur slowly (e.g., over months). Sarcoidosis does not usually cause sudden illness. However, some symptoms may occur suddenly. They include disturbed heart rhythms, arthritis in the ankles, and eye symptoms.

In some serious cases in which vital organs are affected, sarcoidosis can result in death.

Sarcoidosis is not a form of cancer.

There is no known way to prevent sarcoidosis.

Sarcoidosis was once thought to be an uncommon condition. It's now known to affect tens of thousands of people throughout the United States. Because many people who have sarcoidosis have no symptoms, it's hard to know how many people have the condition.

Sarcoidosis was identified in the late 1860s. Since then, scientists have developed better tests to diagnose it and made advances in treating it.

What Causes Sarcoidosis?

The cause of sarcoidosis is not known. There may be more than one thing that causes it.

Scientists think that sarcoidosis develops when your immune system responds to something in the environment (e.g., bacteria, viruses, dust, chemicals) or perhaps to your own body tissue (autoimmunity).

Normally, your immune system defends your body against things that it sees as foreign and harmful. It does this by sending special cells to the organs that are being affected by these things. These cells release chemicals that produce inflammation around the foreign substance or substances to isolate and destroy them.

In sarcoidosis, this inflammation remains and leads to the development of granulomas or lumps.

Scientists have not yet identified the specific substance or substances that trigger the immune system response in the first place. They also think that sarcoidosis develops only if you have inherited a certain combination of genes.

You can't catch sarcoidosis from someone who has it.

More research is needed to discover what causes sarcoidosis.

Who Gets Sarcoidosis?

Sarcoidosis affects people of all ages and races worldwide.
It occurs mostly in the following groups:

- Adults between the ages of twenty and forty
- African Americans (especially women)
- People of Asian, German, Irish, Puerto Rican, and Scandinavian origin.

In the United States, sarcoidosis affects African Americans somewhat more often and more severely than Caucasians.

Studies have shown that sarcoidosis is more likely to affect certain organs in certain populations. For example, sarcoidosis of the heart and eye appears to be more common in Japan, while painful skin lumps on the legs occur more often in people from Northern Europe.

People who are more likely to get sarcoidosis include the following:

- Health care workers
- Nonsmokers
- Elementary and secondary school teachers
- People exposed to agricultural dust, insecticides, pesticides, or mold
- Firefighters

Brothers and sisters, parents, and children of people who have sarcoidosis are more likely than others to have sarcoidosis.

What Are the Signs and Symptoms of Sarcoidosis?

Many people who have sarcoidosis have no symptoms. Often, the condition is discovered by accident only because a person has a chest x-ray for another reason, such as a pre-employment x-ray.

Some people have very few symptoms, but others have many.

Symptoms usually depend on which organs the disease affects.

Lung Symptoms

- Shortness of breath
- A dry cough that doesn't bring up phlegm, or mucus
- Wheezing
- Pain in the middle of your chest that gets worse when you breathe deeply or cough (rare)

Lymph Node Symptoms

- Enlarged and sometimes tender lymph nodes—most often those in your neck and chest but sometimes those under your chin, in your arm pits, or in your groin

Skin Symptoms

- Various types of bumps, ulcers, or, rarely, flat areas of discolored skin, that appear mostly near your nose, eyes, back, arms, legs, and scalp. They usually itch but aren't painful. They usually last a long time.

- Painful bumps that usually appear on your ankles and shins and can be warm, tender, red or purple-to-red in color, and slightly raised. This is called erythema nodosum. You may have fever and swollen ankles and joint pain along with the bumps. The bumps often are an early sign of sarcoidosis, but they occur in other diseases too. The bumps usually go away in weeks to months, even without treatment.

- Disfiguring skin sores that may affect your nose, nasal passages, cheeks, ears, eyelids, and fingers. This is called lupus pernio. The sores tend to be ongoing and can return after treatment is over.

Eye Symptoms

- Burning, itching, tearing, pain
- Red eye
- Sensitivity to light
- Dryness
- Floaters (i.e., seeing black spots)
- Blurred vision

- Reduced color vision
- Reduced visual clearness
- Blindness (in rare cases)

Heart Symptoms

- Shortness of breath
- Swelling in your legs
- Wheezing
- Coughing
- Irregular heartbeat, including palpitations (a fluttering feeling of rapid heartbeats) and skipped beats
- Sudden loss of consciousness
- Sudden death

Joint and Muscle Symptoms

- Joint stiffness or swelling—usually in your ankles, feet, and hands.
- Joint pain.
- Muscle aches (myalgias).
- Muscle pain, a mass in a muscle, or muscle weakness.
- Painful arthritis in your ankles that results from erythema nodosum. It may need treatment but usually clears up in several weeks.
- Painless arthritis that can last for months or even years. It should be treated.

Bone Symptoms

- Painless holes in your bones.
- Painless swelling, most often in your fingers.
- Anemia that results from granulomas affecting your bone marrow. This usually should be treated.

Liver Symptoms

- Fever

- Fatigue
- Itching
- Pain in the upper right part of your abdomen, under the right ribs
- Enlarged liver

Parotid and Other Salivary Gland Symptoms

- Swelling, which makes your cheeks look puffy
- Excessive dryness in your mouth and throat

Blood, Urinary Tract, and Kidney Symptoms

- Increased calcium in your blood or urine, which can lead to painful kidney stones
- Confusion
- Increased urination

Nervous System Symptoms

- Headaches.
- Vision problems.
- Weakness or numbness of an arm or leg.
- Coma (rare).
- Drooping of one side of your face that results from sarcoidosis affecting a facial nerve. This can be confused with Bell palsy, a disorder that may be caused by a virus.
- Paralysis of your arms or legs that results from sarcoidosis affecting your spinal cord.
- Weakness, pain, or a "stinging needles" sensation in areas where many nerves are affected by sarcoidosis.

Pituitary Gland Symptoms (Rare)

- Headaches
- Vision problems
- Weakness or numbness of an arm or leg
- Coma (rare)

Other Symptoms

- Nasal obstruction or frequent bouts of sinusitis.

- Enlarged spleen, which leads to a decrease in platelets in your blood and pain in your upper left abdomen. Platelets are needed to help your blood clot.

Sarcoidosis may also cause more general symptoms, including the following:

- Uneasiness, feeling sick (malaise), an overall feeling of ill health

- Tiredness, fatigue, weakness

- Loss of appetite or weight

- Fever

- Night sweats

- Sleep problems

These general symptoms are often caused by other conditions. If you have these general symptoms but don't have symptoms from affected organs, you probably do not have sarcoidosis.

How Is Sarcoidosis Diagnosed?

Your doctor will find out if you have sarcoidosis by taking a detailed medical history and conducting a physical exam and several diagnostic tests. The purpose is to:

- Identify the presence of granulomas in any of your organs;

- Rule out other causes of your symptoms;

- Determine the amount of damage to any of your affected organs;

- Determine whether you need treatment.

Medical History

Your doctor will ask you for a detailed medical history. He or she will want to know about any family history of sarcoidosis and what jobs you have had that may have increased your chances of getting sarcoidosis.

Your doctor may also ask whether you have ever been exposed to inhaled beryllium metal, which is used in aircraft and weapons manufacture, or organic dust from birds or hay. These things can produce granulomas in your lungs that look like the granulomas that are caused by sarcoidosis but are actually signs of other conditions.

Physical Exam

Your doctor will look for symptoms of sarcoidosis, such as red bumps on your skin; swollen lymph nodes; an enlarged liver, spleen, or salivary gland(s); or redness in your eyes. He or she will also listen for abnormal lung sounds or heart rhythm. Your doctor also will check for other likely causes of your symptoms.

Diagnostic Tests

There is no one specific test for diagnosing sarcoidosis. It is harder to diagnose sarcoidosis in some organs (e.g., heart, nervous system) than in others. Your doctor will probably conduct a variety of tests and procedures to help in the diagnosis.

These include:

- **Chest x-ray:** A chest x-ray takes a picture of your heart and lungs. It may show granulomas or enlarged lymph nodes in your chest. About ninety-five out of every one hundred people who have sarcoidosis have an abnormal chest x-ray. Doctors usually use a staging system for chest x-rays taken to detect sarcoidosis. In general, the higher the stage of the x-ray, the worse your symptoms and lung function are. But there are a lot of differences among people. If your x-ray results show stages 0, 1, 2, or 3, you may not have symptoms or need treatment, and you may get better and have normal chest x-rays again over time. The stages are as follows:

  - *Stage 0:* Normal chest x-ray
  - *Stage 1:* Chest x-ray showing enlarged lymph nodes but otherwise clear lungs
  - *Stage 2:* Chest x-ray showing enlarged lymph nodes and shadows in your lungs
  - *Stage 3:* Chest x-ray showing shadows in your lungs, but the lymph nodes are not enlarged
  - *Stage 4:* Chest x-ray showing scars in the lung tissue.

- **Blood tests:** These tests can show the number and type of cells in your blood. They also will show whether there are increases in your calcium levels or changes in your liver, kidney, and bone marrow that can occur with sarcoidosis.

- **Lung function tests:** One test uses a spirometer, a device that measures how much and how fast you can blow air out of your lungs after taking a deep breath. If there is a lot of inflammation or scarring in your lungs, you will not be able to move normal amounts of air in and out. Another test measures how much air your lungs can hold. Sarcoidosis can cause your lungs to shrink, and they will not be able to hold as much air as healthy lungs.

- **Electrocardiogram (EKG):** This test will help show if your heart is affected by sarcoidosis.

- **Pulse oximetry:** A small clip attached to your fingertip can show how well your heart and lungs are moving oxygen into your blood.

- **Arterial blood gas test:** This test is more accurate than pulse oximetry for checking the level of oxygen in your bloodstream. Blood is taken from an artery (usually in your wrist). It is then analyzed for its oxygen and carbon dioxide levels.

- **Fiberoptic bronchoscopy:** In this procedure, your doctor inserts a long, narrow, flexible tube with a light on the end through your nose or mouth into your lungs to look at your airways. This tube is called a bronchoscope. You most likely would have this procedure as an outpatient in a hospital under local anesthesia.

- **Bronchoalveolar lavage (BAL):** During bronchoscopy, your doctor may inject a small amount of salt water (saline) through the bronchoscope into your lungs. This fluid washes the lungs and helps bring up cells and other material from the air sacs deep in your lungs where the inflammation usually starts to develop. The cells and fluid are then examined for signs of inflammation.

- **Biopsy:** Your doctor may take a small sample of tissue from one of your affected organs. For example, when breathing tests or chest x-rays show signs of sarcoidosis in your lungs, your doctor may do a fiberoptic bronchoscopy biopsy. This will help confirm the diagnosis. Your doctor inserts a tiny forceps through the bronchoscope to collect tissue that will be examined. Because the granulomas may be spread out in your lungs, the bronchoscope may miss some of them. Biopsies of your skin and liver are sometimes done to detect granulomas in these organs. You may have sarcoidosis in other organs as well and multiple biopsies may be necessary. However, every organ involved does not need to be biopsied for a diagnosis to be made.

- **Computerized tomography (CT) scan:** This test provides a computer-generated image of your organs that has more detail than a regular chest x-ray. It can provide more information about how sarcoidosis has affected an organ. Your doctor may do a CT scan to:
  - Obtain more information about how much of your lung is affected by sarcoidosis;
  - Detect sarcoidosis in your liver. A CT scan of your abdomen will show if your liver is enlarged and if there is a pattern suggesting granulomas.

- **Magnetic resonance (MR) scan:** This test is also called nuclear magnetic resonance (NMR) scanning or magnetic resonance imaging (MRI). This scan uses powerful magnets and radio waves to make images of some of your organs that your doctor doesn't want to risk doing a biopsy on. For example, an MR scan can be used to diagnose sarcoidosis in your brain, spinal cord, nerves, or heart.

- **Thallium and gallium scans:** These scans are often done to see if sarcoidosis is affecting your heart. Thallium and gallium are radioactive elements. Your doctor injects a small amount of one of them into a vein in your arm. The elements collect at places in your body where there is inflammation. After awhile, your body is scanned for radioactivity. Increased radioactivity at any place may be a sign of inflammation. This test gives information on the tissue in your body that has been affected by sarcoidosis and the amount of damage to it. But since this test shows all inflammation in your body, even inflammation caused by conditions other than sarcoidosis, it does not give a definite diagnosis of sarcoidosis.

- **Positron emission tomography (PET) scan:** This test also uses radioactive injections. It may be more sensitive than gallium in detecting areas of inflammation. Some doctors are using it instead of gallium scans.

Your doctor may not need to find every one of your organs affected by sarcoidosis, only those that cause symptoms. Often the organs affected by the condition continue to function well and don't need to be treated.

How Is Sarcoidosis Treated?

The goals of treatment are to improve how the organs affected by sarcoidosis work, relieve symptoms, and shrink the granulomas.

Treatment may shrink the granulomas and even cause them to disappear, but this may take many months. If scars have formed, treatment may not help, and you may have ongoing symptoms.

Your treatment depends on:

• What symptoms you have;

• How severe your symptoms are;

• Whether any of your vital organs (e.g., your lungs, eyes, heart, or brain) are affected;

• How the organ is affected.

Some organs must be treated, regardless of your symptoms. Others may not need to be treated. Usually, if you don't have symptoms, you don't need treatment, and you probably will recover in time.

Drugs

The main treatment for sarcoidosis is prednisone. Prednisone is a corticosteroid, or anti-inflammatory drug. Sometimes it is used with other drugs. Sometimes other corticosteroids are used.

Prednisone almost always relieves symptoms of inflammation. If a symptom doesn't improve with prednisone treatment within a couple of months, consult your physician.

Prednisone is usually given for many months, sometimes for a year or more.

Low doses of prednisone can often relieve symptoms without causing major side effects.

When used at high doses, prednisone can cause serious side effects. Side effects can include:

• Weight gain.

• Diabetes.

• High blood pressure.

• Mood swings (depression).

• Difficulty sleeping at night.

• Heartburn.

- Acne.

- Thinning of the skin and bones (called osteoporosis).

- Cataracts.

- Glaucoma.

- Adrenal gland insufficiency, which occurs when these glands don't make enough of certain hormones. This requires treatment by an endocrinologist, a doctor who specializes in the diagnosis and treatment of the endocrine glands. The endocrine glands include your adrenal and pituitary glands.

- Aseptic or avascular necrosis of the hip, the development of cysts and hardened and dead tissue in the hip.

Your doctor can usually help you manage these side effects.

When it is time to stop taking prednisone, you should cut back slowly, with your doctor's help. This will help prevent flare-ups of sarcoidosis and allow your body to adjust to life without the drug.

You may also want to see an endocrinologist to make sure that your endocrine glands are making enough hormones. The endocrinologist may prescribe certain hormones for you to take until your endocrine glands are working well again.

Other Drugs Used to Treat Sarcoidosis

Other drugs are sometimes used to treat sarcoidosis. Your doctor may prescribe one of them if your condition gets worse while you are taking prednisone or you can't stand the side effects of prednisone.

Most of these other drugs are immune system suppressants. This means that they prevent your immune system from fighting things like bacteria and viruses. As a result, you may have a greater chance of getting infections.

Most of these drugs also can cause serious side effects. Some also could increase your chances of getting cancer, especially if you take them at high doses.

You and your doctor must weigh living with the symptoms of sarcoidosis against the side effects of the drugs.

Some drugs work better than others for different people.

You may be given more than one drug.

Some drugs used to treat sarcoidosis are taken by mouth. Others are applied locally to an affected area.

Local therapy is the safest way to treat sarcoidosis. The drug is applied directly to the affected area. As a result, only small amounts of the drug reach other parts of your body.

Drugs used for local therapy include eye drops, inhaled drugs for your lungs, and skin creams.

Drugs can be used locally only if the affected area is easily reached. For instance, inhaled steroids can ease coughing and wheezing in the upper airways, but they don't seem to relieve these symptoms when the affected lung tissue is deep within your chest.

Talk with your doctor about these treatments and the side effects that may occur.

Other drugs used to treat sarcoidosis include:

- **Hydroxychloroquine (Plaquenil®):** This drug can usually help people who have sarcoidosis in the skin or a high level of calcium in their blood. This drug can irritate your stomach. It also can cause eye problems. Before starting on this drug, you should see an ophthalmologist, or eye doctor, for some baseline tests. Once you start taking it, you should have your eyes examined every six months.

- **Methotrexate:** This drug is taken once a week by mouth or injection and usually takes up to six months to relieve symptoms. This drug may cause side effects, especially if you take high doses. If you are pregnant, you should not take this drug. Taking folic acid can help you reduce your chances of having bad side effects from methotrexate. These include:

  - Nausea.

  - Mouth sores.

  - A decrease in infection-fighting white blood cells. You then have a greater chance of getting an infection. If you take this drug, you should have regular blood tests to check the levels of your white blood cells.

  - An allergic reaction in your lungs that goes away when you stop taking the drug. This is extremely rare.

  - Liver damage. This is the most serious side effect. If you take methotrexate you should be followed regularly by your physician.

- **Azathioprine (Imuran®):** This drug may work in about half of the people who have sarcoidosis. You usually take it for at least 6 months. Side effects include nausea and reduced white blood cell levels, which increases your chances of getting an infection. This drug has caused cancer in some people, especially when they have taken it at high doses. If you are pregnant, you should not take this drug.

- **Cyclophosphamide (Cytoxan®):** This is a very toxic drug. It is rarely used to treat sarcoidosis. It is given only to people who have serious forms of sarcoidosis, such as sarcoidosis in their central nervous system (neurosarcoidosis). This drug is more likely to cause nausea and reduce your white blood cell levels than either methotrexate or azathioprine. Your doctor should check your white blood cell levels often while you are taking this drug to make sure you have a high enough level to fight infection. Cyclophosphamide can also irritate your bladder. Some people who have taken it for more than two years have developed bladder cancer. If you are pregnant, you should not take this drug. Cyclophosphamide can be given intravenously (through one of your veins), which lessens some of its side effects, but this doesn't reduce the risk of cancer.

Treatments for Specific Types of Sarcoidosis

Eyes: Sarcoidosis in your eyes almost always responds well to treatment. Often, the only treatment you need is eye drops containing corticosteroids. You should have yearly eye exams, even if you think your eyes are doing well.

Spleen: Sarcoidosis can cause your spleen to become larger. This can lead to a decrease in your red or white blood cells or platelets and increase your chances of infection and blood clotting disorders. Treatment is usually given to increase the number of your blood cells and ease your pain. In rare cases, your spleen may need to be removed.

Liver: Sarcoidosis rarely causes permanent liver damage. As a result, your liver usually isn't treated unless it's causing major symptoms (e.g., fever). Drug treatment can usually reduce granulomas in your liver. Liver transplantation has been successful in those rare cases in which the condition has become worse. Follow-up care includes regular blood tests to find out how well your liver is working. You should check with your doctor to find out how often you need these tests.

Nervous system: Sarcoidosis in your nervous system (neurosarcoidosis) usually needs treatment. Nerve tissue heals slowly, so treatment often takes a long time. You may need to take several drugs at high doses.

Erythema nodosum: These painful bumps on your shins often go away in weeks to months without treatment. Your doctor probably will not give you medication unless you are very uncomfortable. Aspirin or ibuprofen, an anti-inflammatory drug that you can buy without a prescription, will usually help.

Heart: Sarcoidosis in your heart is usually treated with steroids. You may also be given heart drugs to improve your heart's pumping ability or to correct a disturbed heart rhythm.

If you have a severe heart rhythm disturbance, your doctor may prescribe one of these devices:

- A cardiac pacemaker, a small battery-operated device, often put under your skin, that regulates your heartbeat

- A defibrillator, an implanted device that shocks your heart into a normal heartbeat or, if it has stopped, into beating.

If your heart is severely affected and doesn't respond to treatment, a transplant may be done. But this is rarely needed.

Lupus pernio: This rash on your face, especially your cheeks and nose, can be distressing because it's in a very visible area. It often occurs with loss of your sense of smell, nasal stuffiness, and sinus infections. Options for treatment include local treatment with skin creams, oral drugs (Plaquenil or prednisone, for example), or local injections of steroid preparations. Lupus pernio is often treated by dermatologists, doctors who specialize in skin diseases, working with a sarcoidosis specialist.

Because sarcoidosis varies so much among different people, your doctor may find it hard to tell whether the treatment is helping.

Other Drugs Being Studied for Possible Use in Treating Sarcoidosis

Scientists also are studying drugs that are used for other conditions to see if they can help people who have sarcoidosis. These drugs include:

- **Etanercept (Enbrel®):** This drug is an immune system suppressant. It's injected under the skin to reduce symptoms of rheumatoid arthritis. It may also be used to treat psoriasis or ankylosing spondylitis, a type of arthritis that affects the joints in the spine. Early studies suggest that it will not be useful in treating sarcoidosis, but research is ongoing.

- **Infliximab (Remicade®):** This drug is an immune system suppressant. It's injected into a vein in your arm. It's used to treat Crohn disease, rheumatoid arthritis, and ankylosing spondylitis. Some studies have shown it to help sarcoidosis patients who also have lupus pernio, eye disease, or neurosarcoidosis. This drug has serious side effects but may improve lung function in some people who aren't helped by corticosteroids. More research is needed.

- **Pentoxifylline:** This drug is an immune system suppressant. Stomach and gastrointestinal side effects are common. Early studies show that it has helped some people who have sarcoidosis in their lungs reduce their doses of prednisone while taking it. More research is needed.

- **Tetracycline:** Tetracycline antibiotics are used to treat Lyme disease, some types of pneumonia, and acne. A few small studies suggest that they may help in treating sarcoidosis in the skin. Research is ongoing.

- **Thalidomide:** This immune system suppressant can cause bad side effects. It is effective against other conditions that involve granulomas of the skin (e.g., leprosy, tuberculosis). Scientists are studying this drug to see if it can be used to treat sarcoidosis in the skin. More studies are needed.

What Does the Future Hold?

Scientists worldwide are trying to learn more about sarcoidosis and how to improve its diagnosis and treatment. Some recent studies have led to possible new treatments, which, in turn, are being studied. Current research includes studies of:

- The agent or agents that cause sarcoidosis;
- Why sarcoidosis seems to act differently in people of different races;
- Why sarcoidosis appears in some families;
- How genes, passed from one generation to another, may make some people more likely than others to develop sarcoidosis;
- How cells act and communicate with each other to cause sarcoidosis symptoms.

Living with Sarcoidosis

You should take steps to stay healthy. Don't smoke. Avoid substances like dusts and chemicals that can harm your lungs. Try to follow a healthy eating plan. Be as active as you can but don't strain yourself.

Joining a patient support group may help you adjust to living with sarcoidosis. Talking to others who have the same symptoms can help you see how they have coped with them. To find a local support group, check your telephone directory.

Your regular doctor may be able to diagnose and treat your sarcoidosis, but diagnosis and treatment by a doctor who specializes in sarcoidosis is recommended. If you prefer to use your regular doctor, you should see a doctor who specializes in the organs that are affected by your sarcoidosis at least once. For example, see an ophthalmologist if your eyes are affected or a pulmonologist if you have sarcoidosis in your lungs. These specialists are often found at major medical centers. They will work with your regular doctor to help make a diagnosis, develop a treatment plan, and schedule periodic exams and lab tests.

Pregnancy

Many women give birth to healthy babies while being treated for sarcoidosis. Pregnancy usually doesn't affect the course of sarcoidosis, and you can continue corticosteroid treatment through your pregnancy. None of the other drugs are recommended for use during pregnancy.

Sometimes your sarcoidosis may get worse after the baby is delivered.

Women with severe sarcoidosis, especially if they are older, may have trouble becoming pregnant.

It's important for you to discuss this issue with your doctor. If you become pregnant, you should be sure to get both good prenatal care and regular sarcoidosis checkups during and after pregnancy.

Follow-up Care

Regular follow-up care is important, even if you aren't taking medication for your sarcoidosis. New symptoms can occur at any time, and your condition can get worse slowly, without your noticing.

Follow-up exams usually include:

- A review of your symptoms;
- A physical exam;

- A chest x-ray and CT scan;
- Breathing tests
- An eye exam
- Blood tests
- An electrocardiogram (EKG).

How often you have your examinations and tests depends on how severe your symptoms are, which organs were affected at diagnosis, what treatment you are using, and any complications that may develop during treatment.

You will probably need routine follow-up care for several years. Whether you see your regular doctor or a sarcoidosis specialist for this depends on your symptoms during the first year of follow-up.

Here are some examples of how your follow-up care can be managed. They are based on either your condition when you were diagnosed with sarcoidosis or the treatment used.

Follow-up after initial diagnosis: If at diagnosis, you have no symptoms, a normal breathing test, and an abnormal chest x-ray, you should plan on having a follow-up exam every six to twelve months until your condition is stable or improving. Your breathing test may need to be repeated. The need to repeat it depends on your symptoms and ability to be active. If at your first follow-up visit, you have no new symptoms and your chest x-ray is normal, you can go to your regular doctor for future follow-up care.

If at diagnosis, you have some symptoms and an abnormal chest x-ray, but you don't need treatment, you should plan on having a follow-up exam in three to six months. If at your follow-up exam your condition has gotten worse (i.e., you now have more symptoms, an abnormal x-ray, or abnormal lab tests) you may need treatment. If treatment is started, you may need follow-up tests more often.

Follow-up based on your drug treatment: If treatment is begun with prednisone, you should be checked for the side effects of high blood pressure, too much weight gain, diabetes, loss of calcium from your bones, and pain in one or both hips. If treatment is begun with hydroxychloroquine, you should have an eye exam every six months while taking this drug. If treatment is begun with methotrexate, you should have blood tests every month or every other month to see if you have anemia, low white blood cell or platelet levels, or liver inflammation.

Other Follow-up Tests

Depending on how serious your condition is and what organs are affected, you may also need to have certain tests done regularly.

Eye tests: Everyone who is diagnosed with sarcoidosis, even if they don't have eye symptoms, should see an ophthalmologist (eye doctor) for eye tests. This is important because you may have eye damage even if you don't have symptoms.

These tests may include:

- A slit lamp examination. Your doctor uses an instrument with a high-intensity light source to look at the front of your eyes.

- A visual fields examination. Your doctor will ask you to you to look at a light through an instrument.

- Inspection of your retina and optic nerve.

If you develop eye symptoms, your doctor will have you repeat the tests.

You should also have regular eye exams if you are being treated with chloroquine or hydroxychloroquine (Plaquenil®) or corticosteroids.

Breathing tests: These tests are used to check the course of sarcoidosis in your lungs. The results are compared over time.

Blood tests: A blood test for calcium should be done. If your calcium level is high, you probably will need to be treated. You also should not take vitamin and mineral supplements containing calcium or vitamin D, and you should avoid too much exposure to the sun.

Electrocardiogram: This test is needed to make sure that your heart is still not affected by sarcoidosis. The heart can be affected at any time if the sarcoidosis is active.

Chapter 21

Occupational Lung Diseases

Chapter Contents

Section 21.1

Asbestosis

Reprinted from "Asbestos and Health: Frequently Asked Questions,"
Agency for Toxic Substances and Disease Registry, U.S. Centers for
Disease Control and Prevention, 2005.

Asbestos

What is asbestos?

Asbestos is the name given to a group of six different fibrous minerals that occur naturally in the environment. Asbestos fibers are too small to be seen by the naked eye. They do not dissolve in water or evaporate. They are resistant to heat, fire, and chemical or biological degradation.

Asbestos is also used in many commercial products, including insulation, brake linings, and roofing shingles.

What are the types of asbestos?

The two general types of asbestos are amphibole and chrysotile (fibrous serpentine). Chrysotile asbestos has long, flexible fibers. This type of asbestos is most commonly used in commercial products. Amphibole fibers are brittle, have a rod or needle shape, and are less common in commercial products. Although exposure to both types of asbestos increases the likelihood of developing asbestos-related diseases, amphibole fibers tend to stay in the lungs longer. They also are thought to increase the likelihood of illness, especially mesothelioma, to a greater extent than chrysotile asbestos.

What is naturally occurring asbestos?

Naturally occurring asbestos refers to those fibrous minerals that are found in the rocks or soil in an area and released into the air by routine human activities or weathering processes.

If naturally occurring asbestos is not disturbed and fibers are not released into the air, then it is not a health risk. Asbestos is commonly found in ultramafic rock, including serpentine rock, and near fault zones. The amount of asbestos that is typically present in these rocks ranges from less than 1 percent up to about 25 percent, and sometimes more. Asbestos can be released from ultramafic and serpentine rock if the rock is broken or crushed.

In California, ultramafic rock, including serpentine rock, is found in the Sierra foothills, the Klamath Mountains, and the Coast Ranges. This type of rock is present in at least forty-four of California's fifty-eight counties. Not all ultramafic rock contains asbestos; it has the potential to contain asbestos. Environmental testing can determine if a rock contains asbestos.

Asbestos Exposure

What is asbestos exposure?

Asbestos exposure results from breathing in asbestos fibers. If rocks, soil, or products containing asbestos are disturbed, they can release asbestos fibers into the air. These fibers can be breathed into your lungs and could remain there for a lifetime. Asbestos exposure is not a problem if solid asbestos is left alone and not disturbed.

Who is at risk for asbestos exposure?

Almost everyone has been exposed to asbestos at some time in their life. Higher levels of asbestos are more common near: an asbestos mine or factory, a building being torn down or renovated that contains asbestos products, a waste site where asbestos is not properly covered up or stored to protect it from wind erosion, or an area containing naturally occurring asbestos that has been disturbed through activities that crush asbestos-containing rock or stir up dust in soils that contain asbestos fibers.

In indoor air, the concentration of asbestos depends on the following:

- Whether asbestos was used for insulation, ceiling or floor tiles, or other purposes, and whether these asbestos-containing materials are in good condition or are deteriorated and easily crumbled

- Whether activities in the house, such as repairs and home improvements, have disturbed asbestos-containing materials, or

- Whether asbestos has been brought into the home on shoes, clothes, hair, pet fur, or other objects.

Outdoor air concentrations of asbestos can also contribute to indoor air asbestos levels.

Health Effects of Asbestos Exposure

What is the likelihood of developing health problems from asbestos exposure?

Being exposed to asbestos does not mean you will develop health problems. Many things need to be considered when evaluating whether you are at risk for health problems from asbestos exposure. The most important of these are as follows:

- How long and how frequently you were exposed

- How long it has been since your exposure started

- How much you were exposed

- If you smoke cigarettes (cigarette smoking with asbestos exposure increases your chances of getting lung cancer)

- The size and type of asbestos you were exposed to

- Other pre-existing lung conditions

A doctor can help you find out whether you are at risk for health problems from asbestos exposure.

Are children at greater risk for asbestos-related diseases?

Children have more time to be exposed and develop asbestos-related diseases. Medical experts do not know whether lung differences may cause a greater amount of asbestos fibers to stay in the lungs of a child who breaths in asbestos compared with the amount that stays in the lungs of an adult.

What are the symptoms of asbestos-related disease?

Most people don't show any signs or symptoms of asbestos-related disease for ten to twenty years or more after exposure. When symptoms do appear, they can be similar to those of other health problems. Only a doctor can tell if your symptoms are asbestos-related.

What are some types of asbestos-related diseases?

Asbestos-related diseases can be:

- Noncancerous:

  - **Asbestosis** is scarring of the lungs. It is typically caused by very high exposure levels over a prolonged period of time, as seen in work-related asbestos exposure. Smoking increases the risk of developing asbestosis. Some late-stage symptoms include progressive shortness of breath, a persistent cough, and chest pain.

  - **Pleural changes or pleural plaques** include thickening and hardening of the pleura (the lining that covers the lungs and chest cavity). Most people will not have symptoms, but some may have decreased lung function. Some people may develop persistent shortness of breath with exercise or even at rest if they have significantly decreased lung function.

- Cancerous:

  - **Lung cancer** is cancer of the lungs and lung passages. Cigarette smoking combined with asbestos exposure greatly increases the likelihood of lung cancer. Lung cancer caused by smoking or asbestos looks the same. Symptoms for lung cancer can vary. Some late-stage symptoms can include chronic cough, chest pain, unexplained weight loss, and coughing up blood.

  - **Mesothelioma** is a rare cancer mostly associated with asbestos exposure. It occurs in the covering of the lungs and sometimes the lining of the abdominal cavity. Some late-stage symptoms include chest pain, persistent shortness of breath, and unexplained weight loss. Coughing up blood is not common.

Can asbestos-related disease be serious?

Asbestos-related disease can be serious, though not everyone exposed to asbestos gets health problems. Health problems that develop may range from manageable to severe—and some may cause death.

How common are asbestos-related diseases?

Mesothelioma is relatively rare. According to the American Cancer Society, there are about two to three thousand new cases per year in this country. It is most common in asbestos-related work exposure though it has been observed in certain communities worldwide where people have had lifetime exposures to naturally occurring asbestos.

Lung cancer from all causes affects about 61 out of every 100,000 Americans a year. According to the American Cancer Society, it is the leading cause of cancer-related death in both men and women and accounts for about 29 percent of all cancer deaths. Asbestos exposure is only one of many potential causes of lung cancer. Cigarette smoking is by far the most important risk factor for lung cancer. Cigarette smoking combined with asbestos exposure greatly increases the likelihood of lung cancer.

Tests to Diagnose Asbestos-Related Disease

What will my doctor typically do?

Your doctor will first take your medical history and perform a physical exam. He or she will then decide if you need additional testing.

What are some tests to help diagnose asbestos-related disease?

On the basis of your medical history and physical exam, your doctor may or may not recommend any of these tests for you:

- **A chest x-ray** is the most common test used to determine whether you have received sustained exposure to asbestos. The x-ray cannot detect the asbestos fibers themselves, but it can detect early signs of lung changes caused by asbestos. If the chest x-ray shows spots on the lungs, they may or may not be asbestos-related. They may be normal variations or related to infections and different types of diseases. Only a doctor trained in reading x-rays can determine if a spot is asbestos-related or something else.

- **A lung function test also known as a pulmonary function test (PFT)** is a simple breathing test to see how well your lungs are working. In this test, a person blows big breaths into a machine. Based on your medical history and physical exam, your doctor may or may not recommend this test for you.

- **A computerized tomography scan (CT)** is a type of x-ray machine that usually delivers a much higher dose of radiation than a chest x-ray. A CT scan may be more sensitive than a chest x-ray in detecting early changes of disease. A CT scan is recommended only when the chest x-ray is inconclusive.

- For a test called **bronchoalveolar lavage (BAL)**, a small flexible tube is inserted through the nose and down the airway. A small amount of saline solution is injected into the tube and then sucked back up. The fluid obtained contains saline plus material from the lung. Illness from asbestos exposure generally cannot be predicted from this test. This test is performed only under special circumstances.

- For a **lung biopsy**, samples of lung tissue are taken through a needle while the patient is sedated. This tissue is examined under a microscope. Lung biopsies are rarely performed. This is because diagnosis is usually based on findings from the medical evaluation and other tests. A lung biopsy is not needed for most people who are diagnosed with an asbestos-related disease.

What about urine and sputum tests?

Sputum is the material that is brought up from the lungs by coughing. Urine and sputum tests are not reliable for determining how much asbestos may be in the lungs. Nearly everyone has low levels of asbestos in these materials. These tests cannot predict the risk of illness. More research may improve the reliability and predictability of these tests.

Should I have my children tested?

Taking x-rays of children's lungs to look for asbestos-related disease is not currently recommended because changes to the lung usually take years to develop. In addition, x-ray radiation may pose a higher risk for children.

Treatment of Asbestos-Related Disease

What are some preventive health guidelines?

If you have an asbestos-related disease or history of significant asbestos exposure, your doctor may recommend that you follow the preventive care guidelines listed below:

- Regular medical examinations
- Regular vaccinations against flu and pneumococcal pneumonia shots
- Quit smoking if you are a smoker
- Limit further asbestos exposure

387

Following these preventive care guidelines may help reduce complications from asbestos-related disease or exposure. Your doctor may recommend other supportive care for complications and, if needed, treatment.

Supportive care includes interventions that may help the symptoms of the disease, but does not reverse the disease process. Supportive care is tailored to the symptoms and the disease. For example, a severe cough may be treated with a cough suppressant so that a person can rest or sleep at night.

What is the treatment for asbestosis?

Preventive and supportive care are the primary treatments for asbestosis. Preventive care guidelines are given in the previous section. Asbestosis can remain stable or increase in severity, but rarely gets better. Scarring of the lungs is permanent and no method exists to remove it from the lungs.

What is the treatment for pleural changes?

Treatment for pleural changes involves preventive and supportive care. Preventive care guidelines are given in the previous section.

What is the treatment for lung cancer?

Lung cancer treatment depends on location of the cancer, stage of the disease, age of the patient, and general health of the patient.

Treatment options include: chemotherapy, radiation therapy, a combination of chemotherapy and radiation therapy, or removing the diseased part of the lung through surgery.

What is the treatment for mesothelioma?

Depending on the stage of the disease, mesothelioma treatment options include chemotherapy, radiation, and surgery.

Reducing Your Exposure to Asbestos

Can asbestos be removed from the lungs?

No known method exists to remove asbestos fibers from the lung once they are inhaled. Some types of asbestos are cleared naturally by the lung or break down in the lung.

What can I do to reduce my exposure to asbestos?

Limit exposure by taking the following steps if you live in an area where naturally occurring asbestos has been disturbed and is likely to become airborne:

- Walk, run, hike, and bike only on paved trails.

- Play only in outdoor areas with a ground covering such as wood chips, mulch, sand, pea gravel, grass, asphalt, shredded rubber, or rubber mats.

- Pave over unpaved walkways, driveways, or roadways that may have asbestos-containing rock or soil.

- Cover asbestos-containing rock or soil in gardens and yards with asbestos-free soil or landscape covering.

- Pre-wet garden areas before digging or shoveling soil.

- Keep pets from carrying dust or dirt on their fur or feet into the home.

- Remove shoes before entering your home to prevent tracking in dirt.

- Use doormats to lower the amount of soil that is tracked into the home.

- Keep windows and doors closed on windy days and during nearby construction.

- Drive slowly over unpaved roads.

- Use a wet rag instead of a dry rag or duster to dust.

- Use a wet mop on noncarpeted floors.

- Use washable area rugs on your floors and wash them regularly.

- Vacuum carpet often using a vacuum with a high-efficiency particulate air (HEPA) filter.

- Inspect your home for deteriorating asbestos-containing insulation, ceiling, or floor tiles.

- Do not disturb asbestos-containing insulation, ceiling, or floor tiles; hire a trained and certified asbestos contractor to remove the materials.

- Ask your employer if you are working with materials or in an environment containing asbestos. If you are, make sure you are properly protected from asbestos exposure.

Section 21.2

Beryllium Disease

Reprinted from "ToxFAQs for Beryllium," Agency for
Toxic Substances and Disease Registry, U.S. Centers for
Disease Control and Prevention, September 2007.

People working or living near beryllium industries have the greatest potential for exposure to beryllium. Lung damage has been observed in people exposed to high levels of beryllium in the air. About 1 to 15 percent of all people occupationally exposed to beryllium in air become sensitive to beryllium and may develop chronic beryllium disease (CBD), an irreversible and sometimes fatal scarring of the lungs. CBD may be completely asymptomatic or begin with coughing, chest pain, shortness of breath, weakness, and/or fatigue. Beryllium has been found in at least 535 of the 1,613 National Priorities List sites identified by the Environmental Protection Agency (EPA).

What is beryllium?

Beryllium is a hard, grayish metal naturally found in mineral rocks, coal, soil, and volcanic dust. Beryllium compounds are commercially mined, and the beryllium is purified for use in nuclear weapons and reactors, aircraft and space vehicle structures, instruments, x-ray machines, and mirrors. Beryllium ores are used to make specialty ceramics for electrical and high-technology applications. Beryllium alloys are used in automobiles, computers, sports equipment (golf clubs and bicycle frames), and dental bridges.

What happens to beryllium when it enters the environment?

Beryllium dust enters the air from burning coal and oil. This beryllium dust will eventually settle over the land and water.

It enters water from erosion of rocks and soil, and from industrial waste. Some beryllium compounds will dissolve in water, but most stick to particles and settle to the bottom.

Most beryllium in soil does not dissolve in water and remains bound to soil.

Beryllium does not accumulate in the food chain.

How might I be exposed to beryllium?

The general population is exposed to normally low levels of beryllium in air, food, and water.

People working in industries where beryllium is mined, processed, machined, or converted into metal, alloys, and other chemicals may be exposed to high levels of beryllium. People living near these industries may also be exposed to higher than normal levels of beryllium in air.

People living near uncontrolled hazardous waste sites may be exposed to higher than normal levels of beryllium.

How can beryllium affect my health?

Beryllium can be harmful if you breathe it. The effects depend on how much you are exposed to and for how long. If beryllium air levels are high enough (greater than 1,000 $\mu g/m^3$), an acute condition can result. This condition resembles pneumonia and is called acute beryllium disease Occupational and community air standards are effective in preventing most acute lung damage.

Some people (1 to 15 percent) become sensitive to beryllium. These individuals may develop an inflammatory reaction in the respiratory system. This condition is called chronic beryllium disease (CBD), and can occur many years after exposure to higher than normal levels of beryllium (greater than 0.5 $\mu g/m^3$). This disease can make you feel weak and tired, and can cause difficulty in breathing. It can also result in anorexia and weight loss, and may also lead to right side heart enlargement and heart disease in advanced cases. Some people who are sensitized to beryllium may not have any symptoms. The general population is unlikely to develop acute or chronic beryllium disease because ambient air levels of beryllium are normally very low (0.00003–0.0002 $\mu g/m^3$).

Swallowing beryllium has not been reported to cause effects in humans because very little beryllium is absorbed from the stomach and intestines. Ulcers have been seen in dogs ingesting beryllium in the diet. Beryllium contact with skin that has been scraped or cut may cause rashes or ulcers.

How likely is beryllium to cause cancer?

Long-term exposure to beryllium can increase the risk of developing lung cancer in people.

The Department of Health and Human Services (DHHS) and the International Agency for Research on Cancer (IARC) have determined that beryllium is a human carcinogen. The EPA has determined that beryllium is a probable human carcinogen. EPA has estimated that lifetime exposure to 0.04 µg/m³ beryllium can result in a one in a thousand chance of developing cancer.

How can beryllium affect children?

There are no studies on the health effects of children exposed to beryllium. It is likely that the health effects seen in children exposed to beryllium will be similar to the effects seen in adults. We do not know whether children differ from adults in their susceptibility to beryllium.

We do not know if exposure to beryllium will result in birth defects or other developmental effects in people. The studies on developmental effects in animals are not conclusive.

How can families reduce the risk of exposure to beryllium?

Most families will not be exposed to high levels of beryllium.

Children should avoid playing in soils near uncontrolled hazardous waste sites where beryllium may have been discarded.

Is there a medical test to show whether I've been exposed to beryllium?

Beryllium can be measured in the urine and blood. The amount of beryllium in blood or urine may not indicate how much or how recently you were exposed. Beryllium levels can also be measured in lung and skin samples. These tests are not usually available at your doctor's office, but your doctor can send the samples to a laboratory that can perform the tests.

Another blood test, the blood beryllium lymphocyte proliferation test (BeLPT), identifies beryllium sensitization and has predictive value for CBD.

Has the federal government made recommendations to protect human health?

The EPA restricts the amount of beryllium that industries may release into the air to 0.01 µg/m³, averaged over a thirty-day period.

The Occupational Safety and Health Administration (OSHA) sets a limit of 2 µg/m³ of workroom air for an eight-hour work shift.

References

Agency for Toxic Substances and Disease Registry (ATSDR). 2002. *Toxicological Profile for Beryllium*. Atlanta, GA: U.S. Department of Health and Human Services, Public Health Service.

Section 21.3

Black Lung

Reprinted from "Coal Workers' Pneumoconiosis (Black Lung)," U.S. Department of Labor, Mine Safety and Health Administration. The text of this document is available online at http://www.msha.gov/S&HINFO/ BlackLung/blacklung.pdf; accessed October 2007.

Coal workers' pneumoconiosis (black lung) continues to occur among coal miners. Preventing the disease requires the commitment of both miners and mine operators to ensure exposures to harmful levels of coal mine dust are limited.

What is black lung?

Black lung is a job-related disease caused by continued exposure to excessive amounts of respirable coal mine dust. This dust becomes imbedded in the lungs, causing them to harden, making breathing very difficult.

Silicosis is another job-related lung disease included in black lung. Miners develop silicosis when they are overexposed to dust containing silica. Respirable particles of silica embed in the lungs, causing scar tissue to form, reducing the lung's ability to extract oxygen from the air.

What are the symptoms of black lung?

In the early stage of the illness, there may be no immediate symptoms. However, the latter stages of the disease, known as progressive massive fibrosis or PMF, will cause shortness of breath, coughing, and pain during breathing. PMF may result in permanent disability and early death.

How can I find out if I have black lung?

Black lung can be detected by x-ray and pulmonary function tests. Every operator of an underground coal mine is required to have an x-ray plan approved by the National Institute for Occupational Safety and Health (NIOSH). At intervals not to exceed five years, x-rays must be offered to employees at no cost. Results must be kept confidential.

There is no requirement for x-rays to be offered to surface coal miners by mine operators. Surface coal miners should notify their doctor that they may be exposed to coal mine dust which may contain silica, so that appropriate tests may be performed.

What happens if NIOSH discovers black lung on my x-ray?

If you are determined to have black lung, you will be notified by the Mine Safety and Health Administration (MSHA) of the results of your x-ray and of the right to work in a low-dust area under the requirements of 30 CFR Part 90. If you choose to exercise this right, your mine environment will be evaluated by dust sampling. If it is found to be too dusty, controls may be put into place to lower dust concentrations, or you may be moved to a less dusty area of the mine.

What can I do to reduce the potential of developing black lung?

You should be familiar with your mine's ventilation plan dust control provisions, make use of dust controls such as scrubbers and dry dust collectors, utilize respirators when necessary, and at underground coal mines ensure that a respirable dust control on-shift examination is conducted.

Section 21.4

Byssinosis

Alternative Names: Cotton worker's lung; Cotton bract disease; Mill fever; Brown lung

Definition: Byssinosis is a disease of the lungs caused by breathing in cotton dust or dusts from other vegetable fibers such as flax, hemp, or sisal while at work.

Causes: Breathing in the dust produced in the textile industry can cause byssinosis. People who are sensitive can have an asthma-like condition after being exposed to dust. In those with asthma, being exposed to the dust makes breathing more difficult, but in byssinosis, the symptoms usually go away by the end of the workweek. After long periods of exposure, symptoms can continue throughout the week without improving.

Methods of prevention in the U.S. have reduced the number of cases, but byssinosis is still common in developing countries. Smoking increases the risk for this disease. Being exposed to the dust many times can lead to chronic lung disease and shortness of breath or wheezing.

Symptoms:

- Chest tightness
- Cough
- Wheezing

Symptoms will get worse at the beginning of the workweek, and then improve while you are away from the workplace, or later in the workweek.

Exams and tests: Your health care provider will take a detailed medical history, and will ask many questions to try to find out whether your symptoms relate to certain exposures or times of exposure. The health care provider will also do a physical exam, with special attention to the lungs. Other tests include: chest x-ray; pulmonary function tests.

Treatment: The most important treatment is to stop exposure to the dust. Reducing dust levels in the factory (by improving machinery or ventilation) will help prevent byssinosis. Some people may have to change jobs to avoid further exposure.

Medications such as bronchodilators will usually improve symptoms. Corticosteroids may be prescribed in more severe cases.

Stopping smoking is very important for people with this condition. Respiratory treatments, including nebulizers and postural drainage, may be prescribed if the condition becomes chronic. Home oxygen therapy may also be needed if blood oxygen levels are low.

Physical exercise programs, breathing exercises, and patient education programs are often very helpful for people with a chronic lung disease.

Support Groups: Attending support groups with others who are affected by similar diseases can often help you understand your disease and adjust to the treatments and lifestyle changes required.

Outlook (prognosis): Symptoms usually improve after stopping exposure to the dust. Continued exposure can lead to damaged lung function. In the U.S., worker's compensation may be available to people with byssinosis.

Possible complications: Chronic lung disease may develop.

When to contact a medical professional: Call your health care provider if you have symptoms of byssinosis.

Prevention: Controlling dust, using face masks, and other measures can reduce the risk. Stop smoking, especially if you work in textile manufacturing.

Section 21.5

Farmer's Lung (Hypersensitivity Pneumonitis)

Reprinted from "Hypersensitivity Pneumonitis," © 2008 A.D.A.M., Inc. Reprinted with permission. Updated March 16, 2007.

Alternative names: Extrinsic allergic alveolitis; Farmer's lung; Mushroom picker's disease; Humidifier or air-conditioner lung; Bird breeder's lung

Definition: Hypersensitivity pneumonitis is inflammation of the lungs due to breathing in a foreign substance, usually certain types of dust, fungus, or molds.

Causes: Hypersensitivity pneumonitis usually occurs in those who work in places where there are high levels of organic dusts, fungus, or molds. For example, farmer's lung is the most common type of hypersensitivity pneumonitis. Repeated or intense exposure to dust from moldy hay, straw, and grain can lead to lung inflammation and acute lung disease. Over time, this acute condition may turn into long-lasting (chronic) lung disease.

The condition may also result from fungus present in humidifiers, heating systems, and air conditioners found in homes and offices. Exposure to certain bird droppings (for example, among bird owners) can also lead to hypersensitivity pneumonitis.

Symptoms: Symptoms of acute hypersensitivity pneumonitis may occur four to six hours after you have left the area where the foreign substance is found. These symptoms may include: cough; fever; chills; shortness of breath; malaise (feeling ill).

Symptoms of chronic hypersensitivity pneumonitis may include: breathlessness, especially with exertion; cough, often dry; loss of appetite; unintentional weight loss.

Exams and tests: Your doctor may hear abnormal lung sounds called crackles (rales) when listening to your chest with a stethoscope.

Lung changes due to chronic hypersensitivity pneumonitis may be seen on chest x-ray. Other tests may include:

- Pulmonary function tests;
- Complete blood count (CBC);
- Hypersensitivity pneumonitis antibody panels;
- Aspergillus precipitins test;
- High-resolution computed tomography (CT) scan of the chest;
- Bronchoscopy with washings and biopsy;
- Video-assisted or open-lung biopsy.

Treatment: First, the foreign substance must be identified. Treatment involves avoiding this substance in the future. Some people may need to change jobs if they cannot avoid the substance at work.

If you have a chronic form of this disease, your doctor will give you glucocorticoids (power anti-inflammatory medicines).

Outlook (prognosis): Most symptoms go away when you avoid or limit your exposure to the material that caused the problem.

Possible complications: The chronic form of this disease may lead to pulmonary fibrosis (a scarring of the lung tissue that is often not reversible).

When to contact a medical professional: Call your health care provider if symptoms of hypersensitivity pneumonitis develop.

Prevention: The chronic form can be prevented by avoiding the material that causes the lung inflammation.

References

Hoppin JA, Umbach DM, Kullman GJ, et al. Pesticides and other Agricultural Factors Associated with Self-reported Farmer's lung among Farm Residents in the Agricultural Health Study. *Occup Environ Med.* 2006 Dec 20;[Epub ahead of print].

Lacasse Y, Cormier Y. Hypersensitivity pneumonitis. *Orphanet J Rare Dis.* 2006 Jul 3;1:25.

Section 21.6

Flavorings-Related Lung Disease

Reprinted from "Flavorings-Related Lung Disease Health Effects,"
U. S. Department of Labor, Occupational Safety and Health Administration, August 10, 2006.

What are the health effects of flavorings-related lung disease?

Exposure to certain airborne flavorings is associated with higher rates of respiratory symptoms such as cough, fatigue, and difficulty breathing with exertion or exercise. Studies have shown an association with occupational exposure to certain flavorings and the development of lung disease characterized by fixed airways obstruction. Some employees exposed to these flavorings have developed permanent lung damage including a rare disease called bronchiolitis obliterans.[1,2]

How is flavorings-related lung disease diagnosed?

Individuals with flavorings-related lung disease may have respiratory symptoms and/or abnormal spirometry findings of fixed airways obstruction. Spirometry is a test that evaluates lung function. Fixed airways obstruction is diagnosed when the person tested has difficulty blowing air out of the lungs (obstruction) and this difficulty does not improve with asthma medication, indicating a fixed obstruction.

Employees exposed to certain airborne flavorings may complain of respiratory symptoms such as cough, fatigue, and difficulty breathing with exertion. These symptoms may vary in range from mild to severe. Usually symptoms progress gradually, but in some cases severe symptoms can occur suddenly. The symptoms usually do not get better when employees leave the workplace or go on vacation.[1]

What is the treatment for flavorings-related lung disease?

Employers and employees need to make sure that healthcare providers are aware of potential airborne exposures to flavorings in the

399

workplace. The finding of fixed airways obstruction in an exposed employee, especially in a symptomatic individual, should be investigated for possible occupational lung disease, including bronchiolitis obliterans.

Healthcare providers should advise employees about workplace exposures that may possibly aggravate or worsen existing lung disease. Recommendations and options for restricting employee exposure should be discussed.[1] Affected employees may notice a gradual improvement in their cough after they are removed from the flavoring exposure, but this may take years. Unfortunately, the shortness of breath with exertion often persists even after the cough has improved.

Patients with severe lung disease including bronchiolitis obliterans are usually treated with steroid medication, although most have not experienced significant improvement of their illness with this treatment. Patients with severe disease may require a lung transplant.

Can exposure to flavorings cause any other adverse health effects?

Employees may experience eye, nose, throat, and skin irritation after occupational exposure to certain flavorings. Chemical eye burns have also been noted. Additionally, there is some evidence that occupational asthma may be associated with workplace exposure to certain flavorings.[1]

What is bronchiolitis obliterans?

Bronchiolitis obliterans is a very rare lung disease that occurs when the smallest airways of the lung become inflamed and scarred, resulting in thickening and narrowing (obstruction) of the airways. This obstruction interferes with ventilation, the movement of air in the lungs.[3]

How is bronchiolitis obliterans diagnosed?

There are several diagnostic tools available to diagnose bronchiolitis obliterans. Spirometry is a test that evaluates lung function. Patients with bronchiolitis obliterans often have spirometry findings of fixed airways obstruction. Some patients also show restriction on spirometry, which means that the lungs have decreased ability to expand.

Additional tests include chest x-rays, which are often normal, but may show hyperinflation (too much air trapped in the lungs). Another imaging test, high resolution computerized tomography scans (CT or CAT scans), may also show air trapping and thickening of the airway walls. If a biopsy or tissue sample of the lungs is performed, narrowing or complete obstruction of the small airways may be seen when the tissue is examined with a microscope.[1,2,3]

What causes bronchiolitis obliterans?

Bronchiolitis obliterans has been diagnosed in employees with occupational exposures to certain flavorings or certain irritant gasses such as ammonia, chlorine, or sulfur dioxide. People who have had organ transplants or who have connective tissue disorders such as rheumatoid arthritis and lupus can develop bronchiolitis obliterans. Some respiratory infections caused by viruses or bacteria and certain medications are also associated with the development of bronchiolitis obliterans. Although many diseases or occupational exposures are associated with bronchiolitis obliterans, it is actually a rare disease.[1,2,3]

References

1. *Preventing Lung Disease in Workers Who Use or Make Flavorings.* US Department of Health and Human Services (DHHS), National Institute for Occupational Safety and Health (NIOSH) Publication No. 2004-110, (2003).

2. Kreiss, K., et al. "Clinical bronchiolitis obliterans in workers at a microwave-popcorn plant." *New England Journal of Medicine* 347.5(2002): 330–38.

3. Lazarus, S. *Murray & Nadel's Textbook of Respiratory Medicine.* "Chapter 41: Disorders of Intrathoracic Airways". 4th ed. Saunders: Philadelphia, (2005): 1295–1310.

4. Akpinar-Elci M., et al. "Bronchiolitis obliterans syndrome in popcorn production plant workers." *European Respiratory Journal* 24(2004): 298–302.

Section 21.7

Flock Worker's Lung

Excerpted from "Industrial Lung Disease," by Jennifer Vavra, *RT for Decision Makers in Respiratory Care*, December 2000. © Ascend Media. Reprinted with permission. Reviewed by David A. Cooke, M.D., March 2008.

Flock worker's lung is another current industrial lung disease. While the name may imply avian involvement, this is actually not the case. Flock worker's lung is exclusive to employees of the rotary cut synthetic materials industry. Rotary cut nylon, polyester, rayon, textile waste, and other synthetic fibers produce a powder of short fibers that are then adhesive coated to fabrics and other objects to produce a velvety surface.[1] Producing flock has been associated with an increased risk of workers developing chronic interstitial lung disease characterized by a lymphocytic bronchiolitis, bronchiolocentric nodular and diffuse lymphocytic interstitial infiltrates, and variable interstitial fibrosis.[1]

There are two methods for cutting flock. All but two companies, located in the United States, cut the long cables (tow) of nylon, rayon, and polyester with guillotines that produce precision-cut flock of a defined length.[1] The American companies use rotary cutters that are much faster but produce less precisely cut flock.[1] The twenty-four reported cases of identified flock worker's lung arose among workers using rotary cutting methods.[1] While guillotine blades emit a certain sound when the blade becomes dull, it is much more difficult to detect a dull blade on a rotary cutter.[1] Dull rotary blades are more likely to produce flock with tiny protrusions, which during further processing may be released as respirable-sized particles.[1] Kern et al.[1] refer to recent studies that suggest that respirable-sized nylon particles have substantial pulmonary toxicity.

Symptoms of flock worker's lung include a persistent dry cough and dyspnea with or without abnormal pain in the chest.[1] Chest radiographs may reveal diffuse patchy infiltrates.[1] High-resolution computed tomography (HRCT) scans may show scattered areas of consolidation, patchy ground glass opacity, and peripheral honeycombing.[1] To date, HRCT scans are the most effective noninvasive tests when detecting flock worker's lung in the early stages.[1] Pulmonary function tests (PFTs) may show restrictive, or occasional obstructive or normal, physiology.[1] Flock exposure may cause different lung injury to different people.[2] Ratios of interstitial lung disease have been reported to be 48 to 250 times greater for flock workers than for the general population.[1]

Kern et al.[1] believe that the accompanying diffuse interstitial inflammation that is presumably responsible for the severely reduced diffusing capacity and interstitial fibrosis should be included in the diagnostic criteria proposed by the National Institute for Occupational Safety and Health (NIOSH). NIOSH emphasized the central role of a lymphocytic bronchiolitis and peribronchiolitis with associated lymphoid nodules in the histopathologic recognition of flock worker's lung.[1] Kern et al.,[1] however, believe that the case definition for flock worker's lung should focus on previous or ongoing work in the flock industry, constant respiratory symptoms, and histologic proof of interstitial lung disease without better explanation. Further, they propose an atypical dispersal of cell types on bronchoalveolar lavage (BAL), restrictive lung function, and HRCT findings of ground glass opacity or clear fibrosis as a substitute for the histologic standard. The efficacy of corticosteroids and other immunosuppressants remains undetermined to date. Removal from the environment is the only intervention that has been shown to make a positive and noticeable improvement.[1]

Contrary to Kern et al., Kuschner[2] has a different belief about the requirements and efficacy of diagnosis. In an editorial responding to the research by Kern et al., Kuschner[2] notes that diagnosis may be difficult because biomarkers of exposure and susceptibility and a 100 percent accurate flock disease marker are lacking. It is also suggested that the same criteria for diagnosis be applied to flock worker's lung that are applied to diagnosing other industrial lung diseases. Namely, clinicians should look for evidence that helps to establish a causal association between exposure and disease by considering data representing pulmonary health before exposure to the toxicant in question, past data and industrial hygiene data that help distinguish the probable dose and extent of exposure to the toxicant, evaluation of other likely toxicants, data signifying that the inception and progression of lung damage are temporally connected to the toxicant exposure, stabilization or the end of lung disease following termination of exposure, and decline in respiratory health during an exposure-free period. Kuschner[2] warns that stringent terminology used to describe health and illness may make a comprehensive understanding of such terms elusive.

Kern et al.[1] acknowledge that the causative role for rotary cut flock and the relatively high concentrations of air contaminants (or both) remains unclear and the possibility of rotary cut flock—specifically nylon—being a carcinogen is suggested but not proven. However, NIOSH studies appear to implicate respirable-sized nylon particulates as a source for industrial lung disease.[1] Kuschner agrees[2] that a growing body of evidence links respirable flock exposure with disease and believes a careful medical history, PFT, physical examination, industrial hygiene data, radiographic studies, and possibly BAL should garner enough information to make a diagnosis. Further, it has been proposed that a lung biopsy may be more helpful in ruling out other lung diseases than identifying flock worker's lung.[2]

To better understand flock worker's lung and relevant terminology, Kern et al.[1] suggest that further laboratory and field studies are needed to assess the prevalence of this condition. This research may need to concentrate on the role that heat, dull cutting blades, and mechanical shearing play in the development of flock worker's lung. Also of interest may be alternate current versus direct current flocking in the origination of respirable-sized flock particulates. In addition, guillotine versus rotary cut flock should be examined, as well as air concentration of respirable dust. The relative toxicity of nylon, polyester, rayon, and textile waste fragments should be considered and air concentrations of respirable particulates and corresponding higher rates of interstitial lung disease should be investigated.[1]

References

1. Kern DG, Kuhn C III, Ely EW, et al. Flock worker's lung: broadening the spectrum of clinicopathology, narrowing the spectrum of suspected etiologies. *Chest*. 2000;117:251–59.

2. Kuschner WG. What exactly is flock worker's lung? *Chest*. 2000;117:10–13.

Section 21.8

Occupational Asthma

"OSH Answers: Asthma," http://www/ccpjs/ca/psjamswers/diseases/asthma
.html, Canadian Centre for Occupational Health and Safety (CCOHS),
2005. Reproduced with permission of CCOHS, 2007. [Editor's Note: British spellings for drug and chemical names have been retained; please talk to your physician if you have questions about equivalent spellings in other countries.]

What is occupational asthma?

Asthma is a respiratory disease. It creates narrowing of the air passages that results in difficult breathing, tightness of the chest, coughing, and breath-sounds such as wheezing.

Occupational asthma refers to asthma that is caused by breathing in specific agents in the workplace. An abnormal response of the body to the presence of an agent in the workplace causes occupational asthma.

The abnormal response, called "sensitization," develops after variable periods of workplace exposure to certain dusts, fumes, or vapours.

This sensitization may not show any symptoms of disease or it may be associated with skin rashes (urticaria), hay fever-like symptoms, or a combination of these symptoms.

Not all workers react with an asthmatic response when exposed to industrial agents. Asthma strikes only a fraction of workers. Asthmatic attacks can be controlled either by ending exposure to the agent responsible or by medical treatment.

How does asthma develop?

Asthma is triggered in several ways and most of them are not completely understood. For simplicity, we categorize them into two groups: allergic and non-allergic.

Allergic asthma: Allergic asthma involves the body's immune system. This is a complex defense system that protects the body from harm caused by foreign substances or microbes. Among the most important

405

elements of the defense mechanism are special proteins called "antibodies." These are produced when the human body contacts an alien substance or microbe. Antibodies react with substances or microbes to destroy them. Antibodies are often very selective, acting only on one particular substance or type of microbe.

But antibodies can also respond in a wrong way and cause allergic disorders such as asthma. After a period of exposure to an industrial substance, either natural or synthetic, a worker may start producing too many of the antibodies called "immunoglobulin E" (IgE). These antibodies attach to specific cells in the lung in a process known as "sensitization."

When re-exposure occurs, the lung cells with attached IgE antibodies react with the substance. This reaction results in the release of chemicals such as "leukotrienes" that are made in the body. Leukotrienes provoke the contraction of some muscles in the airways. This causes the narrowing of air passages which is characteristic of asthma.

Non-allergic asthma: Following repeated exposure to an industrial chemical, substances such as leukotrienes are released in the lungs. Again, the leukotriene causes narrowing of air passages typical of asthma. The reasons for such release are still not clear because no antibody reaction seems to be involved.

Other types of asthma: In certain circumstances, symptoms of asthma may develop suddenly (within twenty-four hours) following exposure to high airborne concentrations of respiratory irritants such as chlorine. This condition is known as reactive airways dysfunction syndrome (RADS). The symptoms may persist for months or years when the sensitized person is re-exposed to irritants. RADS is controversial because of its rarity and the lack of good information on how the lungs are affected and the range of substances which cause it.

How long does asthma take to develop?

There is no fixed period of time in which asthma can develop. Asthma as a disease may develop from a few weeks to many years after the initial exposure. Studies carried out on some platinum refinery workers show that in most cases asthma develops in six to twelve months. But it may occur within ten days or be delayed for as long as twenty-five years.

Analysis of the respiratory responses of sensitized workers has established three basic patterns of asthmatic attacks, as follows:

- **Immediate:** Typically develops within minutes of exposure and is at its worst after approximately twenty minutes; recovery takes about two hours.

- **Late:** Can occur in different forms. It usually starts several hours after exposure and is at its worst after about four to eight hours with recovery within twenty-four hours. However, it can start one hour after exposure with recovery in three to four hours. In some cases, it may start at night, with a tendency to recur at the same time for a few nights following a single exposure.

- **Dual or combined:** Is the occurrence of both immediate and late types of asthma.

How common is asthma?

The frequency of occupational asthma is unknown, although various estimates are available. In Japan, 15 percent of asthma in males is believed to be occupational. In the United States, 2 percent of all cases of asthma are thought to be of occupational origin. The number of cases of occupational asthma varies from country to country and from industry to industry. About 6 percent of animal handlers develop asthma due to animal hair or dust. Between 10 and 45 percent of workers who process subtilisins, the "proteolytic enzymes" like "Bacillus subtilis" in the detergent industry develop asthma. However, preparations of the enzymes in granulated form, which is less readily inhaled, have reduced the likelihood of asthma. Approximately 5 percent of workers exposed to such chemicals as isocyanates and certain wood dusts develop asthma.

What factors increase the chances of developing asthma?

Some workplace conditions seem to increase the likelihood that workers will develop asthma, but their importance is not fully known. Factors such as the properties of the chemicals, and the amount and duration of exposure are obviously important. However, because only a fraction of exposed workers are affected, factors unique to individual workers can also be important. Such factors include the ability of some people to produce abnormal amounts of IgE antibodies. The contribution of cigarette smoking to asthma is not known. But smokers are more likely than nonsmokers to develop respiratory problems in general.

How does the doctor know if a worker has asthma?

Sufferers from occupational asthma experience attacks of difficult breathing, tightness of the chest, coughing, and breath sounds such as wheezing, which is associated with air-flow obstruction. Such symptoms should raise the suspicion of asthma. Typically these symptoms are worse on working days, often awakening the patient at night, and improving when the person is away from work. While off work, sufferers from occupational asthma may still have chest symptoms when exposed to airway irritants such as dusts, or fumes, or upon exercise. Itchy and watery eyes, sneezing, stuffy and runny nose, and skin rashes are other symptoms often associated with asthma.

Lung function tests and skin tests can help to confirm the disease. But some patients with occupational asthma may have normal lung function as well as negative skin tests.

The diagnosis of work-related asthma needs to be confirmed objectively. This can be done by carrying out pulmonary function tests at work and off work. Specific inhalation challenges can demonstrate the occupational origin of asthma and may identify the agents responsible when the cause is uncertain. Specific inhalation challenge tests require breathing in small quantities of industrial agents that may induce an attack of asthma. But they are safe when performed by experienced physicians in specialized centres.

How can we control occupational asthma?

Although there are drugs that may control the symptoms of asthma, it is important to stop exposure. If the exposure to the causal agent is not stopped, treatment will be needed continuously and the breathing problems may become permanent. People may continue to suffer from occupational asthma even after removal from exposure. For example, a follow-up study of seventy-five patients with asthma caused by red cedar dust showed that only half the patients recovered. The remaining half continued to have asthmatic attacks for a period of one to nine years after the termination of exposure.

Dust masks and respirators can help to control workplace exposure. However, these protective devices, in order to be effective, must be carefully selected, properly fitted, and well maintained. Preventing further exposure might involve a change of job. If a job change is not feasible, relocation to another area of the plant with no exposure may be essential.

How can we prevent occupational asthma?

The best way to prevent occupational asthma is to replace dangerous substances with less harmful ones. Where this is not possible, exposure should be minimized through engineering controls such as ventilation and enclosures of processes.

Education of workers is also very important. Proper handling procedures, avoidance of spills, and good housekeeping reduce the occurrence of occupational asthma.

What occupations are at risk for asthma?

Some of the occupations where asthma has been seen are listed in the following tables. It should be noted that the lists of occupational substances and microbes which can cause asthma are not complete. New causes continue to be added. New materials and new processes introduce new exposures and create new risks.

Table 21.1. Causes of Occupational Asthma: Grains, Flours, Plants, and Gums

Occupation	Agent
Bakers, millers	Wheat
Chemists, coffee bean baggers and handlers, gardeners, millers, oil industry workers, farmers	Castor beans
Cigarette factory workers	Tobacco dust
Drug manufacturers, mold makers in sweet factories, printers	Gum acacia
Farmers, grain handlers	Grain dust
Gum manufacturers, sweet makers	Gum tragacanth
Strawberry growers	Strawberry pollen
Tea sifters and packers	Tea dust
Tobacco farmers	Tobacco leaf
Woolen industry workers	Wool

Table 21.2. Causes of Occupational Asthma: Animals, Insects, and Fungi (continued on next page)

Occupation	Agent
Bird fanciers	Avian proteins
Cosmetic manufacturers	Carmine
Entomologists	Moths, butterflies
Feather pluckers	Feathers

Table 21.2. Causes of Occupational Asthma: Animals, Insects, and Fungi (continued from previous page)

Occupation	Agent
Field contact workers	Crickets
Fish bait breeders	Bee moths
Flour mill workers, bakers, farm workers, grain handlers	Grain storage mites, alternaria, aspergillus
Laboratory workers	Locusts, cockroaches, grain weevils, rats, mice, guinea pigs, rabbits
Mushroom cultivators	Mushroom spores
Oyster farmers	Hoya
Pea sorters	Mexican bean weevils
Pigeon breeders	Pigeons
Poultry workers	Chickens
Prawn processors	Prawns
Silkworm sericulturers	Silkworms
Zoological museum curators	Beetles

Table 21.3. Causes of Occupational Asthma: Chemicals/Materials (continued on next page)

Occupation	Agent
Aircraft fitters	Triethyltetramine
Aluminum cable solderers	Aminoethylethanolamine
Aluminum pot room workers	Fluorine
Auto body workers	Acrylates (resins, glues, sealants, adhesives)
Brewery workers	Chloramine-T
Chemical plant workers, pulp mill workers	Chlorine
Dye weighers	Levafix brilliant yellow, drimarene brilliant yellow and blue, cibachrome brilliant scarlet
Electronics workers	Colophony
Epoxy resin manufacturers	Tetrachlorophthalic anhydride
Foundry mold makers	Furan-based resin binder systems
Fur dyers	Para-phenylenediamine
Hairdressers	Persulphate salts
Health care workers	Glutaraldehyde, latex

410

Table 21.3. Causes of Occupational Asthma: Chemicals/Materials (continued from previous page)

Occupation	Agent
Laboratory workers, nurses, phenolic resin molders	Formalin/formaldehyde
Meat wrappers	Polyvinyl chloride vapour
Paint manufacturers, plastic molders, tool setters	Phthalic anhydride
Paint sprayers	Dimethylethanolamine
Photographic workers, shellac manufacturers	Ethylenediamine
Refrigeration industry workers	chlorofluorocarbons (CFCs)
Solderers	Polyether alcohol, polypropylene glycol

Table 21.4. Causes of Occupational Asthma: Isocyanates and Metals

Occupation	Agent
Boat builders, foam manufacturers, office workers, plastics factory workers, refrigerator manufacturers, (TDI) manufacturers/users, printers, laminators, tinners, toy makers	Toluene diisocyanate
Boiler cleaners, gas turbine cleaners	Vanadium
Car sprayers	Hexamethylene diisocyanate
Cement workers	Potassium dichromate
Chrome platers, chrome polishers	Sodium bichromate, chromic acid, potassium chromate
Nickel platers	Nickel sulphate
Platinum chemists	Chloroplatinic acid
Platinum refiners	Platinum salts
Polyurethane foam manufacturers, printers, laminators	Diphenylmethane diisocyanate
Rubber workers	Naphthalene diisocyanate
Tungsten carbide grinders	Cobalt
Welders	Stainless steel fumes

411

Table 21.5. Causes of Occupational Asthma: Drugs and Enzymes

Occupation	Agent
Ampicillin manufacturers	Phenylglycine acid chloride
Detergent manufacturers	Bacillus subtilis
Enzyme manufacturers	Fungal alpha-amylase
Food technologists, laboratory workers	Papain
Pharmacists	Gentian powder, flaviastase
Pharmaceutical workers	Methyldopa, salbutamol, dichloramine, piperazine dihydrochloride, spiramycin, penicillins, sulphathiazole, sulphonechloramides, chloramine-T, phosdrin, pancreatic extracts
Poultry workers	Amprolium hydrochloride
Process workers, plastic polymer production workers	Trypsin, bromelin

Table 21.6. Causes of Occupational Asthma: Woods

Occupation	Agent
Carpenters, timber millers, woodworkers	Western red cedar, cedar of Lebanon, iroko, California redwood, ramin, African zebrawood
Sawmill workers, pattern makers	Mansonia, oak, mahogany, abiruana
Wood finishers	Cocabolla
Wood machinists	Kejaat

Section 21.9

Silicosis

Excerpted from "Silicosis: Learn the Facts!"
National Institute for Occupational Safety and Health, U.S.
Centers for Disease Control and Prevention, August 2004.

Do you work in construction or do abrasive blasting? If so, here are some important facts you need to know:

- Since 1968, more than fourteen thousand workers in the United States have died from a disease called silicosis.

- In the United States each year more than two hundred workers die with this disease while hundreds more become disabled.

- Many workers with silicosis are only in their thirties; some are as young as twenty-two years old. Many of them are unable to take care of themselves and their families.

What Is Silicosis and How Can You Avoid or Prevent It?

Silicosis is a disabling and often fatal lung disease caused by breathing dust that has very small pieces of crystalline silica in it. Crystalline silica is found in concrete, masonry, sandstone, rock, paint, and other abrasives. The cutting, breaking, crushing, drilling, grinding, or abrasive blasting of these materials may produce fine silica dust. It can also be in soil, mortar, plaster, and shingles. The very small pieces of silica dust get in the air that you breathe and become trapped in your lungs. Even the very small pieces of dust that you cannot see will harm you. As the dust builds up in your lungs, the lungs are damaged and it becomes harder to breathe.

Are You Breathing Silica Dust?

If you do one of the following jobs, you are at risk for breathing silica dust:

- Removal of paint and rust with power tools;

- Abrasive blasting of bridges, pipes, tanks, and other painted surfaces especially while using silica sand;
- Grinding mortar;
- Abrasive blasting of concrete (many bridges and buildings are made of concrete);
- Crushing, loading, hauling, chipping, hammering, drilling, and dumping of rock or concrete;
- Chipping, hammering, drilling, sawing, and grinding concrete or masonry;
- Demolition of concrete and masonry structures;
- Dry sweeping or pressurized air-blowing of concrete or dust; or
- Jackhammering on various materials.

Who Is at Risk?

Workers in the following occupations are at risk for developing silicosis:

- Highway and bridge construction and repair
- Building construction, demolition, and repair
- Abrasive blasting
- Masonry work
- Concrete finishing
- Drywall finishing
- Rock drilling
- Mining
- Sand and gravel screening
- Rock crushing (for road base)

Types of Silicosis

There are three types of silicosis:

1. **Chronic silicosis:** Usually occurs after ten or more years of exposure to crystalline silica at low levels. This is the most common type of silicosis.

2. **Accelerated silicosis:** Results from exposure to higher levels of crystalline silica and occurs five to ten years after exposure.

3. **Acute silicosis:** Can occur after only weeks or months of exposure to very high levels of crystalline silica. Death occurs within months. The lungs drown in their own fluids.

Symptoms

Symptoms may not appear in the early stages of chronic silicosis. In fact, chronic silicosis may go undetected for fifteen to twenty years after exposure. As silicosis progresses, symptoms may include:

- Shortness of breath;
- Severe cough;
- Weakness.

Because the body's ability to fight infections may be weakened by silica in the lungs, other illnesses (such as tuberculosis) may result and can cause:

- Fever;
- Weight loss;
- Night sweats;
- Chest pains;
- Respiratory failure.

These symptoms can become worse over time, leading to death.

What Can I Do to Protect Myself and My Family?

Silicosis is a disabling and often fatal disease that prevents hundreds of workers from being able to care for their families. It could also prevent you from providing for your family. If your work causes you to breathe silica dust, there are things you can do to prevent silicosis from happening to you:

- Be aware of the health effects of breathing air that has silica dust in it.
- Avoid working in dust whenever possible.
- Know what causes silica dust at your workplace.
- Remember if there is no visible dust, you could be at risk. If there is visible dust, you are almost definitely at risk.

- Reduce the amount of silica dust by using water sprays and ventilation when working in confined structures. For example, use a water hose to wet dust before it becomes airborne, use saws that add water to the blade, use drills that add water through the stem or have dust collection systems, and use blast cleaning machines or cabinets to control dust.

- When water sprays and ventilation alone are not enough to reduce silica dust levels, your employer must provide you with a properly fitted and selected respirator (e.g., particulate filter or airline supplied air respirator) designated for protection against crystalline silica.

- Changes should not be made to the respirator.

- Workers who use tight-fitting respirators cannot have beards or mustaches because they do not let the respirator properly seal to the face.

- Take health (or lung screening) programs offered by your employer.

- Sandblasting or abrasive blasting requires the highest level of protection, which is a type CE abrasive blasting respirator.

- Practice good personal hygiene at the workplace:

- Do not eat, drink, or use tobacco products in dusty areas.

- Wash hands and face before eating, drinking, or smoking outside dusty areas.

- Park cars where they will not be contaminated with silica.

- Change into disposable or washable work clothes at the worksite.

- Shower (if possible) and change into clean clothes before leaving the worksite to prevent contamination of other work areas, cars, and homes.

It is your employers' legal responsibility to provide a safe workplace. If you think you are not protected call OSHA at 800-321-OSHA (6742) or go to the OSHA website: www.osha.gov.

Your employer must make sure that you have the proper protective equipment for reducing silica dust levels; but, it's up to you to use them! Taking time to protect yourself on the job is worth it. After all, nothing is more important than your health and the health of your family!

What Type of Respirator Should I Use?

Choosing the right respirator that fits you snugly is important for protecting your health. Your employer will help you choose the type of respirator you need. Always use NIOSH-approved respirators. The type of respirator you need depends on:

- The amount of silica dust to which you are exposed; and

- The kind of work you need to do.

If you must do abrasive blasting, use only a type CE pressure demand abrasive blasting respirator.

Respirators used for protection from crystalline silica should not cause undue discomfort. If you have problems with your respirators, report immediately to your supervisor.

Chapter 22

Other Inflammatory Lung Diseases

Chapter Contents

Section 22.1

Bronchiolitis Obliterans Organizing Pneumonia

What is bronchiolitis obliterans organizing pneumonia (BOOP)?

BOOP is a swelling of the small airways in the lung. The swelling causes blockages in the outermost parts of the lung. BOOP gets its name from the fact that it closely mimics pneumonia infections. It affects men and women equally, usually beginning in their forties or fifties, but has been reported in children with underlying cancer. It occurs in six to seven in every one hundred thousand people.

What causes BOOP?

BOOP can be classified according to whether the cause is known, it is unknown but occurs in a specific or relevant context, or, in approximately half the cases, has no apparent cause (this is called "idiopathic").
BOOP has many causes, including:

- Infection;

- Toxic and fume exposure (most commonly nitrogen dioxide);

- Collagen vascular disease (rheumatoid arthritis, systemic lupus erythematosus);

- Bone marrow and heart-lung or lung transplantation;

- Drug reaction (penicillin).

How is BOOP diagnosed?

In almost three-quarters of people symptoms last less than two months. Few people have symptoms for less than six months before diagnosis. A flu-like illness, characterized by cough, fever, malaise, fatigue, and weight loss, signals the onset of BOOP in two-fifths of people. Inspiratory crackles are frequently heard on chest examination. Diagnosis may involve pulmonary function tests, chest x-rays, a computed tomography (CT) scan, or a lung biopsy.

What is the treatment for BOOP?

If you have an underlying infection, your health professional will give you antibiotics. If a toxin causes BOOP, you should stop all contact with it straight away. In most cases, you will need steroids. Corticosteroid therapy results in clinical recovery in two-thirds of people. Prednisone is the most common steroid treatment. If you do not respond well to steroids (usually people with nonidiopathic BOOP) your health professional will prescribe immunosuppressants.

Can you recover from BOOP?

Sixty-five percent of idiopathic BOOP people are completely cured. Twenty percent are left with fibrous (scarred) tissues in the lungs. Approximately 30 percent relapse after treatment. Only between 3 and 10 percent of people die from BOOP.

Section 22.2

Empyema

What Is Empyema?

The lung is lined by two thin membranes of pleura (inner visceral and outer parietal), which allows the lung to expand and shrink with each breath with minimal friction.

An empyema represents a collection of pus in the pleural space. This is the potential space between the two layers (parietal and visceral) of pleura.

Who Gets It?

It is difficult to calculate the incidence of empyema, but it most commonly occurs as a complication in pneumonia due to *Staphylococcus aureus*.

Predisposing Factors

A number of conditions are risk factors for the development of an empyema. Unresolved pneumonia, usually due to *S. aureus* (and particularly a lung abscess) can lead to infection that spreads to the pleural space (space between the lining of the chest cavity and the lung).

Other conditions such as bronchiectasis, airway-obstructing cancer, thoracic surgery, penetrating wounds, and secondary spread from a distant focus (particularly a subphrenic abscess) are all possible mechanisms of disease development.

Occasionally an empyema may arise as primary pathology (especially if due to mycobacteria or nocardia infection).

Progression

The natural course depends on the exact cause of the empyema. Possible complications include a bronchopleural fistula (which is a permanent communication between a bronchus and the pleural space)—allowing for air to enter the pleural space as well as the pus—leading to a pyopneumothorax (air or pus in the plural cavity).

Probable Outcomes

Usually empyema does not result in permanent pulmonary damage.

How Is It Diagnosed?

- A full blood count will demonstrate a high white cell count with raised platelets, C-reactive protein (CRP), and erythrocyte sedimentation rate (ESR).

- The chest x-ray will show a pleural effusion or a pleural mass. Loculations may be visible on the x-ray.

- Sputum and blood cultures are usually done to look for the causative organism.

How Is It Treated?

The basis of treatment is to drain the pus out with a chest drain. This should preferably be inserted underneath radiological guidance. If the effusion is organized and loculated then agents can be injected to break down the adhesions and allow free drainage (e.g., streptokinase or urokinase). Appropriate antibiotics should also be given. Antibiotics should continue for at least two weeks after the empyema is drained.

Surgery may be required if there are thick adhesions present that do not respond to fibrinolytic agents.

Section 22.3

Goodpasture Syndrome

Reprinted from "Goodpasture's Syndrome," National Institute of Diabetes and Digestive and Kidney Diseases, National Institutes of Health, NIH Publication No. 07-4558, April 2007.

What is Goodpasture syndrome?

Goodpasture syndrome is a rare disease that can affect the lungs and kidneys. Also called anti-glomerular basement antibody disease, it is an autoimmune disease—a condition in which the body's own defense system reacts against some part of the body itself. When the immune system is working normally, it creates antibodies to fight off germs. In Goodpasture syndrome, the immune system makes antibodies that attack the lungs and kidneys. Why this happens is not fully understood. Researchers have identified a number of possible causes, among them the presence of an inherited component; exposure to certain chemicals, including hydrocarbon solvents and the weed killer Paraquat; and viral infections.

What are the symptoms of Goodpasture syndrome?

Goodpasture syndrome can cause people to cough up blood or feel a burning sensation when urinating. But its first signs may be vague, such as fatigue, nausea, difficulty breathing, or paleness. These signs are followed by kidney involvement, represented first by small amounts of blood in the urine, protein in the urine, and other clinical and laboratory findings.

How is Goodpasture syndrome diagnosed?

To diagnose Goodpasture syndrome, doctors use a blood test, but a kidney or lung biopsy may be necessary to check for the presence of the harmful antibodies.

How is Goodpasture syndrome treated?

Goodpasture syndrome is treated with oral immunosuppressive drugs—cyclophosphamide and corticosteroids—to keep the immune system from making antibodies. Corticosteroid drugs may be given intravenously to control bleeding in the lungs. A process called plasmapheresis may be helpful and necessary to remove the harmful antibodies from the blood. In plasmapheresis, a patient's blood is drawn, about 300 milliliters at a time, and placed in a centrifuge to separate the red and white blood cells from the plasma. The cells are then placed in a plasma substitute and returned to the body. This procedure is usually done in combination with immunosuppressive drug treatment.

Goodpasture syndrome may last only a few weeks or as long as two years. Bleeding in the lungs can be very serious and even fatal in some cases. But Goodpasture syndrome does not usually lead to permanent lung damage. Damage to the kidneys, however, may be long lasting. If the kidneys fail, dialysis to remove waste products and extra fluid from the blood, or kidney transplantation, may become necessary.

Section 22.4

Lymphangioleiomyomatosis (LAM)

Reprinted from "LAM," National Heart Lung and Blood Institute,
National Institutes of Health, July 2006.

What Is LAM?

LAM, or lymphangioleiomyomatosis (lim-FAN-je-o-LI-o-MI-o-ma-TO-sis), is a rare lung disease that mostly affects women in their mid-forties.

In LAM, an unusual type of cell begins to grow out of control throughout your body, including in the lungs, lymph nodes and vessels, and kidneys.

Over time, these LAM cells form cysts and clusters of cells, which grow throughout the lungs and slowly block the airways. They also destroy the normal lung tissue and replace it with cysts. As a result, air cannot move freely in and out of the lungs, and the lungs cannot supply enough oxygen to the body's other organs.

More than one out of every three people with LAM also develops growths called angiomyolipomas (AN-je-o-my-o-li-PO-mas), or AMLs, in their kidneys. People with LAM also may develop growths in other organs, including the liver and brain and large tumors on their lymph nodes. There currently is no cure for LAM. The most common cause of death from LAM is respiratory failure.

There are two forms of LAM: sporadic LAM, which occurs for unknown reasons, and an often milder form of LAM that occurs in people with a rare inherited disease called tuberous sclerosis complex

The term "lymphangioleiomyomatosis" comes from the Greek. "Lymph" and "angio" refer to the lymph vessels, and "leiomyomas" refers to the type of cells involved in LAM.

Doctors have learned a lot about LAM in recent years. They are now able to diagnose the condition earlier and provide support services that improve patients' quality of life. Not too long ago, doctors thought that the life expectancy for women with LAM was less than ten years following diagnosis. We now know that some patients with LAM may survive for more than twenty years.

What Causes LAM?

Researchers do not know what causes LAM, or why it affects mostly women. They have recently discovered that LAM has some of the same features as another rare disease called tuberous sclerosis complex (TSC). This discovery has begun to provide some valuable clues about what causes LAM.

The common features of LAM and TSC are as follows:

- People with TSC develop growths in their kidneys that are the same as the angiomyolipomas that many people with LAM develop in their kidneys.

- About one out of every three women who has TSC develops cysts in her lungs that are the same as the ones women with LAM develop in their lungs.

TSC is a genetic disease. It is caused by abnormalities, or defects, in one of two genes. These genes are called TSC1 and TSC2. Normally, they make proteins that control the growth of the cells in the body. In people with TSC, the genes are abnormal, and the proteins that they make cannot control cell growth and movement.

LAM patients also have abnormal versions of the TSC1 and TSC2 genes, and researchers have discovered that these genes play a role in the development of LAM. More research on the TSC genes and the proteins that they make should shed new light on the causes of LAM.

Since LAM mostly affects women in their mid-forties, many doctors think that estrogen also plays a role in causing LAM.

Who Is at Risk for LAM?

LAM mostly affects women in their mid-forties. More than seven out of every ten patients are between the ages of twenty and forty when they begin to have symptoms. But LAM may occur in women as old as seventy to eighty. There are also a few reports of LAM occurring in men.

Today, about 675 women in the United States have been diagnosed with either LAM alone or LAM with tuberous sclerosis complex. Scientists believe that many more women have LAM, but they have been misdiagnosed with another more common lung disease, such as emphysema, asthma, or bronchitis.

Since LAM affects about three out of every ten women with TSC, there may be as many as ten thousand women in the United States who have TSC and undiagnosed LAM. Many of these women may have mild cases of LAM that are not causing symptoms. Not all TSC patients who have LAM have lung problems.

What Are the Signs and Symptoms of LAM?

The signs and symptoms of LAM are caused by the uncontrolled growth of the LAM cells.

The most common signs and symptoms are as follows:

- Shortness of breath, especially following exertion. At first, you may feel short of breath only during strenuous activity. Over time, you may have trouble breathing even during rest.

- Chest pain, usually caused by a collapsed lung.

- Frequent cough, sometimes with bloody phlegm.

LAM also can lead to other serious conditions:

- About six of every seven women with LAM develop a collapsed lung (pneumothorax) at some point. Sometimes one lung will collapse over and over again. Both lungs can collapse too. This is a serious condition that can be life threatening. A lung that is only partly collapsed may slowly re-expand without treatment, but treatment is often required.

- In one out of every three women with LAM, a fluid called lymph leaks into the chest cavity and builds up.

- Nearly half of the women with LAM develop growths called angiomyolipomas in their kidneys.

Many women with LAM also have the following:

- Blood or lymph in their sputum
- Blood in their urine
- Enlarged lymph nodes
- Abdominal swelling

Other diseases can cause many of these signs and symptoms and complications, so it is important that you see a doctor.

How Is LAM Diagnosed?

Methods for diagnosing LAM have improved, and it is now possible to diagnose it at an early stage.

Many of the signs and symptoms of LAM can be caused by other diseases such as asthma, emphysema, and bronchitis. It is important for your doctor to rule out those conditions before making a final diagnosis. Commonly used diagnostic tests include chest x-rays, lung function tests, exercise stress tests, blood tests, pulse oximetry, high-resolution computed tomography scans, and lung biopsies.

Some doctors recommend that once you are diagnosed with LAM, you have magnetic resonance imaging (MRI) of your head. This test can show if you have signs of tuberous sclerosis complex (TSC) or a growth in your brain called a meningioma. About one out of every twenty patients with LAM has this kind of growth. It also appears in people with TSC.

The National Institutes of Health is studying whether blood tests for the TSC1 and TSC2 genes may be helpful in diagnosing LAM patients.

How Is LAM Treated?

There is no treatment available yet to slow or stop the growth of the cell clusters and cysts that are the major feature of LAM.

Most treatments for LAM are aimed at relieving symptoms and preventing complications.

Since many women with LAM are now living so much longer, doctors also focus on treating other health problems that happen with menopause and aging.

The main treatments for LAM are as follows:

- Medicines

- Oxygen therapy

- Procedures to remove fluid from the chest or abdominal cavities and prevent it from building up again

- Procedures to remove angiomyolipomas (AMLs)

- Lung transplantation

Medicines

Some medicines may help open your lungs so that you can breathe more easily:

- Bronchodilators are drugs that relax the muscles around the airways. As a result, the airways can open up, making it easier to breathe. About one out of five women with LAM improves with the use of bronchodilators.

- Octreotide and diuretics are sometimes used to prevent the buildup of fluid in the chest cavity and abdomen. Octreotide may reduce leakage of lymph into the abdominal or chest cavity.

Women with LAM have a greater chance of developing osteoporosis (a condition that causes bones to become weak and brittle) than other women. If you have LAM, your doctor should measure your bone density. If you have lost bone density, your doctor may prescribe drugs that prevent bone loss. He or she also may prescribe calcium and vitamin D supplements.

Physicians who think that estrogen may play a role in the development of LAM usually treat their patients with hormone therapy.

Oxygen Therapy

If the level of oxygen in your blood is low, you may need oxygen therapy. Oxygen is usually given through nasal prongs or a mask. At first, you may need oxygen only while exercising. It also may help to use it while you are sleeping. Over time, you may need full-time oxygen therapy.

Your doctor may give you a standard exercise stress test or a six-minute walk test to find out whether you need oxygen while exercising. A blood test will show what your oxygen level is and how much oxygen you need.

Procedures to Remove Air or Fluid from the Chest or Abdomen

Several procedures help remove air or fluid from your chest and abdominal cavities and prevent them from building up in your chest cavity:

- Removing fluid from your chest or abdominal cavities may help relieve abdominal discomfort and shortness of breath. Your doctor can usually remove this fluid with a needle and syringe. If large amounts of fluid build up in your chest cavity, your doctor may have to insert a tube into your chest to remove it.

- Removing air from your chest cavity may relieve shortness of breath and chest pain caused by a collapsed lung. Your doctor can usually remove the air with a tube that is inserted into your chest cavity between your side ribs. The tube is usually attached to a suction device. If this procedure doesn't work, or if your lungs collapse frequently, you may need surgery.

• If lymph and air leak into your chest cavity often, your doctor may perform a procedure to fuse your lung and chest wall together and remove space for leakage. This procedure is called pleurodesis (ploo-ROD-e-sis). It involves injecting a chemical into the place where the leakage is happening. Your doctor may do it at your bedside, while you are under local anesthesia. It also can be done in the operating room by video-assisted thoracoscopy surgery, while you are under general anesthesia.

Procedures to Remove AMLs

If you have ongoing severe pain or bleeding caused by AMLs, surgery to remove some of the abdominal growths may be helpful. If the bleeding is not too severe, an experienced radiologist can often block the blood vessels feeding the AMLs. This may cause them to shrink.

Lung Transplantation

Surgery to replace one or both of your lungs with healthy lungs from a human donor may be helpful. Survival after a lung transplant for LAM is probably better than survival after a lung transplant for another condition, such as emphysema.

Lung transplantation has a high risk of complications.

In a few cases, doctors have found LAM cells in the new transplanted lungs and other parts of the body, but the LAM cells do not seem to prevent the transplanted lung from working.

Possible New Treatments for LAM

Researchers are now studying several medicines as possible treatments for LAM, including Rapamycin.

Rapamycin (sirolimus) is the first drug to show promise as a treatment that will slow or stop the development and growth of the LAM cell clusters. Doctors now use it to prevent the immune system from rejecting kidney transplants. Researchers are looking into whether this medicine can reduce the size of kidney AMLs in LAM and tuberous sclerosis complex (TSC) patients. They also are planning a larger study of the effects of Rapamycin, or another drug like it, on TSC and LAM patients. This study will test whether the drug can prevent or reverse the growth of the LAM cell clusters and cysts in other organs and slow the decline of lung function.

Living with LAM

In the early stages of LAM, you usually can go about your daily activities, including attending school, going to work, and performing common physical activities such as walking up a hill. Later on, it may be harder for you to be active. You also may require oxygen full time.

Ongoing medical care is important. Treatment by a pulmonologist who specializes in LAM is recommended. These specialists are usually located at major medical centers.

It is important for you to take good care of your health. This means following the same healthy lifestyle that is recommended for all Americans, including eating a healthy diet, being as physically active as you can, and getting plenty of rest. You also should not smoke.

You should check with your doctor before traveling by air or traveling to remote areas where medical attention is not readily available. You also should ask about travel to places where the amount of oxygen in the air is low.

If your lung function is normal, pregnancy may be an option, but you should discuss it first with both a pulmonologist who specializes in LAM and your obstetrician.

Most doctors do not recommend oral contraceptives (birth control pills) containing estrogen. You also should avoid estrogen-rich foods. Progesterone may be used as a contraceptive.

Section 22.5

Pleurisy and Other Disorders of the Pleura

Reprinted from "Pleurisy and Other Pleural Disorders," National Heart Lung and Blood Institute, National Institutes of Health, August 2007.

What are pleurisy and other disorders of the pleura?

Pleurisy: Pleurisy is inflammation (swelling) of the pleura. The pleura is a large, thin sheet of tissue (membrane) that wraps around the outside of your lungs and lines the inside of your chest cavity.

Between the layer of the pleura that wraps around your lungs and the layer that lines your chest cavity is a very thin space. This is called the pleural space. Normally it's filled with a small amount of fluid—about four teaspoons full. The fluid helps the two layers of the pleura glide smoothly past each other as your lungs breathe air in and out.

Pleurisy occurs when the two layers of the pleura become red and inflamed. Then they rub against each other every time your lungs expand to breathe in air. This can cause sharp pain with breathing.

Infections like pneumonia are the most common cause of swelling, or inflammation, of the pleura and pleurisy.

Pleural effusion: In some cases of pleurisy, excess fluid builds up in the pleural space. This is called a pleural effusion. The buildup of fluid usually forces the two layers of the pleura apart so they don't rub against each other when you breathe. This can relieve your pain.

However, a large amount of extra fluid can push the pleura against your lung until the lung, or a part of it, collapses. This can make it hard for you to breathe.

In some cases of pleural effusion, the extra fluid gets infected and turns into an abscess. This is called an empyema.

You can develop a pleural effusion if you don't have pleurisy. For example, pneumonia, heart failure, cancer, or a pulmonary embolism can lead to a pleural effusion.

Pneumothorax: Air or gas also can build up in the pleural space. This is called a pneumothorax. It can result from acute lung injury or a lung disease like emphysema. Lung procedures, like surgery, drainage of fluid with a needle, examination of the lung from the inside with a light and a camera, or mechanical ventilation, also can cause it.

The most common symptom is sudden pain in one side of the lung and shortness of breath. A pneumothorax also can put pressure on the lung and cause it to collapse.

If the pneumothorax is small, it may go away on its own. If it's large, you may need to have a tube placed through your skin and chest wall into the pleural space to remove the air.

Hemothorax: Blood also can collect in the pleural space. This is called hemothorax. The most common cause is injury to your chest from blunt force or chest or heart surgery. Hemothorax also can occur in people with lung or pleural cancer.

Hemothorax can put pressure on the lung and force it to collapse. It also can cause shock, a state in which not enough blood and oxygen reach important organs in the body.

Outlook: Pleurisy and other disorders of the pleura can be serious, depending on what caused the inflammation in the pleura.

If the condition that caused the pleurisy or other pleural disorders isn't too serious and is diagnosed and treated early, you usually can expect a full recovery.

What other names are used for pleurisy and other disorders of the pleura?

- **Pleurisy:** Pleuritis and pleuritic chest pain
- **Pleural effusion:** Fluid in the chest and pleural fluid
- **Pneumothorax:** Air around the lung and air outside the lung

What causes pleurisy and other disorders of the pleura?

Pleurisy: Many different conditions can cause pleurisy. Viral infection is the most common cause. Other conditions that can cause pleurisy include the following:

- Bacterial infections like pneumonia and tuberculosis
- Autoimmune disorders like systemic lupus erythematosus and rheumatoid arthritis
- Lung cancer, including lymphoma

- Other lung diseases like sarcoidosis, asbestosis, lymphangioleio-myomatosis, and mesothelioma

- Pulmonary embolism, a blood clot in the blood vessels that go into the lungs

- Inflammatory bowel disease

- Familial Mediterranean fever, an inherited condition that often causes fever and swelling in the abdomen or lung

- Infection from a fungus or parasite

- Heart surgery, especially coronary artery bypass grafting

Other causes of pleurisy include the following:

- Chest injuries.

- Reactions to certain medicines that can cause a condition similar to systemic lupus erythematosus. These medicines include procainamide, hydralazine, and isoniazid.

In some cases, doctors can't find the cause of the pleurisy.

Pleural effusion: The most common cause of pleural effusion, or fluid in the pleural space, is congestive heart failure. Lung cancer, pneumonia, tuberculosis, and other lung infections also can cause swelling of the pleura and lead to a pleural effusion. Asbestosis, sarcoidosis, and reactions to some medicines also can lead to pleural swelling and pleural effusion.

Pneumothorax: A pneumothorax, or air in the pleural space, can be caused by lung diseases like chronic obstructive pulmonary disease (COPD), tuberculosis, and acute lung injury. Surgery or a wound or injury to the chest also may lead to a pneumothorax.

Hemothorax: The most common cause of hemothorax, or blood in the pleural space, is an injury to the chest. Cancer of the lung or pleura and chest or heart surgery also may lead to a hemothorax. Hemothorax also can be a complication of tuberculosis.

What are the signs and symptoms of pleurisy and other disorders of the pleura?

Pleurisy: The main symptom of pleurisy is a sharp or stabbing pain in your chest that gets worse when you breathe in deeply or cough or sneeze.

The pain may stay in one place or it may spread to your shoulder or back. Sometimes it becomes a fairly constant dull ache.

Depending on what's causing the pleurisy, you may have other symptoms, such as shortness of breath, a cough, fever and chills, rapid, shallow breathing, unexplained weight loss, or a sore throat followed by pain and swelling in your joints.

Pleural effusion: Pleural effusion often has no symptoms.

Pneumothorax: The symptoms of pneumothorax include the following:

- Sudden, sharp chest pain that gets worse when you breathe in deeply or cough
- Shortness of breath
- Chest tightness
- Easy fatigue (tiredness)
- A rapid heart rate
- A bluish color of the skin caused by lack of oxygen

Other symptoms of pneumothorax include flaring of the nostrils; anxiety, stress, and tension; and hypotension (low blood pressure).

Hemothorax: The symptoms of hemothorax are often similar to those of pneumothorax. They include the following:

- Chest pain
- Shortness of breath
- Respiratory failure
- A rapid heart rate
- Anxiety
- Restlessness

How are pleurisy and other disorders of the pleura diagnosed?

Your doctor will find out if you have pleurisy or another pleural disorder by taking a detailed medical history and doing a physical exam and several tests. The purpose is to:

- Rule out other causes of your symptoms;

- Find the cause of the pleurisy or other pleural disorder so it can be treated.

Medical history: Your doctor will ask you for a detailed medical history. He or she is likely to ask you to describe the pain, especially:

- What it feels like;
- Where it's located and whether you can feel it in your arms, jaw, or shoulder;
- When it started and how long you've had it;
- What makes it better or worse;
- Whether it goes away and then comes back.

Your doctor will probably also want to know about any other symptoms that you may have, like shortness of breath, cough, or palpitations (a feeling that your heart has skipped a beat or is beating too hard).

Other things your doctor is likely to ask about include whether you've ever:

- Had heart disease;
- Smoked;
- Traveled to places where you may have been exposed to tuberculosis;
- Had a job that exposed you to asbestos;
- Taken nitrofurantoin or amiodarone or a medicine that can cause a condition that's similar to systemic lupus erythematosus (an autoimmune disorder).

Physical exam: Your doctor will listen to your breathing with a stethoscope to find out whether your lungs are making any strange sounds.

When you have pleurisy, the inflamed layers of the pleura make a rough, scratchy sound as they rub against each other when you breathe. Doctors call this a pleural friction rub. If your doctor hears the friction rub, he or she will know that you have pleurisy.

If you have a pleural effusion, fluid has built up in the pleural space and pushed the two layers of the pleura apart so that they don't produce a friction rub. But if you have a lot of fluid, your doctor may hear a dull sound when he or she taps on your chest. Or the doctor may have trouble hearing any breathing sounds.

Reduced breathing sounds also can be a sign of pneumothorax.

Diagnostic tests: Depending on the results of your physical exam, your doctor may recommend other diagnostic tests. Commonly used diagnostic tests include chest x-rays, computerized tomography (CT) scans, ultrasound imaging, magnetic resonance (MR) scans, blood tests, arterial blood gas tests, thoracentesis, fluid analysis, and biopsies.

How are pleurisy and other disorders of the pleura treated?

The goals of treatment are to remove the fluid, air, or blood from the pleural space, relieve symptoms, and treat the underlying condition.

Remove fluid, air, or blood from the pleural space: If large amounts of fluid, air, or blood aren't removed from the pleural space, they may put pressure on your lung and cause it to collapse.

The procedures used to drain fluid, air, or blood from the pleural space are similar:

- During thoracentesis, the doctor inserts a needle or a thin, hollow, plastic tube through the ribs in the back of your chest into your chest wall. A syringe is attached to draw fluid out of your chest. This procedure can remove more than six cups of fluid at a time.

- When larger amounts of fluid must be removed, a chest tube may be inserted through your chest wall. The doctor injects a local painkiller into the area of your chest wall outside where the fluid is. He or she will then insert a plastic tube into your chest between two ribs. The tube is connected to a box that suctions the fluid out. A chest x-ray is taken to check the tube's position.

- A chest tube also is used to drain blood and air from the pleural space. This can take several days. The tube is left in place, and you usually stay in the hospital during this time.

- Sometimes the fluid contains pus that is very thick or blood clots. Or it may have formed a hard skin or peel. This makes it harder to drain the fluid. To help break up the pus or blood clots, the doctor may use the chest tube to put certain medicines into the pleural space. These medicines are called fibrinolytics. If the pus or blood clots still don't drain out, you may need surgery.

Relieve symptoms: For relief of pleurisy symptoms, your doctor may recommend the following:

- Acetaminophen or anti-inflammatory agents, such as ibuprofen, to control pain.

- Codeine-based cough syrups to control a cough.

- Lying on the painful side. This may make you more comfortable.

- Breathing deeply and coughing to clear mucus as the pain eases. Otherwise, you may develop pneumonia.

- Getting plenty of rest.

Treating the underlying condition: Looking at the fluid under a microscope can often tell the doctor what's causing the fluid buildup. Then treatment of the underlying condition can begin.

If the fluid is infected, treatment involves antibiotics and draining the fluid. If the infection is tuberculosis or from a fungus, treatment involves long-term use of antibiotics or antifungal medicines.

If the fluid is caused by tumors of the pleura, it may build up again quickly after it's drained. Sometimes antitumor medicines will prevent further fluid buildup. If they don't, the doctor may seal the pleural space. This is called pleurodesis.

In pleurodesis, the doctor drains all the fluid out of the chest through a chest tube. Then he or she pushes a substance through the chest tube into the pleural space. This substance irritates the surface of the pleura. This causes the two layers of the pleura to squeeze shut so there is no room for more fluid to build up.

Chemotherapy or radiation treatment also may be used to reduce the size of the tumors.

If congestive heart failure is causing the fluid buildup, treatment usually includes diuretics and other medicines.

Chapter 23

Bronchitis

The bronchi are the two main airways that branch down from the trachea (the airway that starts in the back of the throat and goes into the chest). When the parts of the walls of the bronchi become swollen and tender (inflamed), the condition is called bronchitis. The inflammation causes more mucus to be produced, which narrows the airway and makes breathing more difficult.

There are several types of bronchitis:

- Acute bronchitis can last for up to ninety days.

- Chronic bronchitis can last for months or sometimes years. If chronic bronchitis decreases the amount of air flowing to the lungs, it is considered to be a sign of chronic obstructive pulmonary disease.

- Infectious bronchitis usually occurs in the winter due to viruses, including the influenza virus. Even after a viral infection has passed, the irritation of the bronchi can continue to cause symptoms. Infectious bronchitis can also be due to bacteria, especially if it follows an upper respiratory viral infection. It is possible to have viral and bacterial bronchitis at the same time.

- Irritative bronchitis (or industrial or environmental bronchitis) is caused by exposure to mineral or vegetable dusts or fumes from strong acids, ammonia, some organic solvents, chlorine, hydrogen sulfide, sulfur dioxide, and bromine.

Symptoms

Symptoms will vary somewhat depending on the underlying cause of the bronchitis. When the bronchitis is due to an infection the symptoms may include the following:

- A slight fever of 100 to 101°F with severe bronchitis. The fever may rise to 101 to 102°F and last three to five days even after antibiotics are started.

- A runny nose.

- Aches in the back and muscles.

- Chills.

- Coughing that starts out dry is often the first sign of acute bronchitis. Small amounts of white mucus may be coughed up if the bronchitis is viral. If the color of the mucus changes to green or yellow, it may be a sign that a bacterial infection has also set in. The cough is usually the last symptom to clear up and may last for weeks.

- Feeling tired.

- Shortness of breath that can be triggered by inhaling cold, outdoor air or smelling strong odors. This happens because the inflamed bronchi may narrow for short periods of time, cutting down the amount of air that enters the lungs. Wheezing, especially after coughing, is common.

- Sore throat.

Bronchitis does not usually lead to serious complications (e.g., acute respiratory failure or pneumonia) unless the patient has a chronic lung disease, such as chronic obstructive pulmonary disease or asthma.

Causes and Risk Factors

An infection or irritating substances, gases, or particles in the air can cause acute bronchitis. Smokers and people with chronic lung disease are more prone to repeated attacks of acute bronchitis. This is because the mucus in their airways doesn't drain well. Others at risk of getting acute bronchitis repeatedly are people with chronic sinus infections or allergies; children with enlarged tonsils and adenoids; and people who don't eat properly.

Diagnosis

To diagnose bronchitis, a physician performs a physical examination, listens for wheezing with a stethoscope, and evaluates symptoms, making sure they are not due to pneumonia. A sample of sputum from a cough may be examined because its color—clear or white versus yellow or green—may suggest whether the bronchitis is due to a viral infection or a bacterial infection, respectively. A chest x-ray may be needed to rule out pneumonia, and if the cough lasts more than two months, a chest x-ray may be done to rule out another lung disease, such as lung cancer.

Treatment

Depending on the symptoms and cause of the bronchitis, treatment options include the following:

- Antibiotics may be ordered to treat acute bronchitis that appears to be caused by a bacterial infection or for people who have other lung diseases that put them at a greater risk of lung infections.

- Bronchodilators, which open up the bronchi, may be used on a short-term basis to open airways and reduce wheezing.

- Cool-mist humidifiers or steam vaporizers can be helpful for wheezing or shortness of breath. Leaning over a bathroom sink full of hot water with a towel loosely draped over the head can also be help open the airways.

- Corticosteroids given in an inhaler are sometimes prescribed to help the cough go away, reduce inflammation, and make the airways less reactive. They are most often given when the cough remains after the infection is no longer present.

- Cough medicines should be used carefully. While they can be helpful to suppress a dry, bothersome cough, they should not be used to suppress a cough that produces a lot of sputum. When the cough is wet, expectorants can help thin the secretions and make them easier to cough up. When a lot of mucus is present, coughing is important to clear the lungs of fluid.

- For viral bronchitis, antibiotics will not be effective. If influenza causes the bronchitis, treatment with antiviral drugs may be helpful.

- Over-the-counter pain relievers, such as aspirin, acetaminophen, or ibuprofen, can be used for pain relief and fever reduction. Children with bronchitis should not be given aspirin; instead they should take acetaminophen or ibuprofen.

- Plenty of fluids—enough to keep the urine pale (except for the first urination of the day, when it is usually darker).

- Rest, especially if a fever is present.

Chapter 24

Lung Abscess

What Is Lung Abscess: A lung abscess is a localized infection within the lung. An abscess is a pus-containing cavity. It usually occurs as a complication of inadequately treated pneumonia, when the bacteria are able to replicate to large numbers, and cause damage (necrosis) to the lung tissue. This is then walled off by the immune system and becomes an abscess.

Who Gets It? It is difficult to estimate the true incidence of lung abscesses. They are more common with certain bacterial causes of pneumonia (*Klebsiella pneumoniae, Staphylococcus aureus*) and they are also common in alcoholics—where they are usually caused by aspiration.

Aspiration is when somebody inhales mouth contents—often seen in impaired conscious states and in alcoholism.

Predisposing Factors: There are a number of possible predisposing factors, including: aspiration, bronchial obstruction, pulmonary infarction, direct traumatic inoculation, or spread of an extra-pulmonary septic focus (endocarditis, intravenous drug use (IVDU), subphrenic abscess).

Progression: If pneumonia is not sufficiently treated then an infective focus can remain (other triggers are described above), causing an abscess. Complications of a lung abscess include hemorrhage, septic emboli, and amyloidosis. Extension across interlobar fissures and into the pleural cavity (empyema) develops in 20 to 30 percent of people with a lung abscess.

Probable Outcomes: Most patients with abscesses will recover with antibiotic treatment alone. Others, however, may need some minor surgery to aid in resolving the abscess.

How Will It Affect Me? Generally the development of an abscess will require hospitalization and diagnostic testing. Some may be treated on an outpatient basis, but the possible need for radiology, ultrasound services, or body posture for drainage may require some time in the hospital. Most patients will fully recover.

How Is It Diagnosed?

- A full blood count will show increased white cells. Platelets, erythrocyte sedimentation rate (ESR), and C-reactive protein (CRP) will be raised.
- Blood and sputum cultures should be performed to help isolate the organism.
- A chest x-ray will demonstrate a rounded, cavitating, walled opacity with a fluid level.

How Is It Treated? Other diagnoses such as tuberculosis, fungal infections, carcinoma, pulmonary infarction, and pulmonary vasculitis should be ruled out.

Regular postural drainage and chest physiotherapy will help to drain the purulent secretions. Antibiotic therapy can be started. It should continue for a considerable length of time (four to six weeks)—longer than for a usual lung infection.

Bronchoscopy can allow drainage of pus and further diagnostic options. Aspiration or open surgical excision may be required.

Symptoms of This Disease:

- Cough

Chapter 25

Pneumonia

Pneumonia is a potentially fatal infection that causes inflammation (redness and swelling) inside the lungs, resulting in breathing difficulty.

Among the most vital organs, the lungs pump air in and out of the body so that blood can exchange carbon dioxide for the oxygen that it circulates through the body. When breathing in, air flows through the trachea (windpipe) and then into two branches called bronchi inside the lungs. In turn the bronchi subdivide almost twenty times into smaller and smaller passages creating numerous bronchioles (smaller airways). Each of these airways ends in a cluster of tiny air sacs called alveoli. This creates a vast amount of surface where the blood can collect oxygen inside a small space, the chest cavity.

When certain foreign materials, bacteria, fungi, or viruses enter the body through the lungs and penetrate the natural defenses in the lungs, pneumonia can develop. What is commonly referred to as pneumonia is actually more than fifty variations of the condition, ranging from mild (such as "walking pneumonia") to life threatening. It may affect only one lung or both lungs (sometimes called double pneumonia). Pneumonia can occur independently, after certain illnesses (e.g., colds or influenza), or along with other illnesses.

445

More than sixty thousand Americans die each year from pneumonia. It can strike people of any age, but it is of greatest risk to the elderly, infants and very young children, and persons with chronic illnesses.

Symptoms

Although early treatment is the best way to recover fully and quickly, pneumonia is challenging to diagnose. It sometimes seems like a simple cold or the flu, and its signs can vary depending on what is causing the pneumonia. Symptoms include:

- a persistent cough;
- an unexplained fever, especially one of 102° F or higher for several days in a row;
- chest pain that changes with breathing;
- chills and sweats;
- shortness of breath;
- suddenly feeling worse after a cold or influenza.

Anyone with these symptoms should not hesitate to call a doctor. People who should be especially concerned with these symptoms include older adults and individuals who are undergoing chemotherapy, have a suppressed immune system, are taking drugs that suppress the immune system (e.g., prednisone), are affected by alcoholism, have been injured, are confined to bed, or have heart conditions or other conditions that affect the ability to breathe.

Pneumonia can turn fatal within twenty-four hours under certain conditions. Seeking early treatment is important to ensure that the condition does not become life threatening. Some complications that can occur with pneumonia are as follows:

- The lungs may swell because the disease can fill up the air spaces inside the lungs, making breathing difficult.
- The infection that causes the pneumonia can spread into the bloodstream and then to other organs.
- Fluid can collect between the lining (pleurae) of the lungs and the lining of the inside of the chest. When fluid collects inside it is called pleural effusion. This fluid can become infected (a condition known as empyema) and may need to be drained through a tube inserted between the ribs.

Causes

Some of the organisms that cause pneumonia are commonly found in the air. The lung's natural defenses normally protect against infection from these organisms, but they sometimes break through these defenses. Pneumonia may be caused by any of the following:

- **Bacteria:** The most common cause of pneumonia is bacterial infection, and many different bacteria can cause the condition, producing mild to severe cases. Bacterial pneumonia can occur independently or following illnesses, such as colds, flu, or upper respiratory infections.

- **Fungi:** Certain types of fungus can cause pneumonia. When the fungus is inhaled, some people develop symptoms of acute pneumonia, others develop a form that lasts for months, although most people experience few if any symptoms. *Pneumocystis carinii*, a yeast-like fungi that is known as an opportunistic infection because it usually affects individuals with compromised immune systems, such as those with acquired immunodeficiency syndrome (AIDS) or undergoing chemotherapy.

- **Viruses:** Several different viruses can cause pneumonia, including some of the same viruses that cause influenza. This type of pneumonia usually hits in the fall and winter and is more serious in people with heart or lung disease. People who have viral pneumonia can also develop bacterial pneumonia.

- **Other microorganisms:** In rare cases, other living organisms may be responsible for pneumonia. These organisms include amoebas and mycoplasmas (which have characteristics of both bacteria and virus).

- **Other foreign materials:** Pneumonia can occur when food, mucus, vomit, chemicals, or other substances enter the lungs. Called aspiration pneumonia, this condition can develop from accidentally inhaling substances during a seizure, unconsciousness, or stroke.

Risk Factors

Persons who are at greater risk of developing pneumonia include those who:

- abuse alcohol (alcohol interferes with the action of the white blood cells, which fight infections);

- abuse drugs (injection of illegal drugs can put you at greater risk of getting infections that can affect your lungs);

- are age sixty-five or older;

- are smokers (smoke damages the air passages inside the lungs);

- are very young children (whose immune systems are not fully developed);

- have an impaired immune system due to chemotherapy, immunosuppressant drugs, or illness;

- have been exposed to certain chemicals or pollutants;

- have certain diseases, such as human immunodeficiency virus (HIV)/AIDS, heart disease, emphysema, or diabetes;

- have had the spleen removed;

- live in areas where exposure to types of fungus is greater (An example is valley fever, which is widespread throughout Southern California and the desert of the Southwest. This fungus does not affect everyone who is exposed to it, but a few develop severe pneumonia.)

Diagnosis

To diagnose pneumonia, doctors usually begin with a medical history and a physical examination. Often the medical history may indicate a risk of having pneumonia. During the examination, the doctor uses a stethoscope to listen for abnormal bubbling, crackling, or rumbling sounds that may indicate thick liquid in the lungs or inflammation (swelling) from an infection.

The doctor may recommend a blood test to check the white blood cell count and to detect viruses, bacteria, or other organisms. A phlegm sample may be tested to help determine the cause of the pneumonia.

The doctor may also recommend a chest x-ray to confirm the diagnosis and to note the location and spread of the infection. If the x-ray does not confirm pneumonia, more sophisticated imaging may be needed, such as computed tomography (CT) scan.

Treatment

Because pneumonia has different causes and different degrees of seriousness, treatment will vary according to the type of pneumonia a person has. Prescribed treatment may include the following:

- **Antibiotics:** Normally given for bacterial infections, antibiotics may also be prescribed for other types of pneumonia. Antibiotics should be taken for the complete period prescribed to prevent the infection from returning and to reduce the formation of antibiotic-resistant bacteria.

- **Bed rest:** Stress and fatigue can weaken the immune system, which could allow a relapse.

- **Fluids:** Drinking plenty of fluids, especially water, helps prevent dehydration and break up phlegm in the lungs.

- **Over-the-counter medications:** These medications may be recommended to alleviate aches, pains, coughing, and fever.

- **Oxygen:** In severe cases involving breathing difficulty, oxygen may be administered for several days.

About four to six weeks after treatment for pneumonia, the doctor will probably schedule a follow-up visit. Because the lungs may still be infected, the doctor will track the patient's progress to prevent a relapse or complications. Patients who are not feeling better by that time may need more tests to find out why.

Prevention

Pneumonia usually is not something that a person "catches" from other people. People with pneumonia, however, may want to stay away from those with compromised immune systems. People can develop pneumonia due to weakened resistance. The following may be helpful in avoiding pneumonia, especially for those at greater risk of developing it:

- Do not smoke. Smoking damages the lungs' ability to protect against infections.

- Get enough rest and moderate exercise, and eat a die rich in fruits, vegetables, and whole grains. These measures boost strength and help protect against serious illnesses and infections.

- Get vaccinated against pneumococcal pneumonia at least once after the age of sixty-five. People with chronic lung or heart disease, diabetes, or sickle cell anemia and those with the spleen removed, on chemotherapy, or who have a lowered immune system may want to discuss a pneumonia vaccination with their doctor. Prevnar®, a pneumonia vaccine, can help protect young children under the age of two or those who are older and have a special risk of getting pneumonia.

• Get vaccinated against the flu every year because pneumonia can be a complication of having the flu.

• Regularly wash hands, which come in contact every day with many germs, including those that cause pneumonia. Hand washing also helps reduce chances of getting colds and flu.

Part Four

Other Medical Conditions Affecting the Lungs

Chapter 26

Acute Respiratory Distress Syndrome

What Is Acute Respiratory Distress Syndrome?

Acute respiratory distress syndrome (ARDS) is breathing failure that can occur in critically ill persons with underlying illnesses. It is not a specific disease. Instead, it is a life-threatening condition that occurs when there is severe fluid buildup in both lungs. The fluid buildup prevents the lungs from working properly—that is, allowing the transfer of oxygen from air into the body and carbon dioxide out of the body into the air.

In ARDS, the tiny blood vessels (capillaries) in the lungs or the air sacs (alveoli) are damaged because of an infection, injury, blood loss, or inhalation injury. Fluid leaks from the blood vessels into air sacs of the lungs. While some air sacs fill with fluid, others collapse. When the air sacs collapse or fill up with fluid, the lungs can no longer fill properly with air and the lungs become stiff. Without air entering the lungs properly, the amount of oxygen in the blood drops. When this happens, the person with ARDS must be given extra oxygen and may need the help of a breathing machine.

Breathing failure can occur very quickly after the condition begins. It may take only one or two days for fluid to build up. The process that causes ARDS may continue for weeks. If scarring occurs, this will make it harder for the lungs to take in oxygen and get rid of carbon dioxide.

Excerpted from "ARDS," National Heart Lung and Blood Institute, National Institutes of Health, March 2006.

In the past, only about four out of ten people who developed ARDS survived. But today, with good care in a hospital's intensive or critical care unit, many people (about seven out of ten) with ARDS survive. Although many people who survive ARDS make a full recovery, some survivors have lasting damage to their lungs.

How the Lungs Work

To understand acute respiratory distress syndrome (ARDS), it is helpful to understand how your lungs work.

Normal Lung Function

A slice of normal lung looks like a pink sponge—filled with tiny bubbles or holes. Around each bubble is a fine network of tiny blood vessels. These bubbles, which are surrounded by blood vessels, give the lungs a large surface to exchange oxygen (into the blood, where it is carried throughout the body) and carbon dioxide (out of the blood). This process is called gas exchange. Healthy lungs do this very well.

Here's how normal breathing works:

- You breathe in air through your nose and mouth. The air travels down through your windpipe (trachea) through large and small tubes in your lungs called bronchial tubes. The larger tubes are bronchi, and the smaller tubes are bronchioles. Sometimes, we use the word "airways" to refer to the various tubes or passages that air uses to travel from the nose and mouth into the lungs. The airways in your lungs look something like an upside-down tree with many branches.

- At the ends of the small bronchial tubes, there are groups of tiny bubbles called air sacs or alveoli. The bubbles have very thin walls, and small blood vessels called capillaries are next to them. Oxygen passes from the air sacs into the blood in these small blood vessels. At the same time, carbon dioxide passes from the blood into the air sacs.

Effects of ARDS

In ARDS, the tiny blood vessels leak too much fluid into the lungs. This results from toxins (poisons) that the body produces in response to the underlying illness or injury. The lungs become like a wet sponge, heavy and stiffer than normal. They no longer provide the effective surface for gas exchange, and the level of oxygen in the blood falls. If

ARDS is severe and goes on for some time, scar tissue called fibrosis may form in the lungs. The scarring also makes it harder for gas exchange to occur.

People who develop ARDS need extra oxygen and may need a breathing machine to breathe for them while their lungs try to heal. If they survive, ARDS patients may have a full recovery. Recovery can take weeks or months. Some ARDS survivors take a year or longer to recover, and some never completely recover from having ARDS.

Other Names for ARDS

- Adult respiratory distress syndrome
- Stiff lung
- Shock lung
- Wet lung

There is a similar condition in infants called infant respiratory distress syndrome (also called IRDS, RDS, and hyaline membrane disease). It mainly affects premature infants whose lungs are not well developed when they are born.

What Causes ARDS?

The causes of acute respiratory distress syndrome (ARDS) are not well understood. It can occur in many situations and in persons with or without a lung disease.

There are two ways that lung injury leading to ARDS can occur: through a direct injury to the lungs, or indirectly when a person is very sick or has a serious bodily injury. However, most sick or badly injured persons do not develop ARDS.

Direct Lung Injury

A direct injury to the lungs may result from breathing in harmful substances or an infection in the lungs. Some direct lung injuries that can lead to ARDS include the following:

- Severe pneumonia (infection in the lungs)
- Breathing in vomited stomach contents
- Breathing in harmful fumes or smoke
- A severe blow to the chest or other accident that bruises the lungs

Indirect Lung Injury

Most cases of ARDS happen in people who are very ill or who have been in a major accident. This is sometimes called an indirect lung injury. Less is known about how indirect injuries lead to ARDS than about how direct injuries to the lungs cause ARDS. Indirect lung injury leading to ARDS sometimes occurs in the following cases:

- Severe and widespread bacterial infection in the body (sepsis)
- Severe injury with shock
- Severe bleeding requiring blood transfusions
- Drug overdose
- Inflamed pancreas

It is not clear why some very sick or seriously injured people develop ARDS and others do not. Researchers are trying to find out why ARDS develops and how to prevent it.

Who Is At Risk for ARDS?

Acute respiratory distress syndrome (ARDS) usually affects people who are being treated for another serious illness or those who have had major injuries. It affects about 150,000 people each year in the United States. ARDS can occur in people with or without a previous lung disease. People who have a serious accident with a large blood loss are more likely to develop ARDS. However, only a small portion of people who have problems that can lead to ARDS actually develop it.

In most cases, a person who develops ARDS is already in the hospital being treated for other medical problems. Some illnesses or injuries that can lead to ARDS include the following:

- Serious, widespread infection in the body (sepsis)
- Severe injury (trauma) and shock from a car crash, fire, or other cause
- Severe bleeding that requires blood transfusions
- Severe pneumonia (infection of the lungs)
- Breathing in vomited stomach contents
- Breathing in smoke or harmful gases and fumes
- Injury to the chest from trauma (such as a car accident) that causes bruising of the lungs

- Nearly drowning
- Some drug overdoses

What Are the Signs and Symptoms of ARDS?

The major signs and symptoms of acute respiratory distress syndrome (ARDS) are as follows:

- Shortness of breath
- Fast, labored breathing
- A bluish skin color (due to a low level of oxygen in the blood)
- A lower amount of oxygen in the blood

Doctors and other health care providers watch for these signs and symptoms in patients who have conditions that might lead to ARDS. People who develop ARDS may be too sick to complain about having trouble breathing or other related symptoms. If a patient shows signs of developing ARDS, doctors will do tests to confirm that ARDS is the problem.

ARDS is often associated with the failure of other organs and body systems, including the liver, kidneys, and the immune system. Multiple organ failure often leads to death.

How Is ARDS Diagnosed?

Doctors diagnose acute respiratory distress syndrome (ARDS) when:

- A person suffering from severe infection or injury develops breathing problems;
- A chest x-ray shows fluid in the air sacs of both lungs;
- Blood tests show a low level of oxygen in the blood;
- Other conditions that could cause breathing problems have been ruled out.

ARDS can be confused with other illnesses that have similar symptoms. The most important is congestive heart failure. In congestive heart failure, fluid backs up into the lungs because the heart is weak and cannot pump well. However, there is no injury to the lungs in congestive heart failure. Since a chest x-ray is abnormal for both ARDS and congestive heart failure, it is sometimes very difficult to tell them apart.

457

How Is ARDS Treated?

Patients with acute respiratory distress syndrome (ARDS) are usually treated in the intensive or critical care unit of a hospital. The main concern in treating ARDS is getting enough oxygen into the blood until the lungs heal enough to work on their own again. The following are important ways that ARDS patients are treated.

Extra Oxygen

The main treatment is giving a higher concentration of oxygen than that found in normal air—that is, enough to raise blood levels of oxygen to safe levels. This can sometimes be done with a facemask. A facemask can deliver oxygen at a concentration of 40 to 60 percent. As the ARDS progresses over hours or days, the patient may need a higher level of oxygen than a facemask can give.

If the patient becomes tired from breathing so hard, it may become necessary to connect the patient to a breathing machine (ventilator). This can be done by placing a tube through the mouth or nose into the windpipe (trachea) in a procedure called endotracheal intubation (or just intubation) and connecting the tube to the ventilator. Sometimes the connecting tube is inserted through a surgical opening in the neck (this procedure is called a tracheotomy). The breathing machine can be set to help or completely control breathing. It will deliver the minimum amount of air every minute. If the extra oxygen and help with breathing are not enough, the breathing machine can be set to positive end expiratory pressure (PEEP) to maintain the surface for gas exchange.

PEEP keeps some air in the lungs at the end of each breath. It helps keep the air sacs open instead of collapsing. The setting on the breathing machine can be adjusted to fit the needs of the patient. Other settings on the breathing machine control the number of breaths per minute (rate control) and the amount of air the ventilator uses to inflate the lungs in each breath (tidal volume).

Medicines

Many different kinds of medicines are used to treat ARDS patients. Some kinds of medicines often used include:

- Antibiotics to fight infection;
- Pain relievers;
- Drugs to relieve anxiety and keep the patient calm and from "fighting" the breathing machine;

- Drugs to raise blood pressure or stimulate the heart;
- Muscle relaxers to prevent movement and reduce the body's demand for oxygen.

Other Treatment

With breathing tubes in place, ARDS patients cannot eat or drink as usual. They must be fed through a feeding tube placed through the nose and into the stomach. If this does not work, feeding is done through a vein. Sometimes a special bed or mattress, such as an airbed, is used to help prevent complications such as pneumonia or bedsores. If complications occur, the patient may require treatment for them.

Results

With treatment:

- Some patients recover quickly and can breathe on their own within a week or so. They have the best chance of a full recovery.
- Patients whose underlying illness is more severe may die within the first week of treatment.
- Those who survive the first week but cannot breathe on their own may face many weeks on the breathing machine. They may have complications and a slow recovery if they survive.

Recovering From ARDS

Some people who survive acute respiratory distress syndrome (ARDS) heal quickly and recover completely in a relatively short time. Some are able to have the breathing tube and breathing machine removed in a week or so. Survivors often recover much of their lung function in the first three to six months after leaving the hospital, and they continue to recover for up to a year or more.

Others recover more slowly, however. Some ARDS survivors never recover completely, and they have continuing problems with their lungs. Every case is different. People who are younger and healthier when they develop ARDS are more likely to recover quickly than those who are older or who have more health problems.

ARDS patients who survive the first week but cannot breathe on their own may have to be on a breathing machine for several weeks or longer. These patients often develop complications, such as infections or air leaks. While some of these patients will die, others will get better and be able to breathe on their own again. Their recovery is usually slow, and they may have continuing problems.

After leaving the hospital, ARDS survivors need to visit a doctor during recovery to check how well their lungs are doing. Doctors use lung function tests to check the lungs. Spirometry is the most commonly used lung function test. It involves taking a deep breath and blowing hard into a plastic tube. The doctor will also do an oxygen saturation (oximetry) test or a blood test to check the amount of oxygen in the blood.

After going home from the hospital, the ARDS survivor may need only a little or a lot of help. While recovering from ARDS at home, a person may:

- Need to use oxygen at home or when going out of the home, at least for a while;
- Need to have physical, occupational, or other therapy;
- Have shortness of breath, cough, or phlegm (mucus);
- Have hoarseness from the breathing tube in the hospital;
- Feel tired and not have much energy;
- Have muscle weakness.

Complications of ARDS

Anyone who stays in the hospital for a long time can get complications. Common complications in ARDS patients are infections with hospital-acquired bacteria and leaks of air out of the lungs into other body spaces.

Bacterial infections: The lungs or other parts of the body may become infected. These infections are usually treated with antibiotics after a test to see what kind of bacteria is causing the infection.

Air leaks: Leaks of air through holes in the lungs are caused by pressure from the breathing machine that is needed to be sure the patient gets enough air, and from the very stiff lungs. Air from the injured lungs may enter the space between the lungs and the lining around the lungs (the pleura) and cause a pneumothorax (collapsed lung). Treatment involves using a chest tube and suction to remove the air and help the lungs reinflate. Air may also enter the space between the membranes that line the abdomen (pneumoperitoneum) or the soft tissue under the skin (subcutaneous emphysema). These are not usually treated.

Each complication is treated as it arises. Careful hand washing by hospital staff and visitors helps reduce infections, and new breathing machine methods help reduce air leaks.

Chapter 27

Alpha-1 Antitrypsin Deficiency

What Is Alpha-1 Antitrypsin Deficiency?

Alpha-1 antitrypsin deficiency (AATD) is an inherited condition that causes low levels of, or no, alpha-1 antitrypsin (AAT) in the blood. AATD occurs in approximately 1 in 2,500 individuals. This condition is found in all ethnic groups; however, it occurs most often in whites of European ancestry.

Alpha-1 antitrypsin (AAT) is a protein that is made in the liver. The liver releases this protein into the bloodstream. AAT protects the lungs so they can work normally. Without enough AAT, the lungs can be damaged, and this damage may make breathing difficult.

Everyone has two copies of the gene for AAT and receives one copy of the gene from each parent. Most people have two normal copies of the alpha-1 antitrypsin gene. Individuals with AATD have one normal copy and one damaged copy, or they have two damaged copies. Most individuals who have one normal gene can produce enough alpha-1 antitrypsin to live healthy lives, especially if they do not smoke.

People who have two damaged copies of the gene are not able to produce enough alpha- 1 antitrypsin, which leads them to have more severe symptoms.

Excerpted from "Learning about Alpha-1 Antitrypsin Deficiency (AATD)," National Human Genome Research Institute, National Institutes of Health, February 2007.

What Are the Symptoms of Alpha-1 Antitrypsin Deficiency (AATD)?

AATD can present as lung disease in adults and can be associated with liver disease in a small portion of affected children. In affected adults, the first symptoms of AATD are shortness of breath with mild activity, reduced ability to exercise, and wheezing. These symptoms usually appear between the ages of twenty and forty. Other signs and symptoms can include repeated respiratory infections, fatigue, rapid heartbeat upon standing, vision problems, and unintentional weight loss.

Some Individuals with AATD have emphysema, in which the small air sacs (alveoli) in the lungs are damaged. Symptoms of emphysema include difficulty breathing, a hacking cough, and a barrel-shaped chest. Smoking or exposure to tobacco smoke increases the appearance of symptoms and damage to the lungs. Other common diagnoses include COPD (chronic obstructive pulmonary disease), asthma, chronic bronchitis, and bronchiectasis—a chronic inflammatory or degenerative condition of one or more bronchi or bronchioles.

Liver disease, called cirrhosis of the liver, is another symptom of AATD. It can be present in some affected children, about 10 percent, and has also been reported in 15 percent of adults with AATD. In its late stages signs and symptoms of liver disease can include a swollen abdomen, coughing up blood, swollen feet or legs, and yellowing of the skin and the whites of the eyes (jaundice).

Rarely, AATD can cause a skin condition known as panniculitis, which is characterized by hardened skin with painful lumps or patches. Panniculitis varies in severity and can occur at any age.

How Is Alpha-1 Antitrypsin Deficiency Diagnosed?

Alpha-1 antitrypsin deficiency (AATD) is diagnosed through testing of a blood sample, when a person is suspected of having AATD. For example, AATD may be suspected when a physical examination reveals a barrel-shaped chest, or, when listening to the chest with a stethoscope, wheezing, crackles, or decreased breath sounds are heard.

Testing for AATD, using a blood sample from the individual, is simple, quick and highly accurate. Three types of tests are usually done on the blood sample:

- Alpha-1 genotyping, which examines a person's genes and determines their genotype

- Alpha-1 antitrypsin protease inhibitor (PI) type of phenotype test, which determines the type of AAT protein that a person has

- Alpha-1 antitrypsin level test, which determines the amount of AAT in a person's blood

Individuals who have symptoms that suggest AATD or who have a family history of AATD should consider being tested.

What Is the Treatment for Alpha-1 Antitrypsin Deficiency?

Treatment of alpha-1 antitrypsin deficiency (AATD) is based on a person's symptoms. There is currently no cure. The major goal of AATD management is preventing or slowing the progression of lung disease.

Treatments include bronchodilators and prompt treatment with antibiotics for upper respiratory tract infections. Lung transplantation may be an option for those who develop end-stage lung disease. Quitting smoking, if a person with AATD smokes, is essential.

Replacement (augmentation) therapy with the missing AAT protein is available, although it is used only under special circumstances. It is not known how effective this is once disease has developed or which people would benefit most.

Is Alpha-1 Antitrypsin Deficiency Inherited?

Alpha-1 antitrypsin deficiency is inherited in families in an autosomal codominant pattern. Codominant inheritance means that two different variants of the gene (alleles) may be expressed, and both versions contribute to the genetic trait.

The M gene is the most common allele of the alpha-1 gene. It produces normal levels of the alpha-1 antitrypsin protein.

The Z gene is the most common variant of the gene. It causes alpha-1 antitrypsin deficiency. The S allele is another, less common variant that causes AATD.

If a person inherits one M gene and one Z gene or one S gene ("type PiMZ" or "type PiMS"), that person is a carrier of the disorder. While such a person may not have normal levels of alpha-1 antitrypsin, there should be enough to protect the lungs. However, carriers with the MZ alleles have an increased risk for lung disease, particularly if they smoke.

A person who inherits the Z gene from each parent is called "type PiZZ." This person has very low alpha-1 antitrypsin levels, allowing elastase—an enzyme especially of pancreatic juice that digests elastin—to damage the lungs. A person who inherits an altered version called S and Z is also likely to develop AATD.

Chapter 28

Lung Cancer

Cancer Cells

Cancer begins in cells, the building blocks that make up tissues. Tissues make up the organs of the body.

Normal, healthy cells grow and divide to form new cells as the body needs them. When normal cells grow old or become damaged, they die, and new cells take their place.

Sometimes, this orderly process goes wrong. New cells form when the body does not need them, and old or damaged cells do not die as they should. The build-up of extra cells often forms a mass of tissue called a growth or tumor.

Tumor cells can be benign (not cancer) or malignant (cancer). Benign tumor cells are usually not as harmful as malignant tumor cells.

Benign lung tumors:

- Are rarely a threat to life;

- Usually do not need to be removed;

- Do not invade the tissues around them;

- Do not spread to other parts of the body.

Malignant lung tumors:

Excerpted from "What You Need to Know About Lung Cancer," National Cancer Institute, July 26, 2007.

- May be a threat to life;

- May grow back after being removed;

- Can invade nearby tissues and organs;

- Can spread to other parts of the body.

Cancer cells spread by breaking away from the original tumor. They enter blood vessels or lymph vessels, which branch into all the tissues of the body. The cancer cells attach to other organs and form new tumors that may damage those organs. The spread of cancer is called metastasis.

Risk Factors

Doctors cannot always explain why one person develops lung cancer and another does not. However, we do know that a person with certain risk factors may be more likely than others to develop lung cancer. A risk factor is something that may increase the chance of developing a disease.

Studies have found the following risk factors for lung cancer:

- **Tobacco smoke:** Tobacco smoke causes most cases of lung cancer. It's by far the most important risk factor for lung cancer. Harmful substances in smoke damage lung cells. That's why smoking cigarettes, pipes, or cigars can cause lung cancer and why secondhand smoke can cause lung cancer in nonsmokers. The more a person is exposed to smoke, the greater the risk of lung cancer.

- **Radon:** Radon is a radioactive gas that you cannot see, smell, or taste. It forms in soil and rocks. People who work in mines may be exposed to radon. In some parts of the country, radon is found in houses. Radon damages lung cells, and people exposed to radon are at increased risk of lung cancer. The risk of lung cancer from radon is even higher for smokers.

- **Asbestos and other substances:** People who have certain jobs (such as those who work in the construction and chemical industries) have an increased risk of lung cancer. Exposure to asbestos, arsenic, chromium, nickel, soot, tar, and other substances can cause lung cancer. The risk is highest for those with years of exposure. The risk of lung cancer from these substances is even higher for smokers.

- **Air pollution:** Air pollution may slightly increase the risk of lung cancer. The risk from air pollution is higher for smokers.

- **Family history of lung cancer:** People with a father, mother, brother, or sister who had lung cancer may be at slightly increased risk of the disease, even if they don't smoke.

- **Personal history of lung cancer:** People who have had lung cancer are at increased risk of developing a second lung tumor.

- **Age over sixty-five:** Most people are older than sixty-five years when diagnosed with lung cancer.

Researchers have studied other possible risk factors. For example, having certain lung diseases (such as tuberculosis or bronchitis) for many years may increase the risk of lung cancer. It's not yet clear whether having certain lung diseases is a risk factor for lung cancer.

People who think they may be at risk for developing lung cancer should talk to their doctor. The doctor may be able to suggest ways to reduce their risk and can plan an appropriate schedule for checkups. For people who have been treated for lung cancer, it's important to have checkups after treatment. The lung tumor may come back after treatment, or another lung tumor may develop.

Screening

Screening tests may help doctors find and treat cancer early. They have been shown to be very helpful in some cancers such as breast cancer. Currently, there is no generally accepted screening test for lung cancer. Several methods of detecting lung cancer have been studied as possible screening tests. The methods under study include tests of sputum (mucus brought up from the lungs by coughing), chest x-rays, or spiral (helical) computed tomography (CT) scans.

However, screening tests have risks. For example, an abnormal x-ray result could lead to other procedures (such as surgery to check for cancer cells), but a person with an abnormal test result might not have lung cancer. Studies so far have not shown that screening tests lower the number of deaths from lung cancer.

You may want to talk with your doctor about your own risk factors and the possible benefits and harms of being screened for lung cancer. Like many other medical decisions, the decision to be screened is a personal one. Your decision may be easier after learning the pros and cons of screening.

Symptoms

Early lung cancer often does not cause symptoms. But as the cancer grows, common symptoms may include the following:

- A cough that gets worse or does not go away
- Breathing trouble, such as shortness of breath
- Constant chest pain
- Coughing up blood
- A hoarse voice
- Frequent lung infections, such as pneumonia
- Feeling very tired all the time
- Weight loss with no known cause

Most often these symptoms are not due to cancer. Other health problems can cause some of these symptoms. Anyone with such symptoms should see a doctor to be diagnosed and treated as early as possible.

Diagnosis

If you have a symptom that suggests lung cancer, your doctor must find out whether it's from cancer or something else. Your doctor may ask about your personal and family medical history. Your doctor may order blood tests, and you may have one or more of the following tests:

- **Physical exam:** Your doctor checks for general signs of health, listens to your breathing, and checks for fluid in the lungs. Your doctor may feel for swollen lymph nodes and a swollen liver.

- **Chest x-ray:** X-ray pictures of your chest may show tumors or abnormal fluid.

- **CT scan:** Doctors often use CT scans to take pictures of tissue inside the chest. An x-ray machine linked to a computer takes several pictures. For a spiral CT scan, the CT scanner rotates around you as you lie on a table. The table passes through the center of the scanner. The pictures may show a tumor, abnormal fluid, or swollen lymph nodes.

Finding Lung Cancer Cells

The only sure way to know if lung cancer is present is for a pathologist to check samples of cells or tissue. The pathologist studies the sample under a microscope and performs other tests. There are many ways to collect samples.

Your doctor may order one or more of the following tests to collect samples:

- **Sputum cytology:** Thick fluid (sputum) is coughed up from the lungs. The lab checks samples of sputum for cancer cells.

- **Thoracentesis:** The doctor uses a long needle to remove fluid (pleural fluid) from the chest. The lab checks the fluid for cancer cells.

- **Bronchoscopy:** The doctor inserts a thin, lighted tube (a bronchoscope) through the nose or mouth into the lung. This allows an exam of the lungs and the air passages that lead to them. The doctor may take a sample of cells with a needle, brush, or other tool. The doctor also may wash the area with water to collect cells in the water.

- **Fine-needle aspiration:** The doctor uses a thin needle to remove tissue or fluid from the lung or lymph node. Sometimes the doctor uses a CT scan or other imaging method to guide the needle to a lung tumor or lymph node.

- **Thoracoscopy:** The surgeon makes several small incisions in your chest and back. The surgeon looks at the lungs and nearby tissues with a thin, lighted tube. If an abnormal area is seen, a biopsy to check for cancer cells may be needed.

- **Thoracotomy:** The surgeon opens the chest with a long incision. Lymph nodes and other tissue may be removed.

- **Mediastinoscopy:** The surgeon makes an incision at the top of the breastbone. A thin, lighted tube is used to see inside the chest. The surgeon may take tissue and lymph node samples.

Types of Lung Cancer

The pathologist checks the sputum, pleural fluid, tissue, or other samples for cancer cells. If cancer is found, the pathologist reports the type. The types of lung cancer are treated differently. The most common types are named for how the lung cancer cells look under a microscope:

- **Small cell lung cancer:** About 13 percent of lung cancers are small cell lung cancers. This type tends to spread quickly.

- **Non–small cell lung cancer:** Most lung cancers (about 87 percent) are non–small cell lung cancers. This type spreads more slowly than small cell lung cancer.

Staging

To plan the best treatment, your doctor needs to know the type of lung cancer and the extent (stage) of the disease. Staging is a careful attempt to find out whether the cancer has spread, and if so, to what parts of the body. Lung cancer spreads most often to the lymph nodes, brain, bones, liver, and adrenal glands.

When cancer spreads from its original place to another part of the body, the new tumor has the same kind of cancer cells and the same name as the original cancer. For example, if lung cancer spreads to the liver, the cancer cells in the liver are actually lung cancer cells. The disease is metastatic lung cancer, not liver cancer. For that reason, it's treated as lung cancer, not liver cancer. Doctors call the new tumor "distant" or metastatic disease.

Staging may involve blood tests and other tests:

- **CT scan:** CT scans may show cancer that has spread to your liver, adrenal glands, brain, or other organs. You may receive contrast material by mouth and by injection into your arm or hand. The contrast material helps these tissues show up more clearly. If a tumor shows up on the CT scan, your doctor may order a biopsy to look for lung cancer cells.

- **Bone scan:** A bone scan may show cancer that has spread to your bones. You receive an injection of a small amount of a radioactive substance. It travels through your blood and collects in your bones. A machine called a scanner detects and measures the radiation. The scanner makes pictures of your bones on a computer screen or on film.

- **Magnetic resonance imaging (MRI):** Your doctor may order MRI pictures of your brain, bones, or other tissues. MRI uses a powerful magnet linked to a computer. It makes detailed pictures of tissue on a computer screen or film.

- **Positron emission tomography (PET) scan:** Your doctor uses a PET scan to find cancer that has spread. You receive an injection of a small amount of radioactive sugar. A machine makes computerized pictures of the sugar being used by cells in the body. Cancer cells use sugar faster than normal cells, and areas with cancer look brighter on the pictures.

Stages of Small Cell Lung Cancer

Doctors describe small cell lung cancer using two stages:

- **Limited stage:** Cancer is found only in one lung and its nearby tissues.

- **Extensive stage:** Cancer is found in tissues of the chest outside of the lung in which it began. Or cancer is found in distant organs.

The treatment options are different for limited and extensive stage small cell lung cancer.

Stages of Non–Small Cell Lung Cancer

Doctors describe non–small cell lung cancer based on the size of the lung tumor and whether cancer has spread to the lymph nodes or other tissues:

- **Occult stage:** Lung cancer cells are found in sputum or in a sample of water collected during bronchoscopy, but a tumor cannot be seen in the lung.

- **Stage 0:** Cancer cells are found only in the innermost lining of the lung. The tumor has not grown through this lining. A stage 0 tumor is also called carcinoma in situ. The tumor is not an invasive cancer.

- **Stage IA:** The lung tumor is an invasive cancer. It has grown through the innermost lining of the lung into deeper lung tissue. The tumor is no more than three centimeters across (less than 1 ¼ inches). It is surrounded by normal tissue and the tumor does not invade the bronchus. Cancer cells are not found in nearby lymph nodes.

- **Stage IB:** The tumor is larger or has grown deeper, but cancer cells are not found in nearby lymph nodes. The lung tumor has one of the following characteristics:

  - The tumor is more than three centimeters across.

  - It has grown into the main bronchus.

  - It has grown through the lung into the pleura.

- **Stage IIA:** The lung tumor is no more than three centimeters across. Cancer cells are found in nearby lymph nodes.

- **Stage IIB:** The tumor has one of the following characteristics:
  - Cancer cells are not found in nearby lymph nodes, but the tumor has invaded the chest wall, diaphragm, pleura, main bronchus, or tissue that surrounds the heart.
  - Cancer cells are found in nearby lymph nodes, and the tumor is more than three centimeters across, it has grown into the main bronchus, or it has grown through the lung into the pleura.

- **Stage IIIA:** The tumor may be any size. Cancer cells are found in the lymph nodes near the lungs and bronchi, and in the lymph nodes between the lungs but on the same side of the chest as the lung tumor.

- **Stage IIIB:** The tumor may be any size. Cancer cells are found on the opposite side of the chest from the lung tumor or in the neck. The tumor may have invaded nearby organs, such as the heart, esophagus, or trachea. More than one malignant growth may be found within the same lobe of the lung. The doctor may find cancer cells in the pleural fluid.

- **Stage IV:** Malignant growths may be found in more than one lobe of the same lung or in the other lung. Or cancer cells may be found in other parts of the body, such as the brain, adrenal gland, liver, or bone.

Treatment

Your doctor may refer you to a specialist who has experience treating lung cancer, or you may ask for a referral. You may have a team of specialists. Specialists who treat lung cancer include thoracic (chest) surgeons, thoracic surgical oncologists, medical oncologists, and radiation oncologists. Your health care team may also include a pulmonologist (a lung specialist), a respiratory therapist, an oncology nurse, and a registered dietitian.

Lung cancer is hard to control with current treatments. For that reason, many doctors encourage patients with this disease to consider taking part in a clinical trial. Clinical trials are an important option for people with all stages of lung cancer.

The choice of treatment depends mainly on the type of lung cancer and its stage. People with lung cancer may have surgery, chemotherapy, radiation therapy, targeted therapy, or a combination of treatments.

People with limited stage small cell lung cancer usually have radiation therapy and chemotherapy. For a very small lung tumor, a person may have surgery and chemotherapy. Most people with extensive stage small cell lung cancer are treated with chemotherapy only.

People with non–small cell lung cancer may have surgery, chemotherapy, radiation therapy, or a combination of treatments. The treatment choices are different for each stage. Some people with advanced cancer receive targeted therapy.

Cancer treatment is either local or systemic:

- **Local therapy:** Surgery and radiation therapy are local therapies. They remove or destroy cancer in the chest. When lung cancer has spread to other parts of the body, local therapy may be used to control the disease in those specific areas. For example, lung cancer that spreads to the brain may be controlled with radiation therapy to the head.

- **Systemic therapy:** Chemotherapy and targeted therapy are systemic therapies. The drugs enter the bloodstream and destroy or control cancer throughout the body.

Your doctor can describe your treatment choices and the expected results. You may want to know about side effects and how treatment may change your normal activities. Because cancer treatments often damage healthy cells and tissues, side effects are common. Side effects depend mainly on the type and extent of the treatment. Side effects may not be the same for each person, and they may change from one treatment session to the next. Before treatment starts, your health care team will explain possible side effects and suggest ways to help you manage them.

You and your doctor can work together to develop a treatment plan that meets your medical and personal needs.

Surgery

Surgery for lung cancer removes the tissue that contains the tumor. The surgeon also removes nearby lymph nodes.

The surgeon removes part or all of the lung:

- **A small part of the lung (wedge resection or segmentectomy):** The surgeon removes the tumor and a small part of the lung.

- **A lobe of the lung (lobectomy or sleeve lobectomy):** The surgeon removes a lobe of the lung. This is the most common surgery for lung cancer.

- **All of the lung (pneumonectomy):** The surgeon removes the entire lung.

After lung surgery, air and fluid collect in the chest. A chest tube allows the fluid to drain. Also, a nurse or respiratory therapist will teach you coughing and breathing exercises. You'll need to do the exercises several times a day.

The time it takes to heal after surgery is different for everyone. Your hospital stay may be a week or longer. It may be several weeks before you return to normal activities.

Medicine can help control your pain after surgery. Before surgery, you should discuss the plan for pain relief with your doctor or nurse. After surgery, your doctor can adjust the plan if you need more pain relief.

Radiation Therapy

Radiation therapy (also called radiotherapy) uses high-energy rays to kill cancer cells. It affects cells only in the treated area.

You may receive external radiation. This is the most common type of radiation therapy for lung cancer. The radiation comes from a large machine outside your body. Most people go to a hospital or clinic for treatment. Treatments are usually five days a week for several weeks.

Another type of radiation therapy is internal radiation (brachytherapy). Internal radiation is seldom used for people with lung cancer. The radiation comes from a seed, wire, or another device put inside your body.

The side effects depend mainly on the type of radiation therapy, the dose of radiation, and the part of your body that is treated. External radiation therapy to the chest may harm the esophagus, causing problems with swallowing. You may also feel very tired. In addition, your skin in the treated area may become red, dry, and tender. After internal radiation therapy, a person may cough up small amounts of blood.

Your doctor can suggest ways to ease these problems.

Chemotherapy

Chemotherapy uses anticancer drugs to kill cancer cells. The drugs enter the bloodstream and can affect cancer cells all over the body.

Usually, more than one drug is given. Anticancer drugs for lung cancer are usually given through a vein (intravenous). Some anticancer drugs can be taken by mouth.

Chemotherapy is given in cycles. You have a rest period after each treatment period. The length of the rest period and the number of cycles depend on the anticancer drugs used.

You may have your treatment in a clinic, at the doctor's office, or at home. Some people may need to stay in the hospital for treatment.

The side effects depend mainly on which drugs are given and how much. The drugs can harm normal cells that divide rapidly:

- **Blood cells:** When chemotherapy lowers your levels of healthy blood cells, you're more likely to get infections, bruise or bleed easily, and feel very weak and tired. Your health care team gives you blood tests to check for low levels of blood cells. If the levels are low, there are medicines that can help your body make new blood cells.

- **Cells in hair roots:** Chemotherapy may cause hair loss. Your hair will grow back after treatment ends, but it may be somewhat different in color and texture.

- **Cells that line the digestive tract:** Chemotherapy can cause poor appetite, nausea and vomiting, diarrhea, or mouth and lip sores. Ask your health care team about treatments that help with these problems.

Some drugs for lung cancer can cause hearing loss, joint pain, and tingling or numbness in your hands and feet. These side effects usually go away after treatment ends.

When radiation therapy and chemotherapy are given at the same time, the side effects may be worse.

Targeted Therapy

Targeted therapy uses drugs to block the growth and spread of cancer cells. The drugs enter the bloodstream and can affect cancer cells all over the body. Some people with non–small cell lung cancer that has spread receive targeted therapy.

There are two kinds of targeted therapy for lung cancer:

- One kind is given through a vein (intravenous) at the doctor's office, hospital, or clinic. It's given at the same time as chemotherapy. The side effects may include bleeding, coughing up blood, a rash, high blood pressure, abdominal pain, vomiting, or diarrhea.

- Another kind of targeted therapy is taken by mouth. It isn't given with chemotherapy. The side effects may include rash, diarrhea, and shortness of breath.

During treatment, your health care team will watch for signs of problems. Side effects usually go away after treatment ends.

Second Opinion

Before starting treatment, you might want a second opinion about your diagnosis and treatment plan. Many insurance companies cover a second opinion if you or your doctor requests it.

It may take some time and effort to gather your medical records and see another doctor. In most cases, a brief delay in starting treatment will not make treatment less effective. To make sure, you should discuss this delay with your doctor. Sometimes people with lung cancer need treatment right away. For example, a doctor may advise a person with small cell lung cancer not to delay treatment more than a week or two.

There are many ways to find a doctor for a second opinion. You can ask your doctor, a local or state medical society, a nearby hospital, or a medical school for names of specialists. Also, your nearest cancer center can tell you about doctors who work there.

Comfort Care

Lung cancer and its treatment can lead to other health problems. You may need comfort care to prevent or control these problems.

Comfort care is available both during and after treatment. It can improve your quality of life.

Your health care team can tell you more about the following problems and how to control them:

- **Pain:** Your doctor or a pain control specialist can suggest ways to relieve or reduce pain.

- **Shortness of breath or trouble breathing:** People with lung cancer often have trouble breathing. Your doctor may refer you to a lung specialist or respiratory therapist. Some people are helped by oxygen therapy, photodynamic therapy, laser surgery, cryotherapy, or stents.

- **Fluid in or around lungs:** Advanced cancer can cause fluid to collect in or around the lungs. The fluid can make it hard to breathe. Your health care team can remove fluid when it builds up. In some cases, a procedure can be done that may prevent fluid from building up again. Some people may need chest tubes to drain the fluid.

- **Pneumonia:** You may have chest x-rays to check for lung infections. Your doctor can treat infections.

- **Cancer that spreads to the brain:** Lung cancer can spread to the brain. The symptoms may include headache, seizures, trouble walking, and problems with balance. Medicine to relieve swelling, radiation therapy, or sometimes surgery can help. People with small cell lung cancer may receive radiation therapy to the brain to try to prevent brain tumors from forming. This is called prophylactic cranial irradiation.

- **Cancer that spreads to the bone:** Lung cancer that spreads to the bone can be painful and can weaken bones. You can ask for pain medicine, and the doctor may suggest external radiation therapy. Your doctor also may give you drugs to help lower your risk of breaking a bone.

- **Sadness and other feelings:** It's normal to feel sad, anxious, or confused after a diagnosis of a serious illness. Some people find it helpful to talk about their feelings.

Follow-up Care

You'll need regular checkups after treatment for lung cancer. Even when there are no longer any signs of cancer, the disease sometimes returns because undetected cancer cells remained somewhere in your body after treatment.

Checkups help ensure that any changes in your health are noted and treated if needed. Checkups may include a physical exam, blood tests, chest x-rays, CT scans, and bronchoscopy.

If you have any health problems between checkups, contact your doctor.

Sources of Support

Learning you have lung cancer can change your life and the lives of those close to you. These changes can be hard to handle. It's normal for you, your family, and your friends to have many different and sometimes confusing feelings.

You may worry about caring for your family, keeping your job, or continuing daily activities. Concerns about treatments and managing side effects, hospital stays, and medical bills are also common.

Because most people who get lung cancer were smokers, you may feel like doctors and other people assume that you are or were a smoker (even if you weren't). You may feel as though you're responsible for getting cancer (or that others blame you). It's normal for anyone coping with a serious illness to feel fear, guilt, anger, or sadness. It may help to share your feelings with family, friends, a member of your health care team, or another person with cancer.

Chapter 29

Mesothelioma

Mesothelioma is a rare form of cancer in which malignant (cancerous) cells are found in the mesothelium, a protective sac that covers most of the body's internal organs. Most people who develop mesothelioma have worked on jobs where they inhaled asbestos particles.

What is the mesothelium?

The mesothelium is a membrane that covers and protects most of the internal organs of the body. It is composed of two layers of cells: One layer immediately surrounds the organ; the other forms a sac around it. The mesothelium produces a lubricating fluid that is released between these layers, allowing moving organs (such as the beating heart and the expanding and contracting lungs) to glide easily against adjacent structures.

The mesothelium has different names, depending on its location in the body. The peritoneum is the mesothelial tissue that covers most of the organs in the abdominal cavity. The pleura is the membrane that surrounds the lungs and lines the wall of the chest cavity. The pericardium covers and protects the heart. The mesothelial tissue surrounding the male internal reproductive organs is called the tunica

Reprinted from "Mesothelioma: Questions and Answers," National Cancer Institute, May 13, 2002. Revised by David A. Cooke, M.D., March 2008.

vaginalis testis. The tunica serosa uteri covers the internal reproductive organs in women.

What is mesothelioma?

Mesothelioma (cancer of the mesothelium) is a disease in which cells of the mesothelium become abnormal and divide without control or order. They can invade and damage nearby tissues and organs. Cancer cells can also metastasize (spread) from their original site to other parts of the body. Most cases of mesothelioma begin inside the chest, in the pleural membranes surrounding the lungs. Rarely, it may develop inside the abdominal cavity. It is possible for the cancer to arise in other locations, but this is extremely rare.

How common is mesothelioma?

Although reported incidence rates have increased in the past twenty years, mesothelioma is still a relatively rare cancer. About two thousand new cases of mesothelioma are diagnosed in the United States each year. Mesothelioma occurs more often in men than in women and risk increases with age, but this disease can appear in either men or women at any age.

What are the risk factors for mesothelioma?

Working with asbestos is the major risk factor for mesothelioma. A history of asbestos exposure at work is reported in about 70 to 80 percent of all cases. However, mesothelioma has been reported in some individuals without any known exposure to asbestos.

Asbestos is the name of a group of minerals that occur naturally as masses of strong, flexible fibers that can be separated into thin threads and woven. Asbestos has been widely used in many industrial products, including cement, brake linings, roof shingles, flooring products, textiles, and insulation. If tiny asbestos particles float in the air, especially during the manufacturing process, they may be inhaled or swallowed, and can cause serious health problems. In addition to mesothelioma, exposure to asbestos increases the risk of lung cancer, asbestosis (a noncancerous, chronic lung ailment), and other cancers, such as those of the larynx and kidney.

Smoking does not appear to increase the risk of mesothelioma. However, the combination of smoking and asbestos exposure significantly increases a person's risk of developing cancer of the air passageways in the lung.

Who is at increased risk for developing mesothelioma?

Asbestos has been mined and used commercially since the late 1800s. Its use greatly increased during World War II. Since the early 1940s, millions of American workers have been exposed to asbestos dust. Initially, the risks associated with asbestos exposure were not known. However, an increased risk of developing mesothelioma was later found among shipyard workers, people who work in asbestos mines and mills, producers of asbestos products, workers in the heating and construction industries, and other tradespeople. Today, the U.S. Occupational Safety and Health Administration (OSHA) sets limits for acceptable levels of asbestos exposure in the workplace. People who work with asbestos wear personal protective equipment to lower their risk of exposure.

The risk of asbestos-related disease increases with heavier exposure to asbestos and longer exposure time. However, some individuals with only brief exposures have developed mesothelioma. On the other hand, not all workers who are heavily exposed develop asbestos-related diseases.

There is some evidence that family members and others living with asbestos workers have an increased risk of developing mesothelioma, and possibly other asbestos-related diseases. This risk may be the result of exposure to asbestos dust brought home on the clothing and hair of asbestos workers. To reduce the chance of exposing family members to asbestos fibers, asbestos workers are usually required to shower and change their clothing before leaving the workplace.

In certain parts of the world, the local soils may contain a significant amount of naturally occurring asbestos fibers. The rates of mesothelioma appear to be elevated among residents of these areas.

There is some evidence that prior radiation exposure is a risk factor for mesothelioma. However, it appears to be a much weaker risk factor than asbestos exposure.

About 20 to 30 percent of patients with mesothelioma have no history of asbestos exposure. The cause of the cancer in these individuals is unknown.

What are the symptoms of mesothelioma?

Symptoms of mesothelioma may not appear until thirty to fifty years after exposure to asbestos. Shortness of breath and pain in the chest due to an accumulation of fluid in the pleura are often symptoms of pleural mesothelioma. Symptoms of peritoneal mesothelioma include weight loss and abdominal pain and swelling due to a buildup of fluid in the abdomen. Other symptoms of peritoneal mesothelioma may include bowel obstruction, blood clotting abnormalities, anemia, and fever. If the cancer has spread beyond the mesothelium to other parts of the body, symptoms may include pain, trouble swallowing, or swelling of the neck or face.

These symptoms may be caused by mesothelioma or by other, less serious conditions. It is important to see a doctor about any of these symptoms. Only a doctor can make a diagnosis.

How is mesothelioma diagnosed?

Diagnosing mesothelioma is often difficult, because the symptoms are similar to those of a number of other conditions. Diagnosis begins with a review of the patient's medical history, including any history of asbestos exposure. A complete physical examination may be performed, including x-rays of the chest or abdomen and lung function tests. A computed tomography (CT, or computed axial tomography [CAT]) scan or magnetic resonance imaging (MRI) may also be useful. A CT scan is a series of detailed pictures of areas inside the body created by a computer linked to an x-ray machine. In an MRI, a powerful magnet linked to a computer is used to make detailed pictures of areas inside the body. These pictures are viewed on a monitor and can also be printed.

A biopsy is needed to confirm a diagnosis of mesothelioma. In a biopsy, a surgeon or a medical oncologist (a doctor who specializes in diagnosing and treating cancer) removes a sample of tissue for examination under a microscope by a pathologist. A biopsy may be done in different ways, depending on where the abnormal area is located. If the cancer is in the chest, the doctor may perform a thoracoscopy. In this procedure, the doctor makes a small cut through the chest wall and puts a thin, lighted tube called a thoracoscope into the chest between two ribs. Thoracoscopy allows the doctor to look inside the chest and obtain tissue samples. If the cancer is in the abdomen, the doctor may perform a peritoneoscopy. To obtain tissue for examination, the doctor makes a small opening in the abdomen and inserts a special instrument called a peritoneoscope into the abdominal cavity. If these procedures do not yield enough tissue, more extensive diagnostic surgery may be necessary.

If the diagnosis is mesothelioma, the doctor will want to learn the stage (or extent) of the disease. Staging involves more tests in a careful attempt to find out whether the cancer has spread and, if so, to which parts of the body. Knowing the stage of the disease helps the doctor plan treatment.

Mesothelioma is described as localized if the cancer is found only on the membrane surface where it originated. It is classified as advanced if it has spread beyond the original membrane surface to other parts of the body, such as the lymph nodes, lungs, chest wall, or abdominal organs.

How is mesothelioma treated?

Mesothelioma tends to be an aggressive cancer, and is usually difficult to treat. Survival rates for patients with mesothelioma are typically poor, but cures are sometimes seen with aggressive therapy. The cancer may be treated with the intent of curing the cancer (curative therapy), or to extend life and reduce suffering (palliative therapy) in patients for whom cure is not felt to be possible.

Treatment for mesothelioma depends on the location of the cancer, the stage of the disease, and the patient's age and general health. Standard treatment options include surgery, radiation therapy, and chemotherapy. Frequently, these treatments are combined.

Surgery: This is a common treatment for mesothelioma. The doctor may remove part of the lining of the chest or abdomen and some of the tissue around it. For cancer of the pleura (pleural mesothelioma), a lung may be removed in an operation called a pneumonectomy. Sometimes part of the diaphragm, the muscle below the lungs that helps with breathing, is also removed.

Radiation therapy: This treatment, also called radiotherapy, involves the use of high-energy rays to kill cancer cells and shrink tumors. Radiation therapy affects the cancer cells only in the treated area. The radiation may come from a machine (external radiation) or from putting materials that produce radiation through thin plastic tubes into the area where the cancer cells are found (internal radiation therapy).

Chemotherapy: This is the use of anticancer drugs to kill cancer cells throughout the body. Most drugs used to treat mesothelioma are given by injection into a vein (intravenous, or IV). Doctors are also studying the effectiveness of putting chemotherapy directly into the chest or abdomen (intracavitary chemotherapy).

To relieve symptoms and control pain, the doctor may use a needle or a thin tube to drain fluid that has built up in the chest or abdomen. The procedure for removing fluid from the chest is called thoracentesis.

Removal of fluid from the abdomen is called paracentesis. Drugs may be given through a tube in the chest to prevent more fluid from accumulating. Radiation therapy and surgery may also be helpful in relieving symptoms.

Are new treatments for mesothelioma being studied?

Yes. Because mesothelioma is very hard to control, the National Cancer Institute (NCI) is sponsoring clinical trials (research studies with people) that are designed to find new treatments and better ways to use current treatments. Before any new treatment can be recommended for general use, doctors conduct clinical trials to find out whether the treatment is safe for patients and effective against the disease. Participation in clinical trials is an important treatment option for many patients with mesothelioma.

People interested in taking part in a clinical trial should talk with their doctor.

Chapter 30

Pulmonary Edema

Alternative Names

Lung/pulmonary congestion; lung water

Definition

Pulmonary edema is an abnormal buildup of fluid in the lungs, which leads to swelling.

Causes

Pulmonary edema is usually caused by heart failure. As the heart fails, pressure in the vein going through the lungs starts to rise. As the pressure increases, fluid is pushed into the air spaces (alveoli). This fluid interrupts normal oxygen movement through the lungs, resulting in shortness of breath.

Pulmonary edema may be caused by damage directly to the lung, such as that caused by poisonous gas or severe infection. Lung damage and a buildup of body fluid is also seen in kidney failure.

Pulmonary edema may also be a complication of a heart attack, leaking or narrowed heart valves (mitral or aortic valves), or any disease of the heart that either results in weakening or stiffening of the heart muscle (cardiomyopathy).

Symptoms

- Shortness of breath
- Difficulty breathing
- Feeling of "air hunger" or "drowning"
- Grunting or gurgling sounds with breathing
- Wheezing
- Shortness of breath with lying down—you may need to sleep with your head propped up or use extra pillows
- Cough
- Anxiety
- Restlessness
- Excessive sweating
- Pale skin

Additional symptoms that may be associated with this disease:

- Nasal flaring;
- Coughing up blood;
- Inability to speak;
- Decrease in level of awareness.

Exams and Tests

The health care provider will perform a physical exam and use a stethoscope to listen to the lungs and heart. You may have:

- Rapid breathing;
- Increased heart rate;
- Crackles in the lungs or abnormal heart sounds;
- Pale or blue skin color.

Possible tests include:

- **Blood oxygen levels:** Low in patients with pulmonary edema;
- **Chest x-ray:** May reveal fluid in or around the lung space or an enlarged heart;

- **Ultrasound of the heart (echocardiogram):** May show a weak heart muscle, leaky or narrow heart valves, or fluid surrounding the heart.

Treatment

Oxygen is given through a face mask or tiny plastic tubes (prongs) placed in the nose. A breathing tube may be placed into the windpipe (trachea). A breathing machine (ventilator) may be needed.

The cause of the edema should be rapidly identified and treated. For example, if a heart attack has caused the condition, the heart must be treated and stabilized.

Diuretics, such as furosemide (Lasix®) may be given to help excess water pass through the urine. Medications to strengthen the heart muscle or to relieve the pressure on the heart may also be given.

Outlook (Prognosis)

Although pulmonary edema can be a life-threatening condition, it can be treated. How well a patient does depends on what is causing the edema.

Possible Complications

Some patients may need to use a breathing machine for a long time.

When to Contact a Medical Professional

Go to the emergency room or call 911 if you have breathing problems.

Prevention

If you have a disease that can lead to pulmonary edema, you should be sure to take all medicines as instructed. Following a healthy diet, one usually low in salt, can significantly decrease your risk of this condition.

Chapter 31

Pulmonary Embolism

What Is Pulmonary Embolism?

A pulmonary embolism, or PE, is a sudden blockage in a lung artery, usually due to a blood clot that traveled to the lung from a vein in the leg. A clot that forms in one part of the body and travels in the bloodstream to another part of the body is called an embolus.

PE is a serious condition that can cause the following:

- Permanent damage to part of your lung from lack of blood flow to lung tissue

- Low oxygen levels in your blood

- Damage to other organs in your body from not getting enough oxygen

If the blood clot is large, or if there are many clots, PE can cause death.

Overview

In most cases, PE is a complication of a condition called deep vein thrombosis (DVT). In DVT, blood clots form in the deep veins of the body—most often in the legs. These clots can break free, travel through the bloodstream to the lungs, and block an artery.

Excerpted from National Heart Lung and Blood Institute, National Institutes of Health, June 2007.

This is unlike clots in the veins close to the skin's surface, which remain in place and do not cause PE.

Outlook

At least one hundred thousand cases of PE occur each year in the United States. PE is the third most common cause of death in hospitalized patients. If left untreated, about 30 percent of patients with PE will die. Most of those who die do so within the first few hours of the event.

Other Names for Pulmonary Embolism

Pulmonary embolism is also called venous thromboembolism (VTE). This term is used for both pulmonary embolism and deep vein thrombosis.

What Causes Pulmonary Embolism?

Major Causes

In nine out of ten cases, pulmonary embolism (PE) begins as a blood clot in the deep veins of the leg (a condition known as deep vein thrombosis). The clot breaks free from the vein and travels through the bloodstream to the lungs, where it can block an artery.

Clots in the leg can form when blood flow is restricted and slows down. This can happen when you don't move around for long periods of time, such as:

- After some types of surgeries;
- During a long trip in a car or on an airplane;
- If you must stay in bed for an extended time.

Veins damaged from surgery or injured in other ways are more prone to blood clots.

Other Causes

Rarely, an air bubble, part of a tumor, or other tissue travels to the lungs and causes PE. Also, when a large bone in the body (such as the thigh bone) breaks, fat from the marrow inside the bone can travel through the blood to the lungs and cause PE.

Who Is at Risk for Pulmonary Embolism?

Populations Affected

Pulmonary embolism (PE) occurs equally in men and women. Risk increases with age: For each ten years after age sixty, the risk of PE doubles.

Certain inherited conditions, such as factor V Leiden, increase the risk of blood clotting, and, therefore, the risk of PE.

Major Risk Factors

People at high risk for a blood clot that travels to the lungs are those who:

- Have deep vein thrombosis (DVT, a blood clot in the leg) or a history of DVT;

- Have had PE before.

Other Risk Factors

People who recently have been treated for cancer or who have a central venous catheter (a tube placed in a vein to allow easy access to the bloodstream for medical treatment) are more likely to develop DVT. The same is true for people who have been bedridden or have had surgery or suffered a broken bone in the past few weeks.

Other risk factors for DVT, which can lead to PE, include sitting for long periods of time (such as on long car or airplane rides), pregnancy and the six-week period after pregnancy, and being overweight or obese. Women who take hormone therapy or birth control pills also are at increased risk for DVT.

People with more than one risk factor are at higher risk for blood clots.

What Are the Signs and Symptoms of Pulmonary Embolism?

Major Signs and Symptoms

Signs and symptoms of pulmonary embolism (PE) include unexplained shortness of breath, difficulty breathing, chest pain, coughing, or coughing up blood. An arrhythmia (a rapid or irregular heartbeat) also may indicate PE.

In some cases, the only signs and symptoms are related to deep vein thrombosis (DVT). These include swelling of the leg or along the vein in the leg, pain or tenderness in the leg, a feeling of increased warmth in the area of the leg that's swollen or tender, and red or discolored skin on the affected leg. See your doctor at once if you have any symptoms of PE or DVT.

It's possible to have a PE and not have any signs or symptoms of PE or DVT.

Other Signs and Symptoms

Sometimes people who have PE experience feelings of anxiety or dread, lightheadedness or fainting, rapid breathing, sweating, or an increased heart rate.

How Is Pulmonary Embolism Diagnosed?

Specialists Involved

Doctors who treat patients in the emergency room are often the ones to diagnose pulmonary embolism (PE) with the help of a radiologist (a doctor who deals with x-rays and other similar tests).

Medical History and Physical Exam

To diagnose PE, the doctor will ask about your medical history and perform a physical exam to:

- Identify your risk factors for deep vein thrombosis (DVT) and PE;
- See how likely it is that you could have PE;
- Rule out other possible causes for your symptoms.

During the physical exam, the doctor will check your legs for signs of DVT. He or she also will check your blood pressure and your heart and lungs.

Diagnostic Tests

There are many different tests that help the doctor determine whether you have PE. The doctor's decision about which tests to use and in which order depends on how you feel when you get to the hospital, your risk factors for PE, available testing options, and other conditions you may have.

You may have one of the following imaging tests:

- **Ultrasound:** Doctors use this test to look for blood clots in your legs. Ultrasound uses high-frequency sound waves to check the flow of blood in your veins. A gel is put on the skin of your leg. A hand-held device called a transducer is placed on the leg and moved back and forth over the affected area. The transducer gives off ultrasound waves and detects their echoes after they bounce off the vein walls and blood cells. A computer then turns the echoes of the ultrasound waves into a picture on a computer screen, where your doctor can see the blood flow in your leg. If blood clots are found in the deep veins of your legs, you will begin treatment. DVT and PE are both treated with the same medicines.

- **Spiral computed tomography (CT) scan or CT angiogram:** Doctors use this test to look for blood clots in your lungs and in your legs. Dye is injected into a vein in your arm to make the blood vessels in your lungs and legs more visible on the x-ray image. While you lie on a table, an x-ray tube rotates around you, taking pictures from different angles. This test allows doctors to detect PE in most patients. The test takes only a few minutes. Results are available shortly after the scan is completed.

- **Ventilation-perfusion lung scan (VQ scan):** Doctors use this test to detect PE. The VQ scan uses a radioactive material to show how well oxygen and blood are flowing to all areas of the lungs.

- **Pulmonary angiography:** This is another test used to diagnose PE. It's not available at all hospitals, and a trained specialist must perform the test. A flexible tube called a catheter is threaded through the groin (upper thigh) or arm to the blood vessels in the lungs. Dye is injected into the blood vessels through the catheter. X-ray pictures are taken to show the blood flow through the blood vessels in the lungs. If a clot is discovered, the doctor may use the catheter to extract it or deliver medicine to dissolve it.

Certain blood tests may help the doctor find out whether you're likely to have PE:

- A D-dimer test measures a substance in the blood that's released when a clot breaks up. High levels of the substance mean there may be a clot. If your test is normal and you have few risk factors, PE isn't likely.

- Other blood tests check for inherited disorders that cause clots and measure the amount of oxygen and carbon dioxide in your blood (arterial blood gas). A clot in a blood vessel in your lung may lower the level of oxygen in your blood.

To rule out other possible causes of your symptoms, the doctor may use one or more of the following tests:

- Echocardiogram uses sound waves to check heart function and to detect blood clots inside the heart.
- EKG (electrocardiogram) measures the rate and regularity of your heartbeat.
- Chest x-ray provides a picture of the lungs, heart, large arteries, ribs, and diaphragm.
- Magnetic resonance imaging (MRI) uses radio waves and magnetic fields to make pictures of organs and structures inside the body. In many cases, an MRI can provide information that can't be seen on an x-ray.

How Is Pulmonary Embolism Treated?

Goals of Treatment

The main goals of treating pulmonary embolism (PE) are to:

- Stop the blood clot from getting bigger;
- Keep new clots from forming.

Treatment may include medicines to thin the blood and slow its ability to clot. If your symptoms are life threatening, the doctor may give you medicine to dissolve the clot more quickly. Rarely, the doctor may use surgery or another procedure to remove the clot.

Specific Types of Treatment

Medicines: Anticoagulants, which are blood-thinning medicines, decrease your blood's ability to clot. They're used to stop blood clots from getting bigger and to prevent clots from forming. They don't break up blood clots that have already formed. (The body dissolves most clots with time.)

Anticoagulants can be taken either as a pill, as an injection, or through a needle or tube inserted into a vein (called intravenous, or IV, injection). Warfarin is given in a pill form. (Coumadin® is a common brand name for warfarin.) Heparin is given as an injection or through an IV tube.

Your doctor may treat you with both heparin and warfarin at the same time. Heparin acts quickly. Warfarin takes two to three days before it starts to work. Once warfarin starts to work, usually the heparin will be stopped.

Pregnant women usually are treated with heparin only, because warfarin is dangerous for the pregnancy.

If you have deep vein thrombosis, treatment with anticoagulants usually lasts for three to six months.

If you have had blood clots before, you may need a longer period of treatment. If you're being treated for another illness, such as cancer, you may need to take anticoagulants as long as risk factors for PE are present.

The most common side effect of anticoagulants is bleeding. This happens if the medicine thins your blood too much. This side effect can be life threatening. Sometimes, the bleeding can be internal. This is why people treated with anticoagulants usually receive regular blood tests. These tests are called prothrombin time (PT) and partial thromboplastin time (PTT) tests, and they measure the blood's ability to clot. These tests also help the doctor make sure you're taking the right amount of medicine. Call your doctor right away if you have easy bruising or bleeding.

Thrombin inhibitors are a newer type of anticoagulant medicine. They're used to treat some types of blood clots for patients who can't take heparin.

Emergency treatment: When PE is life threatening, doctors may use treatments that remove or break up clots in the blood vessels of the lungs. These treatments are given in the emergency room or in the hospital.

Thrombolytics are medicines given to quickly dissolve a blood clot. They're used to treat large clots that cause severe symptoms. Because thrombolytics can cause sudden bleeding, they're used only in life-threatening situations.

In some cases, the doctor may use a catheter to reach the blood clot. A catheter is a flexible tube placed in a vein to allow easy access to the bloodstream for medical treatment. The catheter is inserted into the groin (upper thigh) or arm and threaded through a vein to the clot in the lung. The catheter may be used to extract the clot or deliver medicine to dissolve it.

Rarely, surgery may be needed to remove the blood clot.

Other Types of Treatment

When you can't take medicines to thin your blood, or when you're taking blood thinners but continue to develop clots anyway, the doctor may use a device called a vena cava filter to keep clots from traveling to your lungs. The filter is inserted inside a large vein called the inferior vena cava (the vein that carries blood from the body back to the heart). The filter catches clots before they travel to the lungs. This prevents PE, but it doesn't stop other blood clots from forming.

Graduated compression stockings can reduce the chronic (ongoing) swelling that may occur after a blood clot has developed in a leg. The leg swelling is due to damage to the valves in the leg veins. Graduated compression stockings are worn on the legs from the arch of the foot to just above or below the knee. These stockings are tight at the ankle and become looser as they go up the leg. This causes a gentle compression (or pressure) up the leg. The pressure keeps blood from pooling and clotting.

How Can Pulmonary Embolism Be Prevented?

Preventing pulmonary embolism (PE) begins with preventing deep vein thrombosis (DVT). Knowing whether you're at risk for DVT and taking steps to lower your risk are important.

If you've never had a deep vein clot, but are at risk for it, these are steps you can take to decrease your risk:

- Exercise your lower leg muscles during long car trips and airplane rides.

- Get out of bed and move around as soon as you're able after having surgery or being ill. The sooner you move around, the lower your chance of developing a clot.

- Take medicines to prevent clots after some types of surgery (as directed by your doctor).

- Follow up with your doctor.

If you already have had DVT or PE, you can take additional steps to help keep new blood clots from forming:

- Visit your doctor for regular checkups.

- Use compression stockings to prevent chronic swelling in your legs after DVT (as directed by your doctor).

Contact your doctor at once if you have any signs or symptoms of DVT or PE.

Living with Pulmonary Embolism

Treatment for PE usually takes place in the hospital. After leaving the hospital you may need to take medicine at home for six months or longer. It's important to do the following:

- Take medicines as prescribed.

- Have blood tests done as directed by your doctor.

- Talk to your doctor before taking anticoagulants with any other medicines, including over-the-counter medicines. Over-the-counter aspirin, for example, can thin your blood. Taking two medicines that thin your blood (even if one is over-the-counter) may increase your risk for bleeding.

- Ask your doctor about your diet. Foods that contain vitamin K can affect how well warfarin (Coumadin®) works. Vitamin K is found in green leafy vegetables and some oils, such as canola and soybean oil. It's best to eat a well-balanced, healthy diet.

- Discuss with your doctor what amount of alcohol is safe for you to drink if you're taking medicine.

Medicines used to treat PE can thin your blood too much. This can cause bleeding in the digestive system or the brain. If you have signs or symptoms of bleeding in the digestive system or the brain, get treatment at once.

Signs and symptoms of bleeding in the digestive system include the following:

- Bright red vomit or vomit that looks like coffee grounds

- Bright red blood in your stool or black, tarry stools

- Pain in your abdomen

Signs and symptoms of bleeding in the brain include the following:

- Severe pain in your head

- Sudden changes in your vision
- Sudden loss of movement in your legs or arms
- Memory loss or confusion

Excessive bleeding from a fall or injury also may mean that your PE medicines have thinned your blood too much. Excessive bleeding is bleeding that will not stop after you apply pressure to a wound for ten minutes. If you have excessive bleeding from a fall or injury, get treatment at once.

Once you have had PE (with or without deep vein thrombosis (DVT)), you have a greater chance of having another one. During treatment and after, continue to do the following things:

- Take steps to prevent DVT.
- Check your legs for any signs or symptoms of DVT, such as swollen areas, pain or tenderness, increased warmth in swollen or painful areas, or red or discolored skin.

If you think that you have DVT or are having symptoms of PE, contact your doctor at once.

Chapter 32

Pulmonary Hypertension

What is pulmonary hypertension?

Pulmonary hypertension (PH) is a rare blood vessel disorder of the lung in which the pressure in the pulmonary artery (the blood vessel that leads from the heart to the lungs) rises above normal levels and may become life-threatening.

What are the symptoms of PH?

Symptoms of pulmonary hypertension include shortness of breath with minimal exertion, fatigue, chest pain, dizzy spells, and fainting.

What causes PH?

When pulmonary hypertension occurs in the absence of a known cause, it is referred to as primary pulmonary hypertension (PPH). This term should not be construed to mean that because it has a single name it is a single disease. There are likely many unknown causes of PPH. PPH is extremely rare, occurring in about two persons per million population per year.

Secondary pulmonary hypertension (SPH) means the cause is known. A common cause of SPH are the breathing disorders emphysema and bronchitis. Other less frequent causes are inflammatory or

---

collagen vascular diseases such as scleroderma, CREST syndrome, or systemic lupus erythematosus (SLE). Congenital heart diseases that cause shunting of extra blood through the lungs like ventricular and atrial septal defects, chronic pulmonary thromboembolism (old blood clots in the pulmonary artery), human immunodeficiency virus (HIV) infection, liver disease, and diet drugs like fenfluramine and dexfenfluramine are also causes of pulmonary hypertension.

How is PH diagnosed?

Pulmonary hypertension is frequently misdiagnosed and has often progressed to late stage by the time it is accurately diagnosed.

The gold standard test for diagnosing PH is right-heart cardiac catheterization, where the doctor places a thin, flexible tube, or catheter, through an arm, leg, or neck vein, then threads the catheter into the right ventricle and pulmonary artery. Most important in PPH is if the doctor gets a precise measure of the blood pressure in the right side of the heart and the pulmonary artery. It is the only way to get this measure, and must be performed in the hospital by a specialist. During catheterization, the doctor can also evaluate the right heart's pumping ability; this is done by measuring the amount of blood pumped out of the right side of the heart with each heartbeat.

Prior to performing this test a number of noninvasive tests may suggest the diagnosis, including the electrocardiogram, chest x-ray, and echocardiogram. The diagnosis of PPH is made by excluding all known causes of SPH.

Pulmonary hypertension has been historically chronic and incurable with a poor survival rate. However, new treatments are available which have significantly improved prognosis. Recent data indicate that the length of survival is continuing to improve, with some people able to manage the disorder for fifteen to twenty years or longer.

What treatments are available?

Current treatments include calcium channel blocking drugs, prostacyclin, and endothelin receptor antagonists. Calcium is an agent that helps cause smooth muscles cells to contract.

Calcium channel blockers (CCBs) block the movement of calcium into the cells of the heart and blood vessels. Blocking the calcium helps to relax blood vessels and increase the supply of blood and oxygen to the heart while reducing its workload. Unfortunately, less than 30 percent of people with PH respond to CCBs. CCBs are also prescribed for systemic hypertension, but in much lower dosages than when they are prescribed for PH. It is not unusual for CCBs to cause fluid retention.

Prostaglandin is a steroid that is produced naturally in the body in a normally healthy person. It causes blood vessels in the lungs to relax and allows blood to flow through them more easily. People with pulmonary hypertension do not produce enough prostaglandin, so the blood vessels in the lungs are constricted. Prostacyclin, also known as epoprostenol, is a synthetic substance that is administered to remedy this deficiency. Prostacyclin therapy was initially used as a bridge to lung transplantation although it has also emerged as an alternative to transplantation in some people.

Endothelin receptor antagonists: These are a new class of drugs for the treatment of a number of major diseases, including pulmonary arterial hypertension. Endothelin is a peptide made by the body in the endothelium (a layer of cells which line the heart and blood vessels). It constricts blood vessels and elevates blood pressure. Endothelin is a potent vasoconstrictor that plays an important role in blood flow. In PH, the body produces excess endothelin, contributing to the constriction of blood vessels and affecting the blood pressure in the lungs. Although endothelin is present in healthy people, high concentrations of the substance have been found in the plasma and lungs of people with PH, suggesting it is capable of causing PH or increasing the symptoms of PH. Endothelin must connect with an endothelin receptor in order to be activated. Endothelin receptor antagonists block endothelin receptors, thereby limiting harmful excess endothelin in the blood vessels.

Lung transplantation: Quality of life can be moderately to substantially improved by lung transplantation, and life may be extended beyond your life expectancy prior to transplantation. It is impossible to predict how long you may survive after transplantation. The most critical period is the year after transplantation; this is the period when surgical complications, rejection, and infection are the greatest threat to survival. People who survive the first year are more likely to survive three years or longer after transplantation. There are people alive today who had lung transplantation five or even more years ago.

Life expectancy after lung transplantation is shorter than for heart, liver, or kidney transplantation, particularly for PPH people. Rejection and infection are the two major complications of lung transplantation. Immunosuppressive (antirejection) medications prescribed by your doctors will help keep the rejection process "turned off." Other medications may be necessary to control and treat rejection if your immune system breaks through the immunosuppressive blockade. Following your doctor's instructions and taking all medications as prescribed help to prevent or control rejection.

Because you will be taking immunosuppressive medications, your immune system will be less able to fight off invading bacteria and viruses. You will be much more susceptible to infections, which are more likely to become severe.

Therapies that may be used in conjunction with treatments include diuretics used to control an excessive amount of watery fluid in cells, tissues, or serous cavities (such as the abdomen). Pulmonary hypertension can lead to right heart failure and an excess of fluid in the lower and upper extremities and abdomen. An excess of fluid can also be caused by high-dose calcium channel blockers. Diuretics will cause frequent urination.

Digitalis medicines (Digoxin, Lanoxin) are used to improve the strength and efficiency of the heart or to control the rate and rhythm of the heartbeat. This leads to better blood circulation and reduced swelling of hands and ankles in people with right heart problems. Its value for people with PH has not yet been fully examined but it is often used with calcium channel blockers because CCBs tend to weaken the pumping effectiveness of the heart.

Supplementary oxygen is sometimes prescribed for PH people when someone has an inadequate amount of available oxygen (hypoxemia) in the blood at rest or with physical activity. Supplementary oxygen, however, is an important addition to treating the symptoms of PH with hypoxemia or under special conditions, such as when hospitalized with a respiratory infection, or at high altitudes or sometimes when traveling by air.

Blood clots are potential complications of PH. Oral anticoagulant therapy (Coumadin, Warfarin) is widely recommended for people with PH because it probably prolongs survival.

Chapter 33

Sleep Apnea

What Is Sleep Apnea?

Sleep apnea is a common disorder that can be very serious. In sleep apnea, your breathing stops or gets very shallow while you are sleeping. Each pause in breathing typically lasts ten to twenty seconds or more. These pauses can occur twenty to thirty times or more an hour.

The most common type of sleep apnea is obstructive sleep apnea. During sleep, enough air cannot flow into your lungs through your mouth and nose even though you try to breathe. When this happens, the amount of oxygen in your blood may drop. Normal breaths then start again with a loud snort or choking sound.

When your sleep is upset throughout the night, you can be very sleepy during the day. With sleep apnea, your sleep is not restful because:

- These brief episodes of increased airway resistance (and breathing pauses) occur many times.

- You may have many brief drops in the oxygen levels in your blood.

- You move out of deep sleep and into light sleep several times during the night, resulting in poor sleep quality.

Reprinted from National Heart, Lung, and Blood Institute, National Institutes of Health, February 2006.

People with sleep apnea often have loud snoring. However, not everyone who snores has sleep apnea. Some people with sleep apnea don't know they snore.

Sleep apnea happens more often in people who are overweight, but even thin people can have it.

Most people don't know they have sleep apnea. They don't know that they are having problems breathing while they are sleeping.

A family member and/or bed partner may notice the signs of sleep apnea first.

Untreated sleep apnea can increase the chance of having high blood pressure and even a heart attack or stroke. Untreated sleep apnea can also increase the risk of diabetes and the risk for work-related accidents and driving accidents.

What Causes Sleep Apnea?

Sleep apnea happens when enough air cannot move into your lungs while you are sleeping. When you are awake, and normally during sleep, your throat muscles keep your throat open and air flows into your lungs. In obstructive sleep apnea, however, the throat briefly collapses, causing pauses in your breathing. With pauses in breathing, the oxygen level in your blood may drop. This happens if the following conditions occur:

- Your throat muscles and tongue relax more than is normal.

- Your tonsils and adenoids are large.

- You are overweight. The extra soft tissue in your throat makes it harder to keep the throat area open.

- The shape of your head and neck (bony structure) results in somewhat smaller airway size in the mouth and throat area.

With the throat frequently fully or partly blocked during sleep, enough air cannot flow into your lungs, even though your efforts to breathe continue. Your breathing may become hard and noisy and may even stop for short periods of time (apneas).

Central apnea is a rare type of sleep apnea that happens when the area of your brain that controls your breathing doesn't send the correct signals to the breathing muscles. Then there is no effort to breathe at all for brief periods. Snoring does not typically occur in central apnea.

Who Is at Risk for Obstructive Sleep Apnea?

Anyone can have obstructive sleep apnea.

It is estimated that more than twelve million Americans have obstructive sleep apnea. More than half the people who have sleep apnea are overweight, and most snore heavily.

Sleep apnea is more common in men. One out of twenty-five middle-aged men and one out of fifty middle-aged women have sleep apnea that causes them to be very sleepy during the day. Sleep apnea is more common in African Americans, Hispanics, and Pacific Islanders than in Caucasians. If someone in your family has sleep apnea, you are more likely to develop it than someone without a family history of the condition.

Adults who are most likely to have sleep apnea have one or more of the following characteristics:

- They snore loudly.

- They are overweight.

- They have high blood pressure.

- The airways in their nose, throat, or mouth are decreased in size. This can be caused by the shape of these structures or by medical conditions causing congestion in these areas, such as hay fever or other allergies.

- They have a family history of sleep apnea.

Obstructive sleep apnea can also occur in children who snore. If your child snores, you should discuss it with your child's doctor or health care provider.

What Are the Signs and Symptoms of Sleep Apnea?

The most common signs of sleep apnea are as follows:

- Loud snoring

- Choking or gasping during sleep

- Fighting sleepiness during the day (even at work or while driving)

Your family members may notice the symptoms before you do. Otherwise, you will likely not be aware that you have problems breathing while you are asleep.

Others signs of sleep apnea may include the following:

- Morning headaches

- Memory or learning problems
- Feeling irritable
- Not being able to concentrate on your work
- Mood swings or personality changes; perhaps feeling depressed
- Dry throat when you wake up
- Frequent urination at night

How Is Sleep Apnea Diagnosed?

Your doctor will do a physical exam and take a medical history that includes asking you and your family questions about how you sleep and how you function during the day. As part of the exam, your doctor will check your mouth, nose, and throat for extra or large tissues; for example, tonsils, uvula (the tissue that hangs from the middle of the back of the mouth), and soft palate (the roof of your mouth in the back of your throat).

Your doctor may order a sleep recording of what happens with your breathing while you sleep. A sleep recording is a test that is often done in a sleep center or sleep laboratory, which may be part of a hospital. You may stay overnight in the sleep center, although sleep studies are sometimes done in the home. The most common sleep recording used to find out if you have sleep apnea is called a polysomnogram, or PSG. This test records the following things:

- Brain activity
- Eye movement
- Muscle activity
- Breathing and heart rate
- How much air moves in and out of your lungs while you are sleeping
- The percentage of oxygen in your blood

A PSG is painless. You will go to sleep as usual. The staff at the sleep center will monitor your sleep throughout the night. The results of your PSG will be analyzed by a sleep medicine specialist to see if you have sleep apnea, how severe it is, and what treatment may be recommended.

In certain circumstances, the PSG can be done at home. A home monitor can be used to record your heart rate, how air moves in and out of your lungs, the amount of oxygen in your blood, and your breathing effort. For this test, a technician will come to your home and help you apply the monitor that you will wear overnight. You will go to sleep as usual, and the technician will come back the next morning to get the monitor and send the results to your doctor.

Once all your tests are completed, the sleep medicine specialist will review the results and work with you and your family to develop a treatment plan. In some cases, you may also need to see another physician for evaluation of one or more of the following:

- Lung problems (treated by a pulmonologist)

- Problems with the brain or nerves (treated by a neurologist)

- Heart or blood pressure problems (treated by a cardiologist)

- Ear, nose, or throat problems (treated by an ear, nose, and throat specialist)

- Mental health issues, such as anxiety or depression (treated by a psychologist or psychiatrist)

How Is Sleep Apnea Treated?

Treatment is aimed at restoring regular nighttime breathing and relieving symptoms such as very loud snoring and daytime sleepiness. Treatment will also help associated medical problems, such as high blood pressure, and reduce the risk for heart attack and stroke.

Changes in Activities or Habits

If you have mild sleep apnea, some changes in daily activities or habits may be all that are needed:

- Avoid alcohol, smoking, and medicines that make you sleepy. They make it harder for your throat to stay open while you sleep.

- Lose weight if you are overweight. Even a little weight loss can improve your symptoms.

- Sleep on your side instead of your back. Sleeping on your side may help keep your throat open.

People with moderate or severe sleep apnea will need to make these changes as well. They also will need other treatments, such as the following.

Continuous Positive Airway Pressure

Continuous positive airway pressure (CPAP) is the most common treatment for sleep apnea. For this treatment, you wear a mask over your nose during sleep. The mask blows air into your throat at a pressure level that is right for you. The increased airway pressure keeps the throat open while you sleep. The air pressure is adjusted so that it is just enough to stop the airways from briefly getting too small during sleep.

Treating sleep apnea may help you stop snoring. Stopping snoring does not mean that you no longer have sleep apnea or that you can stop using CPAP.

Sleep apnea will return if CPAP is stopped or if it is not used correctly. Usually, a technician comes to your home to bring the CPAP equipment. The technician will set up the CPAP machine and make adjustments based on your doctor's orders.

CPAP treatment may cause side effects in some people. Some side effects are as follows:

- Dry or stuffy nose
- Irritation of the skin on your face
- Bloating of your stomach
- Sore eyes
- Headaches

If you are having trouble with CPAP side effects, work with your sleep medicine specialist and technician. Together you can do things, such as the following, to reduce these side effects:

- Use a nasal spray to relieve a dry, stuffy, or runny nose.
- Adjust the CPAP settings.
- Adjust the size or fit of the mask.
- Add moisture to the air as it flows through the mask.
- Use a CPAP machine that can automatically adjust the amount of air pressure to the level that is required to keep the airway open.
- Use a CPAP machine that will start with a low air pressure and slowly increase the air pressure as you fall asleep.

People with severe sleep apnea symptoms generally feel much better once they begin treatment with CPAP. When using CPAP, it is very important that you follow up with your doctor. If you are having side effects, talk to your doctor.

Mouthpiece

A mouthpiece (oral appliance) may be helpful in some people with mild sleep apnea. Some doctors may also recommend this if you snore loudly but do not have sleep apnea.

A custom-fit plastic mouthpiece will be made by a dentist or orthodontist. An orthodontist is a specialist in correcting teeth or jaw problems. The mouthpiece will adjust your lower jaw and your tongue to help keep the airway in your throat open while you are sleeping. Air can then flow easily into your lungs because there is less resistance to breathing.

Possible side effects of the mouthpiece include damage to the following parts of your body:

- Your teeth
- Your gums
- Your jaw

Follow up with your dentist or orthodontist to check for any side effects and to be sure that your mouthpiece fits.

Surgery

Some people with sleep apnea may benefit from surgery. The type of surgery depends on the cause of the sleep apnea:

- Surgery may be done to remove the tonsils and adenoids if they are blocking the airway. This surgery is especially helpful for children.

- Uvulopalatopharyngoplasty (U-vu-lo-PAL-a-to-fa-RIN-go-plas-te) (UPPP) is a surgery that removes the tonsils, uvula (the tissue that hangs from the middle of the back of the roof of the mouth), and part of your soft palate (the roof of your mouth in the back of your throat). This surgery is only effective for some people with sleep apnea.

- Laser-assisted uvulopalatoplasty (U-vu-lo-PAL-a-to-plas-te) (LAUP) is a surgery that can stop snoring but is probably not helpful in treating sleep apnea. A laser device is used to remove the uvula and part of the soft palate. Because this surgery stops the main symptom of sleep apnea (snoring), it is important to have a sleep study first.

- Tracheostomy is a surgery used in severe sleep apnea. A small hole is made in the windpipe and a tube is inserted. Air will flow through the tube and into the lungs. This surgery is very successful but is needed only in patients not responding to all other possible treatments.

Other possible surgeries for some people with sleep apnea include the following:

- Rebuilding the lower jaw
- Surgery on the nose
- Surgery to treat obesity

Currently, there are no medicines for the treatment of sleep apnea.

Living with Sleep Apnea

Getting treatment for sleep apnea and following your doctor's advice can help you and your family members:

- Getting treatment for sleep apnea can help snoring and can improve your sleep.

- Treating sleep apnea helps you feel rested during the day.

- Many people will benefit by making healthy changes, such as stopping smoking and losing weight.

- Some people will need to wear a mask at night to help keep the throat open and improve breathing.

- A few people will need to have surgery to remove tonsils and adenoids, part of the uvula (the tissue that hangs from the middle of the back of the roof of the mouth), and/or the soft palate (the roof of your mouth in the back of your throat) that may block the airway.

- Regular and ongoing follow-up is needed; your sleep medicine specialist will check whether your treatment is working and whether you are having any side effects.

What Can Family Do to Help?

Often, people with sleep apnea do not know they have it. They are not aware that their breathing stops and starts many times while they are sleeping. Family members or bed partners are usually the first ones to notice that the person snores and stops breathing while sleeping.

There are many things family members can do to help a loved one who has sleep apnea, including the following:

- Letting the person know if he or she snores loudly during sleep or has breathing stops and starts

- Encouraging the person to get medical help

- Helping the person follow the doctor's treatment plan, including continuous positive airway pressure (CPAP)

- Making sure the person puts on the CPAP mask before falling asleep

- Providing emotional support

- Helping with insurance paperwork

Sleep apnea can be very serious. People with sleep apnea are at higher risk for car crashes, work-related accidents, and other medical problems due to their sleepiness. It is important that people with sleep apnea see their doctor to treat and control this disorder.

Treatment may improve a person's overall health and happiness as well as the quality of sleep for both the person and the entire family.

Key Points

Sleep apnea is a common breathing disorder that can be very serious.

In sleep apnea, your breathing stops or becomes very shallow for periods of ten to twenty seconds or longer many times during the night.

The most common type of sleep apnea is obstructive sleep apnea.

It is estimated that more than twelve million Americans have sleep apnea.

The most common signs of sleep apnea are loud snoring and choking or gasping during sleep and being sleepy during the day.

Having a physical exam and providing your doctor with information about your sleep will help to diagnose sleep apnea. Your doctor may also want you to have special sleep tests.

Treatment is aimed at restoring regular nighttime breathing and relieving symptoms such as loud snoring and daytime sleepiness. Treatment will also help associated medical problems, such as high blood pressure, and reduce the risk for heart attack and stroke.

Continuous positive airway pressure (CPAP) is the most common treatment for sleep apnea.

Some people with sleep apnea may benefit from surgery.

Family members can help a person who snores loudly or stops breathing while sleeping by encouraging him or her to get medical help.

Treatment for sleep apnea may improve a person's overall health and happiness as well as the quality of sleep for both the person and the entire family.

Chapter 34

Lung Disorders Affecting Infants and Young Children

Chapter Contents

Section 34.1

Bronchopulmonary Dysplasia

Excerpted from National Heart, Lung, and Blood Institute,
National Institutes of Health, May 2007.

What Is Bronchopulmonary Dysplasia?

Bronchopulmonary dysplasia, or BPD, is a serious lung condition that affects mostly babies who:

- Are born more than ten weeks before their due dates;
- Weigh less than 2.5 pounds, or 1,000 grams, at birth;
- Have breathing problems at birth;
- Need long-term breathing support and oxygen.

Many of these babies are born with serious respiratory distress syndrome (RDS). Their lungs haven't yet developed enough to make surfactant. Surfactant is a liquid that coats the inside of the lungs and keeps them open so that the baby can breathe in air once he or she is born.

As a result, these babies are usually put on oxygen and a breathing machine at birth—either a ventilator (also known as a respirator) or a nasal continuous positive airway pressure (NCPAP) machine. This can prevent damage to their brains and other body organs from lack of oxygen. They also are given surfactant.

Most babies with RDS begin to get better within the next two to four weeks. But some get worse and need more oxygen and/or breathing assistance from a machine. These babies have developed BPD.

The lungs of the babies who are born with RDS and go on to develop BPD are less developed than those of babies with RDS who recover. They usually have fewer and larger alveoli, or air sacs, than other newborns. They also may have fewer tiny blood vessels in the alveoli. The blood vessels are needed to move oxygen from the alveoli into the bloodstream.

These babies also are more likely than other infants to have problems in other parts of their bodies that aren't yet fully developed. These include the heart, kidneys, brain, stomach, intestines, and eyes.

With new and better treatments now available, most babies with BPD get better over time, and many go on to live normal, active lives.

How the Lungs Work

The air that you breathe in through your nose or mouth travels down through your windpipe (trachea) into tubes in your lungs called bronchial tubes, or airways.

The airways are shaped like an upside-down tree with many branches. The trachea is the trunk. It splits into tubes, called bronchi. Thinner tubes, called bronchioles, branch out of the bronchi.

The bronchioles end in tiny air sacs called alveoli. The alveoli have very thin walls, and small blood vessels called capillaries run through them. There are about 300 million alveoli in a normal lung.

When the air reaches the alveoli, the oxygen in the air passes through the thin walls of the alveoli into the blood in the capillaries. From there, it flows into larger veins and arteries, which carry it to your heart. The heart then pumps the oxygen-rich blood to all of your body's organs. Your heart and other organs can't do their jobs without an ongoing supply of oxygen.

In babies who develop bronchopulmonary dysplasia, the airways aren't yet fully developed. The alveoli are larger than normal, and there are fewer of them. The capillaries also may not be fully developed. As a result, the lungs can't move enough oxygen into the bloodstream to support the heart and other body organs.

Other Names for Bronchopulmonary Dysplasia

- Neonatal chronic lung disease (CLD)
- Evolving chronic lung disease

What Causes Bronchopulmonary Dysplasia?

The lungs of babies born more than ten weeks before they are due are fragile and easily irritated or injured by things in the outside environment during the first hours or days after birth.

Doctors now believe that a baby gets bronchopulmonary dysplasia (BPD) as a result of the way his or her lungs respond to some of these things, including the following:

- **High levels of oxygen:** Doctors usually give oxygen to newborns with breathing problems. This is to make sure that their

515

brains, hearts, livers, and kidneys receive enough oxygen to do their jobs. But high levels of oxygen can cause inflammation in the lungs. This can result in injury to the breathing passages. High levels of oxygen also can slow the normal development of the lungs in babies born very early.

- **Pressure caused by mechanical ventilation:** In the past, doctors usually put newborns who couldn't breathe on their own on mechanical ventilators. These machines apply pressure to push air into the babies' lungs. This pressure can irritate the lungs and cause them to become more inflamed. Mechanical ventilation is a factor in most cases of BPD. Doctors try to minimize the injury by using ventilation only when absolutely needed. Today, more and more doctors are putting these babies on nasal continuous positive airway pressure (NCPAP) machines, which don't put the same kind of pressure on the babies' lungs.

- **Infections:** Infections in babies born early can cause inflammation in their underdeveloped lungs. This narrows the breathing passages and makes it harder for the baby to breathe. Lung infections also increase the baby's need for extra oxygen and help with breathing.

Some doctors think that heredity may be a factor in the development of BPD.

Who Is at Risk for Bronchopulmonary Dysplasia?

The earlier a baby is born and the lower his or her weight at birth, the greater the chances the baby will develop bronchopulmonary dysplasia (BPD). Most babies who are diagnosed with BPD today weigh less than 3.5 pounds, or 1,500 grams, at birth.

About one of every three newborns who weighs less than 2 pounds, or 1,000 grams, at birth gets BPD.

About five thousand to ten thousand babies born in the United States each year develop BPD. The number of babies who develop BPD is higher than it was thirty years ago because doctors are now able to keep more babies who weigh less than three pounds at birth alive.

BPD develops in some babies who have mild or no respiratory distress syndrome. Most of these babies are born at extremely low birth weights or have patent ductus arteriosus, a problem in the heart that is present at birth, or sepsis, a serious bacterial infection in the bloodstream.

What Are the Signs and Symptoms of Bronchopulmonary Dysplasia?

Most babies who get bronchopulmonary dysplasia (BPD) are born with respiratory distress syndrome (RDS). The signs and symptoms of RDS at birth are as follows:

- Rapid, shallow breathing

- Sharp pulling in of the chest below the ribs with each breath taken in

- Grunting sounds during exhalation

- Flaring of the nostrils during breathing

As a result, these babies usually are put on a breathing machine right away. This is to prevent damage to their brains, hearts, and other body organs from lack of oxygen. These babies also are given surfactant to coat the tiny air sacs and to help prevent their lungs from collapsing.

Doctors can usually diagnose BPD after about two weeks. At this point, the baby hasn't started getting better, and he or she needs more oxygen.

Babies with severe BPD may also develop the following conditions:

- Pulmonary arterial hypertension, continuous high blood pressure in the blood vessels that carry oxygen-poor blood from the right ventricle in the heart to the small arteries in the lungs

- Cor pulmonale, failure of the right side of the heart caused by ongoing high blood pressure in the pulmonary artery and right ventricle

How Is Bronchopulmonary Dysplasia Diagnosed?

It's hard to tell whether a baby with breathing problems has bronchopulmonary dysplasia (BPD) before he or she is about fourteen to thirty days old. At this point, the baby should be showing improvement in the breathing problems. Instead, the baby's condition seems to be getting worse and he or she needs more oxygen or help from a breathing machine.

Doctors usually conduct a number of tests on newborns with breathing problems to make sure they diagnose their condition correctly. These tests include the following:

517

- **Blood tests:** Blood samples are checked to see whether the baby has enough oxygen in his or her blood.

- **Chest x-ray:** A chest x-ray takes a picture of the heart and lungs. It shows larger areas of air and changes from inflammation or infection. It also shows areas of the lung that have collapsed and may help confirm that the lungs aren't developing normally.

- **Echocardiogram:** This test uses sound waves to create a moving picture of the heart. Echocardiogram is used to rule out congenital heart defects or pulmonary arterial hypertension as the cause of the breathing problems.

Doctors grade BPD as mild, moderate, or severe, depending on how much extra oxygen the baby needs and how long he or she needs it.

How Is Bronchopulmonary Dysplasia Treated?

The goals of treatment for babies with bronchopulmonary dysplasia (BPD) are to reduce further injury to the lungs and to provide nutrition and other support to help the lungs grow and recover.

Treatment is done in three stages:

- Treatment for respiratory distress at birth and before doctors know whether the baby has BPD

- Treatment after doctors know the baby has BPD

- Home care after the baby leaves the hospital

Treatment of respiratory distress usually begins as soon as the baby is born, sometimes in the delivery room. Most infants who show signs and symptoms of respiratory distress syndrome (RDS) are quickly moved to a special intensive care unit called a neonatal intensive care unit (NICU). There they receive around-the-clock treatment from a group of health care professionals who specialize in treating premature infants.

The most important treatments for RDS are breathing support and surfactant replacement therapy.

Breathing Support

These babies usually are put on a breathing machine to help them breathe—either a mechanical ventilator or a nasal continuous positive airway pressure (NCPAP) machine. The ventilator is connected to a breathing tube that runs through the baby's mouth or nose into the windpipe. The ventilator can be set to help a baby breathe or to completely control a baby's breathing. It also is set to give the amount of oxygen the baby needs.

Today, more and more babies are receiving breathing support from an NCPAP machine, which pushes air into the baby's lungs through prongs in the nostrils.

With breathing help, the baby's lungs have a chance to develop. Breathing machines today don't cause as much injury to the airways and lungs as those used in the past.

Surfactant Replacement Therapy

The baby is given surfactant to open his or her lungs until the lungs have developed enough to start making their own surfactant. Surfactant is given through a tube that is attached to the breathing machine, which pushes the surfactant directly into the baby's lungs.

Other Types of Treatment

Other treatments for babies who show signs and symptoms of RDS and haven't yet been diagnosed with BPD include medicines, supportive therapy, and treatment for patent ductus arteriosus, a condition that affects some premature infants.

Medicines: Doctors usually give the baby medicines to reduce swelling in the airways and improve the flow of air in and out of the lungs. These medicines include bronchodilators to improve the flow of air in and out of the lungs, diuretics to help remove extra fluid from the lungs, and antibiotics to control infections.

Supportive therapy: Treatment in the NICU is designed to limit stress on the baby and meet his or her basic needs of warmth, nutrition, and protection. Such treatment usually includes the following:

- Using a radiant warmer or incubator to keep your baby warm and reduce the chances of infection.

- Ongoing monitoring of blood pressure, heart rate, breathing, and temperature through sensors taped to the baby's body.

- Using a sensor on a finger or toe to monitor the amount of oxygen in the baby's blood.

- Giving fluids and nutrients through a needle or tube inserted into a vein to prevent malnutrition and promote growth. Nutrition is critical to the growth and development of the lungs. Later, your baby may be given milk through a tube that is passed through his or her nose into the mouth.

- Monitoring fluid intake to make sure that fluid doesn't build up in the baby's lungs.

Once doctors know that the baby has BPD, some or all of these treatments are continued in the NICU:

- Babies with BPD are usually taken off the breathing machine slowly over time. They are often moved from the ventilator to an NCPAP machine until they can breathe on their own. This machine pushes air into the baby's lungs through prongs in the nostrils.

- The baby is likely to continue to need extra oxygen for some time. Once the baby no longer needs help breathing, he or she may get additional oxygen through prongs in the nostrils.

- Babies with moderate to severe BPD have an echocardiogram every two to three months to check their pulmonary artery pressure.

These babies also may need physical therapy to strengthen their muscles and help their lungs clear out mucus.

Today, most babies with BPD recover. They may spend several weeks or months in the hospital. But the best place for the baby's growth and development is at home with the family where he or she can be in a loving and familiar environment.

After the baby goes home:

- It's important for the parents to know about the symptoms and treatments for BPD. Parents and family members play an important role by being loving and involved with their babies and giving care.

- The baby may continue to have some breathing symptoms and may remain in poor health.

- He or she may still need extra oxygen and a breathing machine.

- He or she needs good nutrition and extra calories because of the extra work involved with breathing.

- Regular checkups and timely vaccinations from a pediatrician (a doctor who specializes in treating children) are important. A pediatrician also can treat any other illnesses that the baby may develop.

- The family also may need social services to help them take care of the baby's medical and nonmedical needs.

How Can Bronchopulmonary Dysplasia Be Prevented?

You can do certain things to help ensure that your baby isn't born before his or her lungs have developed completely. They include seeing your doctor regularly during your pregnancy, eating right, avoiding tobacco smoke, alcohol, and illegal drugs, controlling any ongoing medical conditions you have, and preventing infection.

Your doctor may also recommend that you take progesterone if you had a prior preterm birth. This is a hormone that may help delay delivery.

Your doctor may give you injections of a corticosteroid medicine if it looks as though you may give birth too early. This medicine can speed up surfactant production and development of the lungs, brain, and kidneys in the fetus. Usually, within about twenty-four hours after you start taking the medicine, the fetus's lungs will work better. They also will respond better to surfactant treatment so that respiratory distress syndrome will not develop after delivery, or it will be relatively mild.

Living with Bronchopulmonary Dysplasia

Babies with bronchopulmonary dysplasia (BPD) may continue to have problems after they leave the hospital:

- They may continue to need extra oxygen.

- They may need to use a breathing machine throughout early childhood.

- They may be more likely than other infants to get colds, flu, and other infections. This includes viral infections. These infections are usually mild in other children but can be life threatening in babies who have BPD.

- They may have a greater chance of developing complications from the most common childhood infections. Your doctor may want to put your baby in the hospital for treatment of a respiratory infection, to be safe.

- They may grow more slowly than normal during the first year or two of life. Babies who survive BPD usually stay smaller than other children of the same age.

As with most other children, the lungs of babies who had BPD are almost completely grown by age eight. But these children may have some ongoing lung problems, even when they're adults.

Some babies with very severe BPD may develop some long-term problems:

- Poor coordination and muscle tone
- Trouble walking and being active
- Eye and hearing problems
- Frequent breathing problems and infection
- Learning problems

The chances of developing these problems are very low. Parents shouldn't assume that their child will have these problems. If they do occur, parents and families can get information about these problems from the baby's doctors.

Parents can take a number of steps to help their babies recover and grow as normally as possible. These include the following:

- Call your baby's doctor if you see any signs of respiratory infection. The symptoms include irritability, fever, stuffy nose, cough, changes in breathing pattern, and wheezing.

- Keep your baby away from large daycare centers and crowds to avoid germs that cause colds, flu, and other infections.

- Make sure that no one smokes in your home, and keep your baby away from cigarette smoke, dust, pollution, and other things in the air that irritate the lungs.

- Make sure that your baby and other children get all their childhood shots. Doctors now recommend shots to protect against the respiratory syncytial virus.

Caring for a premature infant can be challenging. You may experience any of the following:

- Emotional pain, including feelings of guilt, anger, and depression

- Anxiety about your baby's future
- A feeling of a lack of control over the situation
- Financial stress
- Problems relating to the baby in the neonatal intensive care unit (NICU)
- Fatigue (tiredness)

Things you can do to help yourself during this difficult time include the following:

- Taking care of your health so that you have enough energy to deal with this situation.
- Breast-feeding your baby.
- Learning as much as you can about what goes on in the NICU so that you can help your baby during his or her stay there and begin to bond with the baby before he or she comes home.
- Learning as much as you can about your baby's condition and what is involved in daily care so you can ask the right questions and feel more confident about your ability to care for him or her at home.
- Seeking out support from family and friends, as well as hospital personnel. The hospital case manager or social worker can help you plan for your baby's needs after leaving the hospital. The social worker also may be able to help you find a support group in your community.
- Enjoying your new baby, spending as much time with him or her as you can, and looking forward to a happy future.

Section 34.2

Meconium Aspiration

Every expectant parent hopes for an uncomplicated birth and a healthy baby. But some babies do face delivery room complications. One condition that may affect a newborn's health is meconium aspiration, also referred to as meconium aspiration syndrome (MAS). Although it can be serious, most cases of MAS are not.

About Meconium Aspiration

MAS can happen before, during, or after labor and delivery when a newborn inhales (or aspirates) a mixture of meconium and amniotic fluid (the fluid in which the baby floats inside the amniotic sac). Meconium is the baby's first feces, or poop, which is sticky, thick, and dark green and is typically passed in the womb during early pregnancy and again in the first few days after birth.

The inhaled meconium can partially or completely block the baby's airways. Although air can flow past the meconium trapped in the baby's airways as the baby breathes in, the meconium becomes trapped in the airways when the baby breathes out. And so, the inhaled meconium irritates the baby's airways and makes it difficult to breathe.

MAS can affect the baby's breathing in a number of ways, including chemical irritation to the lung tissue, airway obstruction by a meconium plug, infection, and the inactivation of surfactant by the meconium (surfactant is a natural substance that helps the lungs expand properly).

The severity of MAS depends on the amount of meconium the baby inhales as well as underlying conditions, such as infections within the uterus or postmaturity (when a baby is overdue, or more than forty weeks' gestational age). Generally, the more meconium a baby inhales, the more serious the condition.

Normally, fluid is moved in and out of only the trachea (the upper portion of the airway) when there's breathing activity in the fetus. Meconium can be inhaled into the lungs when the baby gasps while still in the womb or during the initial gasping breaths after delivery. This gasping typically happens when there has been a problem (i.e., an infection or compression of the umbilical cord) that causes the baby to have difficulty getting enough oxygen in the womb.

Incidence

Although 6 to 25 percent of babies delivered have meconium-stained amniotic fluid, not all infants who pass meconium during labor and delivery develop MAS. Of the babies who either pass meconium during birth or are delivered having meconium-stained fluid, 2 to 36 percent either inhale the meconium *in utero* (while still in the uterus) or with the first breath. Of the infants born with meconium-stained amniotic fluid, 11 percent of them experience some degree of MAS.

Causes

MAS is often related to fetal stress. Fetal stress can be caused by problems in the womb, such as infections, or by difficulties during the labor process. A distressed baby may experience hypoxia (decreased oxygen), which may make the baby's intestinal activity increase and may cause relaxation of the anal sphincter (the muscular valve that controls the passage of feces out of the anus). This relaxation then moves meconium into the amniotic fluid that envelops the baby.

But meconium passage during labor and delivery isn't always associated with fetal distress. Occasionally, babies who aren't distressed during the birth process pass meconium before birth. In either case, a baby that gasps or inhales meconium can develop MAS.

Additional risk factors for MAS include:

- A difficult delivery;
- Advanced gestational age (or postmaturity);
- A mother who smokes cigarettes heavily or who has diabetes, hypertension (high blood pressure), or chronic respiratory or cardiovascular disease;
- Umbilical cord complications;

- Poor intrauterine growth (poor growth of the baby while in the uterus).

Prematurity is not a risk factor. In fact, MAS is rare in babies born before thirty-four weeks.

Signs and Symptoms

At birth, the doctor will likely notice one or more symptoms of MAS, including:

- Meconium or dark green streaks or stains in the amniotic fluid;
- Discoloration of the baby's skin—either blue (cyanosis) or green (from being stained by the meconium);
- Problems with breathing—including rapid breathing (tachypnea), labored (difficulty) breathing, or suspension of breathing (apnea);
- Low heart rate in the baby before birth;
- Low Apgar score (the Apgar test is given to newborns just after birth to quickly evaluate color, heartbeat, reflexes, muscle tone, and breathing);
- Limpness in the baby;
- Postmaturity (signs that a baby is overdue, such as long nails).

Diagnosis

If a baby is thought to have inhaled meconium, treatment will begin during delivery. As soon as the baby's head comes out, the doctor will suction out any meconium from the nose and mouth before the baby takes a first breath. This may help prevent the baby from inhaling any more meconium.

The most accurate way to detect MAS is to examine the vocal cords with a laryngoscope after delivery to see whether they're stained with meconium. The doctor will also probably listen to the baby's chest with a stethoscope for sounds in the lungs that are common in infants with MAS.

The doctor may also order tests—a blood test (called a blood gas analysis) that helps determine if the baby is getting enough oxygen and a chest x-ray that can show patches or streaks on the lungs that are found in babies with MAS.

Treatment

Current recommendations say that if an infant has inhaled meconium but looks active, appears well, and has a strong heartbeat (more than 100 beats per minute), the delivery team can watch the baby for MAS symptoms, which typically appear within the first twenty-four hours. So the baby is observed for such signs as increased respiratory rate, grunting, or cyanosis.

For an infant that has inhaled meconium and shows signs of poor activity level, has a lower heart rate (less than 100 beats per minute), is limp, and has poor muscle tone, the goal is to clear the airway as much as possible to decrease the amount of meconium that's aspirated. This is done by putting in an endotracheal tube (a plastic tube that's placed into the baby's windpipe through the mouth or nose) and applying suction as the tube is slowly removed. This allows the infant to receive suctioning of both the upper and lower airways. The doctor will continue trying to clear the airway until there's no meconium in the suctioned fluids.

Most babies with MAS improve within a few days or weeks, depending on the severity of the aspiration. Although a baby's rapid breathing may continue for days after birth, there's usually no severe permanent lung damage. There are studies, however, indicating that those born with MAS are at a higher risk of having reactive airway disease (lungs that are more sensitive and can possibly lead to an asthmatic condition).

Babies with MAS may be sent to a special care nursery or a neonatal intensive care unit (NICU) to be closely monitored for the next few days. Treatments may include:

- Oxygen therapy by oxygen hood or ventilation;
- Antibiotics;
- Use of surfactant;
- Nitric oxide;
- Obtaining blood routinely to determine if the baby is receiving enough oxygen.

Babies who have severe aspiration and require mechanical ventilation are at increased risk for bronchopulmonary dysplasia, a lung condition that can be treated with medication or oxygen. Another complication associated with MAS is a collapsed lung. Also known as pneumothorax, a collapsed lung is treated by reinflating the lung (inserting a tube between the ribs, allowing the lung to gradually re-expand).

Although rare, a small percentage of babies with severe MAS develop aspiration pneumonia. If this occurs, the doctor may recommend advanced lung rescue therapy.

Three therapies are currently used to treat aspiration pneumonia and severe forms of MAS:

- **Surfactant therapy:** An artificial surfactant is instilled into the baby's lungs, which helps to keep the air sacs open.

- **High-frequency oscillation:** This special ventilator vibrates air enriched with extra oxygen into the baby's lungs.

- **Rescue therapy:** Nitric oxide is added to the oxygen in the ventilator. It dilates the blood vessels and allows more blood flow and oxygen to reach the baby's lungs.

If one of these therapies (or a combination of them) doesn't work, there is another alternative. Extra corporeal membrane oxygenation (ECMO) is a form of cardiopulmonary bypass, meaning that an artificial heart and lung will temporarily take over to supply blood flow to the baby's body. ECMO reduces the fatality rate for these severely distressed infants from 80 percent to 10 percent. Not all hospitals are ECMO centers, so babies that require ECMO may need to be moved to another hospital.

Babies with severe cases of MAS may come home from the hospital on oxygen. They may be more likely to have wheezing and lung infections during their first year, but lungs can regenerate new air sacs, so the long-term prognosis for their lungs is excellent.

Severely affected babies are at risk for developing chronic lung disease and may also have developmental abnormalities and hearing loss. Babies diagnosed with MAS will be screened at the hospital for hearing problems or neurological damage. Although very rare, severe cases of MAS may be fatal. Studies have indicated that deaths from MAS have decreased significantly through interventions such as suctioning and reducing the number of post-term births.

Prevention

It's important for a pregnant woman to tell her doctor immediately if meconium is present in the amniotic fluid when her water breaks, or if the fluid has dark green stains or streaks. Doctors also use a fetal monitor during labor to observe the baby's heart rate for any signs of fetal distress. In some cases doctors may recommend amnioinfusion, the dilution of the amniotic fluid with saline, to wash meconium out of the amniotic sac before the baby has a chance to inhale it at birth.

Although MAS is a frightening complication for parents to face during the birth of their child, the majority of cases are not severe. Most infants are monitored for fetal distress during labor, and doctors pay careful attention to any signs that would indicate meconium aspiration. If it does occur, treatment will begin immediately.

For most infants who have inhaled meconium, early treatment can prevent further complications and help to reassure anxious new parents.

Section 34.3

Persistent Pulmonary Hypertension of the Newborn

After you endure labor and delivery, the first few cries of your newborn are a sweet reward that indicates your baby is healthy and strong. After all, a hearty yell means your infant was born with a healthy set of lungs, right?

But some newborns may experience breathing and lung function problems immediately after birth. Most of the time, these babies recover quickly and uneventfully, especially if they are full term. But others continue to have breathing complications that are more serious and require a longer course of treatment and intensive care.

Although persistent pulmonary hypertension of the newborn (PPHN) isn't common, it can seriously compromise a newborn's health and have long-term complications. Fortunately, better understanding of newborn lung function and technology has improved the outcome for infants affected by this serious condition. Keep reading to learn more about causes and treatment of PPHN.

What Is Persistent Pulmonary Hypertension of the Newborn?

In the womb, the pathway of your baby's blood circulation is different than it is after birth.

In the uterus, a baby's circulation bypasses the lungs. The lungs are not needed to exchange oxygen because the placenta (the organ that nourishes and protects your developing baby) supplies the baby with oxygen through the umbilical cord. The pulmonary artery—which, after birth, will carry blood from the heart to the lungs—instead sends blood directly back to the heart through a fetal blood vessel called the ductus arteriosus.

Normally, when a baby is born and begins to breathe air, his circulatory system quickly adapts to the outside world. The pressure in the lungs changes as air enters and inflates the lungs. As a result, the ductus arteriosus, which previously supplied the fetal heart with blood, permanently closes. Blood returning to the heart from the body can now be pumped into the lungs, where oxygen and carbon dioxide are exchanged. The blood is then returned to the heart and pumped back out to the body in an oxygen-rich state.

In a baby with PPHN, however, the fetal circulatory system doesn't "switch over." The ductus arteriosus remains open, and the baby's blood flow continues to bypass the lungs. Even though the baby is breathing, oxygen in the breathed air will not reach the bloodstream. Because the blood returning from the body is unable to enter the lungs properly—and instead flows through the still-open ductus arteriosus—it returns to the heart in an oxygen-poor state. This condition is known as persistent fetal circulation, or PFC.

"The baby's circulation has not made the normal transition from fetal circulation to normal newborn circulation, because pressure in the lungs is increased and this causes distress," says Neal Cohn, M.D., a pediatrician. Depending on the degree of PPHN causing the persistent fetal circulation, the oxygen in the air your baby breathes into his lungs is not adequately picked up and carried by the blood to other areas of the body that need it (such as the brain, kidneys, liver, and other organs). These organs soon become stressed from lack of oxygen.

PPHN sometimes develops as the result of another event during delivery or from a disease or congenital condition affecting the newborn (usually one that either directly affects the lungs or oxygen supply to the baby before or during birth). Often, however, PPHN occurs as an isolated condition, and its cause is not known. It is usually seen soon after birth, often within twelve hours after birth. PPHN occurs in approximately one in seven hundred births.

What Causes PPHN?

In an otherwise healthy newborn, the cause of PPHN is usually unknown. Some researchers believe that stress while the baby is in the uterus (associated with certain pregnancy complications, such as maternal diabetes, high blood pressure or anemia, or delivery after forty weeks) may increase the risk of developing PPHN.

PPHN may occur with certain diseases or congenital conditions of the infant that affect the lungs in some way. Meconium aspiration syndrome, anemia, severe pneumonia, infection, hypoglycemia (low blood sugar), and birth asphyxia (when the baby is deprived of oxygen during a complicated delivery) have all been associated with PPHN.

These conditions may cause the pressure in the blood vessels leading to the lungs to increase to the point where the baby's blood continues to bypass the lungs after birth, resulting in PFC. These conditions are often temporary and reversible, with intensive care and time for the lungs and body to heal. Certain congenital conditions that result in immature or incomplete lung development (such as diaphragmatic hernia) may also be associated with PPHN.

Signs and Symptoms

The following signs and symptoms may indicate a baby has PPHN:

- Rapid breathing (also called tachypnea)
- Rapid heart rate
- Respiratory distress, including signs such as flaring nostrils and grunting
- Cyanosis (when the skin has a bluish tinge), even while the baby is receiving extra oxygen to breathe

Sometimes when examining a baby with PPHN, the doctor will hear a heart murmur (an extra or abnormal heart sound). With PPHN, a baby may also continue to have low oxygen levels in the blood while receiving 100 percent oxygen.

How Is It Diagnosed and Treated?

For any newborn having difficulty breathing and showing signs of poor oxygen delivery to the body's tissues, several tests will be performed to determine possible causes. Various imaging and laboratory tests can help determine if a baby has PPHN.

Imaging tests will be done to get a better look at the lungs, heart, and circulation, and to check for other possible causes of the baby's problems:

- Chest x-rays can show whether the baby has lung disease and whether the heart is enlarged.

- An ultrasound of the heart (an echocardiogram) can show whether the baby has heart or lung disease and can determine the direction of blood flow in those organs. This test is often very helpful in diagnosing PPHN because it will show the doctor the baby's circulating blood flow, including whether the ductus arteriosus is open or closed, and can determine if PFC exists.

- An ultrasound of the head may be used to look for bleeding in the brain.

Laboratory tests can also assist doctors in making a diagnosis of PPHN:

- An arterial blood gas (ABG) determines how much oxygen, carbon dioxide, and acid buildup are in the arterial blood. Arteries normally contain high levels of oxygen, and this test is the most accurate way to determine how well oxygen is being delivered to the body.

- A complete blood count (CBC) measures the number of oxygen-carrying red blood cells, white blood cells (which help fight infection), and platelets (which are involved in blood clotting). A CBC usually shows if anemia or possible infection is causing the baby to be ill.

- Serum electrolyte tests evaluate the balance of minerals in the blood.

- A lumbar puncture (spinal tap) and other blood tests can help determine whether an infection is present.

- Pulse oximetry, which measures oxygen levels in the blood, can help doctors monitor whether the baby's tissues are receiving an adequate amount of oxygen.

A doctor who specializes in newborn problems, called a neonatologist, will direct the treatment for a child with PPHN. Babies with PPHN usually need to be cared for in a neonatal intensive care unit (NICU). NICUs are usually found in larger hospitals or children's hospitals.

The first step in PPHN treatment is to maximize the amount of oxygen delivered to the baby's lungs (and, in turn, to the blood), so 100 percent oxygen will be given through a tube inserted directly into the baby's trachea (windpipe). The oxygen is administered by a mechanical ventilator, which does the work of breathing for the baby. This treatment is given in conjunction with other treatments for the illnesses that may have contributed to the initial development of PPHN (such as low blood sugar, pneumonia, or other infections).

If your child has PPHN caused by a lung problem, his breathing rate may be set at a higher than usual rate and pressure through the mechanical ventilator. This is known as high-frequency oscillatory ventilation (HFOV). This ventilation technique improves oxygen delivery to the lungs, reduces acid buildup in the blood, and often helps open up the blood vessels leading to the lungs—thus allowing more blood to flow to the lungs. Because PPHN is worsened by narrowed lung blood vessels and raised acid levels in the body (a condition called acidosis), sodium bicarbonate may also be given with this form of ventilation to lower acid levels and help dilate blood vessels.

Recent research shows that supplying inhaled nitric oxide to babies with PPHN may also be successful. Nitric oxide has been shown to have a relaxing effect on contracted lung blood vessels, thus improving blood flow to the lungs in some babies with PPHN.

If other methods can't reverse the PPHN and raise the baby's oxygen levels to the necessary range, a type of intensive procedure called extracorporeal membrane oxygenation (ECMO) may be needed. ECMO requires major surgery, is complicated to monitor, and has potentially serious side effects associated with it. It is reserved for the sickest babies who are not responding to other forms of treatment.

The ECMO machine acts as an artificial heart and lung for the baby for several days while the baby's lungs heal and recover. Although ECMO is very successful in treating PPHN, fewer than one hundred hospitals (mostly children's hospitals) in the United States have facilities that can provide this treatment.

Complications and Prognosis

PPHN is a serious condition and intensive monitoring and treatment are critical. Even with prompt recognition and treatment, an infant with

PPHN may continue to supply an inadequate amount of oxygen to the body's tissues, resulting in shock, heart failure, brain hemorrhage, seizures, kidney failure, multiple organ damage, and possibly even death.

Some causes of PPHN are treatable and reversible; others are associated with a poor survival rate, even if nitric oxide and ECMO are used. In some newborns with PPHN, the lungs are too diseased or malformed to heal adequately, even if the baby stays on ECMO for a longer period of time.

Periods of inadequate oxygenation can have long-term effects on infants who survive PPHN, such as bronchopulmonary dysplasia (a chronic lung disease associated with scarred, stiffened lungs) and breathing difficulties. Seizure disorders, developmental delay, and neurological deficits may also be seen.

For several weeks following treatment, infants who've had PPHN may not be able to take feedings by mouth. A temporary feeding tube may have to be inserted into the baby's nose, or for longer-term feeding problems, directly into the stomach through the skin on the abdomen. Feeding tubes will be needed if the baby cannot eat enough to meet his nutritional requirements for growth.

Hearing problems are another common condition associated with PPHN. If your child had PPHN, he will probably need to be evaluated by a hearing specialist during early childhood to check for hearing loss, and the development of his speech will also need to be followed closely.

Medical treatments such as high frequency ventilation, nitric oxide, and ECMO have significantly decreased the percentage of children who die from PPHN. Fifteen years ago, almost half of infants diagnosed with PPHN died; today, less than 20 percent of infants with PPHN die, and only about one-fifth of surviving infants experience long-term physical or developmental complications.

Editor's Note

The underlying cause for most cases of PPHN remains unknown. It is suspected that genetic factors may be important. However, it has been determined that exposure to a class of antidepressants known as serotonin-specific reuptake inhibitors (SSRIs) during the second trimester of pregnancy significantly increases the risk of PPHN. Additionally, use of aspirin or nonsteroidal anti-inflammatory drugs (NSAIDs) such as ibuprofen or naproxen can increase the risk of PPHN.

Surfactant, a substance that improves the ability of the lungs to expand, is routinely used as part of treatment for PPHN, and has been shown to improve outcomes.

Inhaled nitric oxide therapy has significantly improved the outlook for infants with PPHN and severe respiratory failure. This treatment has risks, however, so it is recommended to be used only for severe cases, and preferably in centers with experience using the medication and access to ECMO therapy.

Preliminary research has suggested that sildenafil, the active ingredient in Viagra®, may be useful in treating PPHN. However, larger trials will need to be performed to confirm whether it is safe and effective for this purpose.

Section 34.4

Primary Ciliary Dyskinesia

Excerpted from "Facts About Primary Ciliary Dyskinesia (PCD)," © PCD Foundation. Reprinted with permission.

What is Primary Ciliary Dyskinesia (PCD)?

PCD stands for primary ciliary dyskinesia. The term PCD is used to describe inherited disorders of motile (moving) cilia, including Kartagener syndrome, immotile cilia syndrome, and ciliary aplasia. The estimated incidence of inherited ciliary disorders ranges from 1 in 12,500 to 1 in 25,000. This means that roughly fifteen thousand to twenty thousand Americans have PCD.

What are motile cilia and what do they do?

Motile cilia are microscopic hairlike structures that line many internal body surfaces including the respiratory tract, sinuses, Eustachian tubes of the ear, ventricles of the brain, and the reproductive organs. There are approximately ten billion cilia per square centimeter in the respiratory system, and they beat constantly at a rate of five to fifty beats or cycles per second. Cilia are an essential component of the mucociliary clearance activity required to sustain healthy respiratory tissue. The beating activity of the cilia moves debris-laden mucus out of areas vulnerable to infection or inflammation.

The beating motion of the cilia is also believed to be essential in determining organ placement during embryonic development. Roughly half the people affected by PCD will have a condition called situs inversus, in which their thoracic and abdominal organs are "flipped" to a mirror image position in the body. When situs inversus is present, the patient is diagnosed with Kartagener syndrome, a subcategory of PCD. Other abnormalities of the structure or function of abdominal/ thoracic organs may be present in PCD, as well. Collectively, these unusual organ arrangements are known as situs ambiguous (ambiguus) or heterotaxy.

What happens in PCD?

PCD is an inherited defect of the structure or function of motile cilia. The cilia in people with PCD do not function adequately (sometimes not at all). Respiratory difficulties are present almost from birth. Without functioning cilia, mucociliary clearance activity is profoundly impaired. Respiratory secretions begin to collect, thicken, and promote infection. Without aggressive treatment a form of permanent lung damage called bronchiectasis may develop at an early age. Delays in proper diagnosis and treatment may increase the risk of developing end-stage lung disease.

PCD is also associated with female subfertility and male infertility. Other complications include complex congenital heart defects, pectus deformities, and asplenia/polysplenia syndromes. Rare reports of hydrocephalus and biliary atresia have been published.

How is PCD diagnosed?

Currently, the diagnosis of PCD relies primarily on an assessment of ciliary ultrastructure done at a specialized laboratory or clinic. Clinical history and symptoms, and measurement of exhaled nasal nitric oxide, are also aids in diagnosis.

Is genetic testing available for PCD?

Recently, progress in identifying the genes responsible for PCD has resulted in the development of the first molecular (genetic) test for DNAI1 and DNAH5 mutations associated with PCD. Current genetic testing may only find mutations in one quarter to one third of PCD patients, so it will not replace ultrastructural studies for the majority of patients at this time. However, this testing may be useful as an aid to diagnosis of PCD or in testing family members of patients with known mutations. As more mutations are identified, the test will be modified to reflect new genetic information.

How can I get tested for PCD?

PCD diagnostic testing must be arranged through a medical professional familiar with the disorder and with other conditions that may mimic the symptoms of PCD. The PCD Foundation can help you locate a physician with PCD expertise. Because PCD is a rare and difficult to diagnose disorder, travel to a large academic or specialized center for diagnosis may be required.

How is PCD treated?

The main goal of treatment in PCD is to minimize the damage caused by chronic infection and/or inflammation. Airway clearance therapy, including secretion removal and bronchodilation, and aggressive use of antibiotics are the most common forms of treatment. Other treatments are aimed at reducing or eliminating symptoms such as sinus pain and gastrointestinal upset.

Section 34.5

Respiratory Distress Syndrome of the Newborn

Excerpted from "Respiratory Distress Syndrome," National Heart, Lung, and Blood Institute, National Institutes of Health, May 2007.

What Is Respiratory Distress Syndrome?

Respiratory distress syndrome (RDS) is a breathing problem that sometimes affects babies born about six weeks or more before their due dates. Their lungs aren't developed enough to make surfactant. Surfactant is a liquid that coats the inside of the lungs and keeps them open so that the baby can breathe in air once he or she is born.

Without surfactant, the lungs collapse and the baby has to work hard to breathe. The baby might not be able to breathe in enough oxygen to support the body's organs.

Most infants who develop RDS show signs of breathing problems at birth or within the next few hours. If they're not given the right treatment, their brains and other organs may suffer from the lack of oxygen.

Overview

RDS is one of the most common lung disorders in premature babies. It affects about ten of every one hundred premature infants in the United States, or about forty thousand babies, each year. In fact, nearly all babies born before twenty-eight weeks of pregnancy develop RDS. Full-term infants rarely get it.

RDS is different from bronchopulmonary dysplasia (BPD), another breathing condition that affects premature babies. While RDS usually develops in the first twenty-four hours after birth, BPD usually develops within the next week or two. Doctors aren't sure exactly what causes BPD, but they do know that most babies who develop it are born with serious RDS.

All of these babies lack surfactant. But the babies with RDS who go on to develop BPD have less developed lungs than the babies with

RDS who recover. Their lungs usually have fewer, larger alveoli, with fewer tiny blood vessels than normal. The blood vessels are needed to move oxygen from the alveoli into the bloodstream.

Outlook

Thanks to recent medical advances, most babies with RDS who weigh more than two pounds at birth now survive and have no long-term health or development problems.

Other Names for Respiratory Distress Syndrome

- Hyaline membrane disease (HMD)
- Neonatal respiratory distress syndrome
- Infant respiratory distress syndrome

What Causes Respiratory Distress Syndrome?

A lack of surfactant in a premature baby's lungs causes respiratory distress syndrome (RDS). Surfactant is a liquid that a fetus's lungs start making at around twenty-six to thirty-four weeks of pregnancy. It coats the insides of the lungs and keeps them open so they can breathe in air after birth. Without surfactant, the lungs collapse when the baby exhales. The baby then has to work hard to breathe.

Other factors that can increase the chances your baby will develop RDS include if you have diabetes mellitus, cesarean delivery, stress during delivery, especially hemorrhage (a large blood loss), and infection. Some infants born at term develop RDS because they have abnormal genes for surfactant.

What Are the Signs and Symptoms of Respiratory Distress Syndrome?

Signs and symptoms of respiratory distress syndrome (RDS) usually appear at birth or within the next few hours. They include rapid, shallow breathing, sharp pulling in of the chest below the ribs with each breath taken in, grunting sounds during exhalation, and flaring of the nostrils during breathing. The baby may also stop breathing for a few seconds every now and then. This is called apnea.

Depending on how severe the RDS is, these babies also may develop other serious medical problems, including the following:

- A collapsed lung.

539

- Leakage of air from the lung into the chest cavity. This is rare.

- Bronchopulmonary dysplasia, another lung disease in premature infants.

- Bleeding in the brain, which can lead to delayed mental development, mental retardation, and cerebral palsy.

- Sepsis, an infection of the bloodstream.

- Bleeding in the lung.

- Blindness and other eye problems.

- Kidney failure, only in the most severe cases.

- Necrotizing enterocolitis, a disease of the bowel.

How Is Respiratory Distress Syndrome Diagnosed?

Doctors usually begin treating respiratory distress syndrome (RDS) as soon as the baby is born. At the same time, they do several tests to rule out any other conditions that could be causing the baby's breathing problems. The tests also can confirm that the doctors have diagnosed the condition correctly.

The tests include:

- **Chest x-ray:** A chest x-ray takes a picture of the heart and lungs. It shows signs of RDS. A chest x-ray also can identify complications, such as a collapsed lung, that may require urgent treatment.

- **Blood tests:** Blood samples are checked to see whether the baby has enough oxygen in his or her blood. These tests also can rule out infection and sepsis as a cause of the breathing problems.

- **Echocardiogram:** This test uses sound waves to create a moving picture of the heart. An echocardiogram is used to rule out congenital heart defects as the cause of the breathing problems.

How Is Respiratory Distress Syndrome Treated?

Treatment of respiratory distress syndrome (RDS) usually begins as soon as the baby is born, sometimes in the delivery room. Most infants who show signs of RDS are quickly moved to a special intensive care unit called a neonatal intensive care unit (NICU). There they receive around-the-clock treatment from a group of health care professionals who specialize in treating premature infants.

The most important treatments for RDS are surfactant replacement therapy and breathing support.

Surfactant Replacement Therapy

The baby is given surfactant until his or her lungs have developed enough to start making their own surfactant. Surfactant usually is given through a tube that's attached to a breathing machine. The machine pushes the surfactant directly into the baby's lungs.

Surfactant may be given right after birth in the delivery room to try to prevent or treat RDS. It can be given two to four more times over the next few days, until the baby is able to breathe on his or her own.

Breathing Support

Babies with RDS often are put on a machine that helps them breathe until their lungs have developed enough to start making their own surfactant. Until recently, these babies usually were put on a mechanical ventilator that was connected to a breathing tube that ran through the baby's mouth or nose into the windpipe.

Today, more and more babies are receiving breathing support from a nasal continuous positive airway pressure (NCPAP) machine, which pushes air into the baby's lungs through prongs in the nostrils.

Other Types of Treatment

Other treatments for babies with RDS include medicines, supportive therapy, and treatment for patent ductus arteriosus, a condition that affects some premature infants.

Medicines: Doctors usually give the baby antibiotics to control infections.

Supportive therapy: Treatment in the NICU is designed to limit stress on the baby and meet his or her basic needs of warmth, nutrition, and protection. Such treatment usually includes the following:

- Using a radiant warmer or incubator to keep the baby warm and reduce the chances of infection.

- Ongoing monitoring of blood pressure, heart rate, breathing, and temperature through sensors taped to the baby's body.

- Using a sensor on a finger or toe to monitor the amount of oxygen in the baby's blood.

- Giving fluids and nutrients through a needle or tube inserted into a vein to prevent malnutrition and promote growth. Nutrition is critical to the growth and development of the lungs. Later, your baby may be given milk through a tube that's passed through his or her nose into the mouth.

- Monitoring fluid intake to make sure that fluid doesn't build up in the baby's lungs.

How Can Respiratory Distress Syndrome Be Prevented?

You can do certain things to help ensure that your baby isn't born before his or her lungs have developed completely:

- See your doctor regularly during your pregnancy
- Eat right
- Avoid tobacco smoke, alcohol, and illegal drugs
- Control any ongoing medical conditions you have
- Prevent infection

Your doctor may give you injections of a corticosteroid medicine if it looks as though you may give birth too early. This medicine can speed up surfactant production and development of the lungs, brain, and kidneys in the fetus. Usually, within about twenty-four hours after you start taking the medicine, the fetus's lungs start making enough surfactant, and the baby's chances of developing respiratory distress syndrome (RDS) are reduced. If the baby does develop RDS, it will probably be relatively mild.

If you start taking this medicine at least fifteen hours before you deliver, it also can reduce the chances that your baby will have any bleeding into the brain or develop necrotizing enterocolitis, a serious condition that affects the baby's intestines.

Living with Respiratory Distress Syndrome

Caring for a premature infant can be challenging. You may experience any of the following:

- Emotional pain, including feelings of guilt, anger, and depression

- Anxiety about your baby's future

- A feeling of a lack of control over the situation

- Financial stress

- Problems relating to the baby in the neonatal intensive care unit (NICU)

- Fatigue (tiredness)

There are some things you can do to help yourself during this difficult time:

- Take care of your health so that you have enough energy to deal with this situation.

- Breastfeed your baby.

- Learn as much as you can about what goes on in the NICU so that you can help your baby during his or her stay there and begin to bond with the baby before he or she comes home.

- Learn as much as you can about your baby's condition and what is involved in daily care so you can ask the right questions and feel more confident about your ability to care for him or her at home.

- Seek out support from family and friends, as well as hospital personnel. Ask the case manager or social worker at the hospital about what you'll need after the baby leaves the hospital. The physicians and nursing staff can assist with questions about your infant's care. Also ask whether there is a support group in your community.

- Enjoy your new baby, spend as much time with him or her as you can, and look forward to a happy future.

Your baby also may need special care after leaving the NICU, including special hearing and eye examinations, speech or physical therapy, and specialty care for other medical problems caused by premature birth.

Section 34.6

Sudden Infant Death Syndrome (SIDS)

A lack of answers is part of what makes sudden infant death syndrome (SIDS) so frightening. SIDS is the leading cause of death among infants who are one month to one year old, and claims the lives of about 2,500 infants each year in the United States. It remains unpredictable despite years of research. Even so, you can take steps to help reduce the risk of SIDS in your infant. First and foremost, put your infant to sleep on his or her back if the baby is younger than one year old.

Searching for Answers

As the name implies, SIDS is the sudden and unexplained death of an infant who is younger than one year old. It is a frightening prospect because it can strike without warning, usually in a seemingly healthy infant. Most SIDS deaths are associated with sleep (hence the common reference to "crib death"), and infants who die of SIDS show no signs of suffering.

While most conditions or diseases usually are diagnosed by the presence of specific symptoms, most SIDS diagnoses come only after all other possible causes of death have been ruled out through a review of the infant's medical history and environment. This review helps distinguish true SIDS deaths from those resulting from accidents, abuse, and previously undiagnosed conditions, such as cardiac or metabolic disorders.

When considering which babies could be most at risk, no single risk factor is likely to be sufficient to cause a SIDS death. Rather, several risk factors combined may contribute to cause an at-risk infant to die of SIDS.

Most deaths due to SIDS occur between two and four months of age, and incidence increases during cold weather. African-American infants are twice as likely and Native American infants are about three times more likely to die of SIDS than Caucasian infants. More boys than girls fall victim to SIDS.

Other potential risk factors include:

- Smoking, drinking, or drug use during pregnancy;

- Poor prenatal care;

- Prematurity or low birth-weight;

- Mothers younger than twenty;

- Smoke exposure following birth;

- Overheating from excessive sleepwear and bedding;

- Stomach sleeping.

Stomach sleeping. Foremost among these risk factors is stomach sleeping. Numerous studies have found a higher incidence of SIDS among babies placed on their stomachs to sleep than among those sleeping on their backs or sides. Some researchers have hypothesized that stomach sleeping puts pressure on a child's jaw, therefore narrowing the airway and hampering breathing.

Another theory is that stomach sleeping can increase an infant's risk of "rebreathing" his or her own exhaled air, particularly if the infant is sleeping on a soft mattress or with bedding, stuffed toys, or a pillow near the face. In that scenario, the soft surface could create a small enclosure around the baby's mouth and trap exhaled air. As the baby breathes exhaled air, the oxygen level in the body drops and carbon dioxide accumulates. Eventually, this lack of oxygen could contribute to SIDS.

Also, infants who succumb to SIDS may have an abnormality in the arcuate nucleus, a part of the brain that may help control breathing and awakening during sleep. If a baby is breathing stale air and not getting enough oxygen, the brain usually triggers the baby to wake up and cry. That movement changes the breathing and heart rate, making up for the lack of oxygen. But a problem with the arcuate nucleus could deprive the baby of this involuntary reaction and put him or her at greater risk for SIDS.

Going "Back to Sleep"

The striking evidence that stomach sleeping might contribute to the incidence of SIDS led the American Academy of Pediatrics (AAP) to recommend in 1992 that all healthy infants younger than one year of age be put to sleep on their backs (also known as the supine position). Since the AAP's recommendation, the rate of SIDS has dropped by over 50 percent. Still, SIDS remains the leading cause of death in young infants, so it's important to keep reminding parents about the necessity of back sleeping.

Many parents fear that babies put to sleep on their backs could choke on spit-up or vomit. According to the AAP, however, there is no increased risk of choking for healthy infants who sleep on their backs. (For infants with chronic gastroesophageal reflux disease [GERD] or certain upper airway malformations, sleeping on the stomach may be the better option. The AAP urges parents to consult with their child's doctor in these cases to determine the best sleeping position for the baby.)

Placing infants on their sides to sleep is not a good idea, the AAP said. There is too much risk that the infants will roll over onto their bellies while they sleep.

Some parents may also be concerned about positional plagiocephaly, a condition in which babies develop a flat spot on the back of their heads from spending too much time lying on their backs. Since the Back to Sleep campaign, this condition has become quite common—but it is usually easily treatable by changing your baby's position frequently and allowing for more "tummy time" while he or she is awake.

Of course, once babies can roll over consistently—usually around four to seven months—they may choose not to stay on their backs all night long. At this point, it's fine to let babies pick a sleep position on their own.

Tips for Reducing the Risk of SIDS

In addition to placing healthy infants on their backs to sleep, the AAP suggests the following measures to help reduce the risk of SIDS:

- Place your baby on a firm mattress to sleep, never on a pillow, waterbed, sheepskin, or other soft surface. To prevent rebreathing, do not put blankets, comforters, stuffed toys, or pillows near the baby.

- Make sure your baby does not get too warm while sleeping. Keep the room at a temperature that feels comfortable for an adult in a short-sleeved shirt. Some researchers suggest that a baby who gets too warm could go into a deeper sleep, making it more difficult to awaken.

- Do not smoke, drink, or use drugs while pregnant and do not expose your baby to secondhand smoke. Infants of mothers who smoked during pregnancy are three times more likely to die of SIDS than those whose mothers were smoke-free; exposure to secondhand smoke doubles a baby's risk of SIDS. Researchers speculate that smoking might affect the central nervous system, starting prenatally and continuing after birth, which could place the baby at increased risk.

- Receive early and regular prenatal care.

- Make sure your baby has regular well-baby checkups.

- Breast-feed, if possible. There is some evidence that breast-feeding may help decrease the incidence of SIDS. The reason for this is not clear, though researchers think that breast milk may help protect babies from infections that increase the risk of SIDS.

- If your baby has GERD, be sure to follow your doctor's guide-lines on feeding and sleep positions.

- Put your baby to sleep with a pacifier during the first year of life. If your baby rejects the pacifier, don't force it. Pacifiers have been linked with lower risk of SIDS. If you're breast-feeding, try to wait until after the baby is one month old so that breast-feeding can be established.

- While infants can be brought into a parent's bed for nursing or comforting, parents should return them to their cribs or bassinets when they're ready to sleep. It's a good idea to keep the cribs and bassinets in the room where parents sleep. This has been linked with a lower risk of SIDS.

For parents and families who have experienced a SIDS death, there are many groups, including the Sudden Infant Death Syndrome Alliance, that provide grief counseling, support, and referrals. Growing public awareness of SIDS and the steps to reduce infants' risk of sudden death hopefully will leave fewer parents searching for answers in the future.

Section 34.7

Transient Tachypnea of the Newborn

For some newborns, the breaths during those first hours of life are
more rapid and labored than normal because of a condition called
transient tachypnea of the newborn (TTN). About 1 to 2 percent of
all newborns develop TTN, a lung condition that usually subsides
within a few days with treatment.

Although babies born with TTN need special monitoring and treatment while in the hospital, afterwards they typically make a full recovery, and the TTN has no lasting effect on growth and development.

What Is Transient Tachypnea of the Newborn?

Before birth, the lungs of the fetus are filled with fluid. While a
fetus is inside of its mother, it does not use its lungs to breathe—all
its oxygen comes from the blood vessels of the placenta.

During the birthing process, as a baby passes through the birth
canal, some of the fluid inside the baby's lungs is "squeezed" out. After the birth, during the first breaths that a newborn takes, the lungs
fill with air and more fluid is pushed out of the lungs. Any remaining
fluid is then coughed out or gradually absorbed into the body through
the bloodstream.

In infants with TTN, however, there is extra fluid in the lungs or
the fluid in the lungs is absorbed too slowly. As a result, it is more
difficult for the baby to take in oxygen properly, and the baby breathes
faster and harder to compensate. TTN is also called "wet lungs" or type
II respiratory distress syndrome. Doctors usually can diagnose TTN
in the hours after birth. The condition typically lasts between twenty-
four and seventy-two hours.

What Causes Transient Tachypnea of the Newborn?

It is not possible to detect whether a child will have TTN before the baby is born. TTN occurs in both premature and full-term infants. Premature babies tend to have TTN because their lungs are not yet fully developed.

Newborns at higher risk for TTN include those who are:

- Delivered by cesarean section;

- Born to mothers who smoked during pregnancy;

- Born to mothers with diabetes;

- Small for gestational age (small at birth).

Delivery by cesarean section increases the risk for TTN because during vaginal births, especially with full-term babies, the pressure of passing through the birth canal squeezes some of the fluid out of the lungs. Babies who are small or premature or who are delivered via rapid vaginal deliveries or cesarean births don't experience the usual squeezing that occurs with a more routine vaginal birth. So these babies tend to have more fluid than normal in their lungs when they take their first breaths.

Some doctors have suggested that in babies with TTN, the release of the hormone epinephrine is inhibited during labor. In normal births, epinephrine aids in the clearing of fluids from the lungs. When a smaller amount of epinephrine is released, babies are less effective at clearing the fluid from the lungs.

Signs and Symptoms of TTN

Symptoms of TTN include:

- Rapid, labored breathing (tachypnea) of more than sixty breaths a minute;

- Grunting or moaning sounds when the baby exhales;

- Flaring nostrils or head bobbing;

- Retractions (when the skin pulls in between the ribs or under the ribcage during rapid or labored breathing);

- Cyanosis (when the skin turns a bluish color) around the mouth and nose.

549

Other than the above symptoms, infants who have TTN will look fairly healthy.

How Is TTN Diagnosed?

Because TTN has symptoms that are initially similar to more severe newborn respiratory problems such as pneumonia or persistent pulmonary hypertension, doctors usually use chest x-rays in addition to physical examination to make a diagnosis. Doctors may also use other indicators to make a diagnosis of TTN:

- If an infant has TTN, the x-ray picture of the lungs will appear streaked, and fluid will usually be seen. The x-ray will otherwise appear fairly normal.

- Pulse-oximetry monitoring, which is when a small piece of tape containing an oxygen sensor is placed around a baby's foot or toe and connected to a monitor, can aid in diagnosis. This tells doctors how well the lungs are sending oxygen to the blood and is also useful in monitoring TTN.

- A complete blood count (CBC) may also be drawn from one of the baby's veins or the heel to check for signs of infection.

How Is TTN Treated?

As with any newborn who has a breathing problem, infants diagnosed with TTN are closely observed and monitored. Sometimes they'll be admitted to the neonatal intensive care unit (NICU) for extra care. The babies are typically attached to monitors so that heart rate, breathing rate, and oxygen levels can be closely watched.

Some babies with TTN are simply monitored to ensure that their breathing rates slow down and their oxygen levels remain normal. Sometimes they may need to receive extra oxygen through a mask or under a plastic oxygen hood (called a "headbox").

If a baby struggles to breathe in oxygen, even while under an oxygen hood, continuous positive airway pressure (CPAP) is sometimes used to keep air flowing through the lungs. With CPAP, a baby wears a special oxygen cannula (a type of tubing that is placed directly into the baby's nose) and a machine continuously pushes a stream of pressurized air into the baby's nose to help keep the lungs open as he or she breathes.

In the most severe cases of TTN, a baby would need ventilator support, but this is rare.

Nutrition can be a problem if an infant is breathing so fast that he or she can't suck, swallow, and breathe simultaneously. Intravenous (IV) fluids provide hydration and will prevent the infant's blood sugar from dipping to dangerously-low levels. If your baby has TTN and you want to breast-feed, talk to your doctor or a nurse about maintaining your milk supply by using a breast pump while your infant receives IV fluids.

Within twenty-four to forty-eight hours, the breathing in infants with TTN typically improves and returns to normal, and within seventy-two hours, all symptoms of TTN typically dissipate altogether.

If fluid persists in a baby's lung beyond that time, then doctors will likely look into other medical problems which may be causing the condition.

Bringing Your Baby Home

After babies with TTN receive special monitoring and treatment in the hospital, they usually recover fully and are at no increased risk for other respiratory conditions, or other health problems.

Even though you won't have to worry about TTN after the third day of life, it's a good idea to stay aware of the signs of respiratory distress so you can call your child's doctor if you suspect a problem. If your baby has trouble breathing, appears blue, or if the skin pulls in between the ribs or under the ribcage during rapid or labored breathing, it's important to call your child's doctor or emergency services (911) right away.

Chapter 35

Traumatic Lung Disorders

Chapter Contents

Section 35.1

Atelectasis
(Collapsed Lung)

The lungs are like a pair of balloons inside the chest that fill up with air and then relax to let air leave the body. When a blockage occurs in the airway so the lung cannot fill up with air or if a hole or weakened place develops in the lung, allowing air to escape, the lung can collapse like a balloon that has lost its air.

Symptoms

Symptoms of a collapsed lung vary. They may include:

- falling oxygen levels in the blood, which causes the person to look bluish or ashen and can bring on abnormal heart rhythms (arrhythmias);
- fever, if an infection is present;
- rapid, shallow breathing;
- sharp pain on the affected side, if the symptoms are severe and the blockage occurred quickly;
- shock with a severe drop in blood pressure and a rapid heart rate;
- shortness of breath, which can be sudden and extreme in severe cases.

If the blockages happen slowly, there may be few or no symptoms. Those that do occur may include shortness of breath, an increased heart rate, or a hacking cough that does not seem to go away.

Causes and Risk Factors

A variety of factors can lead to a collapsed lung, including the following:

- A plug of mucus, a tumor, or something breathed into the lungs. Pressure on an airway from outside—a swollen lymph node or fluid between the lining of the lungs and the chest wall, for example—can also cause a lung to collapse. When the airway is blocked, the blood absorbs the air inside the air sacs (alveoli). Without more air, the sac shrinks. The space where the lung was before the collapse fills up with blood cells, fluids, and mucus. It may then become infected.

- Abdominal swelling.

- Experiencing high speeds, such as being a fighter jet pilot.

- Injuries, such as from a car accident, a fall, or a stabbing.

- Lack of the liquid (surfactant) that coats the lining of the alveoli, which helps keep it from collapsing. This can happen in premature babies or in adults who have had too much oxygen therapy or mechanical ventilation.

- Large doses of opioids or sedatives.

- Lying immobilized in bed.

- Scarring and shrinking of the membranes that cover the lungs and line the inside of the chest, which can occur as a result of exposure to asbestos.

- Smoking.

- Surgery, especially involving the chest or abdomen.

- Tight bandages.

Diagnosis

To diagnose a collapsed lung, a physician conducts a physical examination and asks about symptoms and the setting in which they occurred. Other tests that may be performed include:

- bronchoscopy;

- chest x-rays, which may or may not show the airless area of the lung;

- computed tomography (CT), which can help identify an obstruction.

Prevention

Preventing a collapsed lung is as important as treating one. These help avoid a collapsed lung:

- Patients who smoke should stop six to eight weeks before surgery.

- After surgery, patients should breathe deeply, cough regularly, and move about as soon as possible. Certain exercises, such as changing positions to help the lungs drain, or devices to encourage voluntary deep breathing (incentive spirometry), also help.

- Patients with a deformed chest or nerve condition that causes shallow breathing might need help breathing. Continuous positive airway pressure delivers oxygen through the nose or a facemask. This ensures the airways do not collapse even during the pause between breaths. Sometimes a mechanical ventilator is needed.

Treatment

There are several options for treating a collapsed lung:

- If the lung has collapsed because of a blockage, the blockage can be removed by coughing, suctioning the airways, or bronchoscopy.

- Antibiotics can be given to treat an infection.

- Surgery to remove a part of the lung may be needed if chronic infections become disabling or if significant bleeding occurs.

- Surgery, radiation, chemotherapy, or laser therapy may be used if a tumor is causing the blockage.

- Drugs to treat a lack of surfactant may be used. This is a life-saving measure in newborns. In adults with acute respiratory distress syndrome, it is considered experimental. For adults, the amount of oxygen in the blood is raised by continuous positive-pressure oxygen or mechanical ventilation.

Section 35.2

Hemothorax

Definition

Hemothorax is a collection of blood in the space between the chest wall and the lung (the pleural cavity).

Causes

The most common cause of hemothorax is chest trauma. Hemothorax can also occur in patients with lung or pleural cancer, or in patients with a defect of the blood clotting mechanism. The condition is also commonly linked with thoracic or heart surgery, and can also occur in patients who suffer pulmonary infarction (death of lung tissue).

In blunt chest trauma, a rib may lacerate lung tissue or an artery, causing blood to collect in the pleural space. In penetrating chest trauma, a weapon such as a knife or bullet lacerates the lung.

A large hemothorax is often a cause of shock in a trauma victim. Hemothorax may also be associated with pneumothorax (air trapped in the pleural cavity). Depending on the amount of blood or air in the pleural cavity, a collapsed lung can lead to respiratory and hemodynamic failure (tension pneumothorax).

Hemothorax can also be a complication of tuberculosis.

Symptoms

- Chest pain
- Shortness of breath
- Respiratory failure
- Rapid heart rate
- Anxiety
- Restlessness

Exams and Tests

Your doctor may note decreased or absent breath sounds on the affected side. Signs of hemothorax may be seen on the following tests:

- Chest x-ray;
- Thoracentesis;
- Pleural fluid analysis.

Treatment

The goal of treatment is to stabilize the patient, stop the bleeding, and remove the blood and air in the pleural space. A chest tube is inserted through the chest wall to drain the blood and air. It is left in place for several days to re-expand the lung.

The cause of the hemothorax should be also treated. In trauma patients, depending on the severity of the injury, chest tube drainage is often all that is necessary, and surgery is often not required.

Outlook (Prognosis)

The outcome depends on the underlying cause of the hemothorax and the promptness of the treatment.

Possible Complications

- Shock
- Fibrosis or scarring of the pleural membranes
- Death

When to Contact a Medical Professional

Call 911 for any penetrating or serious blunt injury to the chest, or if chest pain or shortness of breath occur.

Go to the emergency room or call the local emergency number (such as 911) if severe chest pain, severe difficulty breathing, absent breathing, and/or other symptoms of hemothorax occur.

Prevention

Use safety measures (such as seatbelts) to avoid injury. Depending on the cause, a hemothorax may not be preventable.

Section 35.3

Pneumothorax

What is pneumothorax?

Your lungs sit within a chest cavity. If you get a lung puncture, air escapes from the lung into the chest cavity ("pneumothorax" means "air in the chest"), and the lung partly collapses. Although this can be caused by an injury from broken ribs or even from some medical procedures, a "spontaneous" pneumothorax happens without any warning.

Who gets pneumothorax?

Mostly healthy young men get pneumothorax. Their lungs are in good shape but they happen to have a weakness at the top of the lung which means it can pop. This defect is often invisible on chest x-rays and is only found during an operation. Even if the lung completely collapses, these people may not be really breathless. Older patients with chronic chest problems are also at risk of an unexpected pneumothorax, which even if small can cause major breathing problems. In both cases it is much more common if you smoke.

What are the symptoms?

In younger people chest pain, worse on breathing, may be the major symptom (this happens because when the lung pops, there is a little bleeding), and some even wonder if they are having a heart attack. However, particularly in older people, the main effect is sudden unexpected breathlessness. The diagnosis is confirmed by a chest x-ray.

How is pneumothorax treated?

If you are only mildly breathless, you may be sent home just with painkillers. For a bigger collapse with more troublesome symptoms, it is often possible to suck the air out of the chest cavity using a small plastic tube inserted using local anesthetic. Occasionally this doesn't work and a large tube will have to be attached to a bottle of water to allow the air to bubble out, which means staying in the hospital. If the lung still fails to heal, then you will have to have an operation. In any case you should be given a follow-up appointment to see the local chest specialist.

Are there any special precautions?

If you have just been sent home from the hospital, you may notice bubbling noises in your chest as you breathe, particularly in bed, as the lung heals. You shouldn't travel by air until told it is safe to do so. You don't need to inform anybody, unless you are a scuba-diver. Since most episodes happen at rest, there is no reason why you can't exercise normally. If you smoke, stop!

Will it happen again?

After one pneumothorax, the chance of it happening again is only one in four, but rises to one in three (second episode) and one in two (third). Recurrence is uncommon after two years. You would easily recognize another episode and should then follow the specialist's advice about whether to telephone the chest clinic or go to the emergency room.

What about surgery?

If it keeps happening, or hospital treatment doesn't work, your health professional will advise you to have an operation. This allows the weakness to be removed, and the lung becomes stuck to the chest so that it can't collapse again. Often this can be achieved using keyhole surgery, so you may only be inactive for a few days.

Chapter 36

Lung Disorders Caused by Bioterrorism and Chemical Agents

Chapter Contents

Section 36.1

Frequently Asked Questions about Bioterrorism

"Bioterrorism: Frequently Asked Questions,"
© 2005 American Medical Association. Reprinted with permission.

What is bioterrorism?

Bioterrorism is the deliberate or threatened use of bacteria, viruses, and toxins to cause disease, death, or fear. Bioterrorism could also be directed against livestock, food crops, and environmental resources such as reservoirs.

What is the likelihood of a large-scale attack on the United States?

The likelihood of a large-scale bioterrorist attack is thought to be low. It is not a simple procedure to spread a biologic agent in a way that could infect massive numbers of people. To do so, an individual or individuals would have to have a high level of technical expertise. In Japan, a terrorist group has dispersed airborne formulations of anthrax and botulism throughout Tokyo on at least eight occasions but for unclear reasons, the attacks failed to produce illness. (*JAMA* 1999;281:1735–45)

The heavy coverage of this story by the media and the widespread prescribing of antibiotics to prevent anthrax emphasizes the need for public education to help people put the risk of bioterrorism in perspective. While a major attack could be devastating, preparations will minimize casualties. The importance of planning and preparation cannot be overstated.

Is the U.S. health system prepared for an act of bioterrorism?

Federal, state, and local health authorities (the Centers for Disease Control and Prevention, the Public Health Service, Cook County Public Health Office) routinely conduct surveillance for a bioterrorist event. If an attack occurs, the local health agency would rapidly advise the medical community (the AMA, state medical society, individual physicians) by phone, fax, and the media with recommendations for diagnosis and treatment, as well as preventive measures for the specific biological agent involved.

Our system is not perfect. Much needs to be done and can be done to strengthen it. Federal, state, and local authorities are working with physicians, hospitals, and the pharmaceutical industry to enhance information and communication systems; ensure the availability and rapid deployment of life-saving pharmaceuticals, vaccines, and antidotes; and provide necessary medical supplies to counter the effects of chemical (e.g., sarin, mustard gas) and biological agents.

What if fear gets the best of me?

Considering all that has happened since September 11th, it is reasonable and normal to feel anxious. Should fear get to the point that it stops you from normal activities or disrupts your sleep, it may be helpful to talk with someone. Your doctor can help you directly or refer you to a qualified psychiatrist or other health care professional that can provide counseling. Many people in New York City and Washington, D.C., have learned how helpful it is to seek counseling services.

Anthrax and Other Disease Threats

What are the major disease (biological agent) threats and how are they spread and treated?

Any infectious agent could theoretically be engineered for deliberate use as a weapon. While no one knows for sure exactly what microbes a terrorist will use, public health officials are most concerned with the following disease threats:

- **Inhalational anthrax** is the most serious form of anthrax and results from breathing bacterial spores into the lungs. Once in the lungs, the spores germinate into live bacteria that release potent toxins. The disease starts with flu-like symptoms, followed by severe respiratory complications. Death may occur within two to three days of symptoms. Exposure to airborne anthrax spores could cause symptoms as soon as two days after exposure or as late as six to eight weeks after exposure. Once symptoms appear, antibiotics may have limited effectiveness for treatment of inhalational anthrax because it is too advanced.

- **Cutaneous anthrax**, the skin form of anthrax, can cause skin or intestinal disease. It is the most common form of anthrax and results from contamination of the skin with anthrax spores (particularly on exposed areas of the hands, arms, or face). The disease begins with a local swelling that may look like an insect bite and progresses to a fluid-filled blister. The blister dries, ulcerates, and then forms a coal-black scab (the word anthrax comes from the Greek word for coal). Without antibiotic treatment, the local infection may spread through the body and can be fatal.

- **Smallpox** is a serious viral disease that starts with fever, aches, fatigue, and vomiting, and progresses to a rash with blisters over much of the body. Initially, the rash may be confused with chickenpox. Smallpox spreads directly from person to person through airborne transmission. Because it is a virus, it does not respond to antibiotics. A vaccine exists but is not available for widespread use.

- **Pneumonic (new-monic) plague** is caused by inhaling the bacteria associated with the "Black Death." It begins as a severe pneumonia with high fever, chills, and cough. Without prescription antibiotics, respiratory failure and death may occur within twelve to twenty-four hours after the initial symptoms appear. It spreads directly from person to person through the air (e.g., cough, sneeze). A vaccine exists for prevention of bubonic plague (when the lymph nodes are infected instead of the lungs) but is not considered effective against the inhaled (pneumonic) form of this disease.

- **Botulism** is caused by a bacterial protein that has been taken by mouth (eaten) or inhaled. It is one of the most potent toxic compounds known. Affected individuals may have difficulty speaking, seeing, and swallowing. Depending on the severity of exposure, symptoms may progress to general muscle weakness and respiratory failure. Without adequate respiratory care and treatment with antitoxin, death can occur within twenty-four to seventy-two hours. Botulism does not spread from person to person. A bioterrorist attack would likely involve airborne or foodborne release of botulinum toxin. Antibiotics are not effective.

- **Tularemia (too-la-ree-mia)** is one of the most infectious bacterial diseases known. A bioterrorist attack would likely involve airborne release of this organism. Fever, headache, and a pneumonia-like illness characterize the disease. Without antibiotic treatment, the disease can progress to respiratory failure, shock, and death. There is no evidence that it can be spread from person to person. A vaccine exists but is not available for widespread use.

- **Viral hemorrhagic fevers** are caused by a diverse group of viruses (e.g., Ebola, Marburg, yellow fever, Lassa, Rift Valley). Illness generally begins with flu-like symptoms such as fever, fatigue, dizziness, headache, and muscle aches. After five days a rash often develops, which is most prominent on the trunk of the body. Severe infection may lead to death due to complications from massive bleeding and shock due to widespread damage to blood vessels. These viruses can be spread from person to person through contact with body fluids (e.g., blood). A vaccine is available for prevention of yellow fever. Other vaccines are under investigation. No antibiotic is effective against these or any viral diseases.

Immunization

Should I be immunized against anthrax?

The anthrax vaccine is only available to military personnel and those who might come in contact with natural anthrax in their work (special-risk groups such as goat-hair mill or goatskin workers, wool or tannery workers, laboratory workers). Vaccination is not one shot but a series of six shots given over eighteen months, followed by yearly boosters. Physicians do not have this vaccine and cannot obtain it. In the event of a bioterrorist attack, health authorities would conduct a rapid investigation, determine the place and time of the release, and identify individuals who need antibiotics rather than vaccine. The anthrax vaccine is only recommended for people between eighteen and sixty-five years of age.

Should I be immunized against smallpox?

The last naturally occurring case of smallpox in the world occurred in 1977. The United States stopped routine smallpox immunizations in 1972 and, consequently, drug companies stopped making the vaccine. The vaccine is not generally available to the public. The CDC says there are approximately twelve to fifteen million doses of vaccine remaining in the United States. Although there is no treatment for the disease, the smallpox vaccine provides excellent protection and serves to stop spread of the disease. While many vaccines must be given weeks or months before a person is exposed to infection, the smallpox vaccine is different. It can be protective when given two to three days after exposure and may prevent death even when given as late as four to five days after exposure.

There is suspicion that some nations or groups have stolen stocks of the smallpox virus from the former Soviet Union. Since we don't know if terrorists have stolen the virus or (if they have) who they would target, we cannot determine who should receive the vaccine. In the event of a smallpox outbreak, the national vaccine stockpile would be used to control the spread of the disease. The federal government has a contractor developing new vaccine for a larger stockpile. Although rare, the smallpox vaccine can have serious side effects (e.g., severe skin reaction, brain infection, and death). Currently, the benefits and risks of reintroducing the vaccine are being carefully evaluated. The only way that health authorities would recommend wide-scale vaccination is if there was clear evidence that the disease had resurfaced and citizens were at risk of becoming infected.

I was vaccinated against smallpox before 1980, can I still get smallpox?

In most people, vaccination wears off after ten to fifteen years but may last longer if the person had been successfully vaccinated on multiple occasions. It is likely that most vaccinated persons are now susceptible to smallpox and would need to be re-vaccinated.

Antibiotics

Should I ask my doctor for antibiotics to have on hand in case of a bioterrorist attack?

No. Indiscriminate use of antibiotics could be harmful, particularly for pregnant women and children. Many antibiotics are effective for a variety of diseases but there is no antibiotic that is effective against all diseases. Antibiotics can cause side effects and should only be taken with medical supervision. This type of inappropriate use of antibiotics may lead to increased antibiotic resistance in bacteria that cause other common infections (e.g., otitis media, pneumonia, urinary tract infections), which can complicate treatment. Keeping a supply of antibiotics on hand poses an additional problem because they have a limited shelf life and will lose potency over time.

What is the "National Pharmaceutical Stockpile" that health officials talk about on the news?

This is a large reserve of antibiotics, chemical antidotes, and other medical supplies set aside for emergencies. The Centers for Disease

Control and Prevention reports that it can move stockpiled material to affected areas in the United States within one to two hours of notification from a state's governor.

Gas Masks

Should I purchase a gas mask?

No. A gas mask provides a false sense of security and would only be protective if you were wearing it at the exact moment of a bioterrorist attack. Since such an attack would be unannounced and initially undetected, the mask would have to be worn continuously to be protective. In other words, in order to be protected, you would have to wear this mask twenty-four hours a day, seven days a week—never removing it. This is impractical, if not impossible. Gas masks can actually be dangerous for persons with preexisting heart or lung problems; there have been reports of accidental suffocation when people have worn masks incorrectly.

Also, to work effectively, a gas mask must be specially fitted to you and you must be trained in its use. This is usually done for the military and for workers in industries and laboratories who are routinely exposed to hazardous chemical and biological agents. Purchasing a gas mask from an Army surplus store or off the Internet carries no guarantee of effectiveness.

Exposure and What to Do

Who do I contact regarding a possible exposure?

If you believe you have been exposed to an infectious bioagent or if you develop symptoms that you believe might be associated with such an exposure, immediately contact a physician. Your physician may choose to contact the local health department to determine the best course of action based on the circumstances of the exposure.

What can I do to protect my family and myself?

Although there is little that you as an individual can do in advance to protect yourself from a bioterrorist attack, there is much we can do as a country. The best protection is a strong and prepared public health system; well-trained physicians and other medical personnel who can recognize an illness caused by a bioterrorist agent; coordinated planning between medical, public health, emergency management, and law enforcement personnel; and an informed public. Government agencies, health care institutions, and public health agencies can and are doing more to improve capacity to protect the public following a bioterrorist attack. We can all educate ourselves about this issue, make family preparations for a disaster, and find out ahead of time what our local communities suggest we do.

Furthermore, in the event of a disaster, every family should have the following emergency supplies on hand:

- A battery-powered radio and flashlight, with plenty of extra batteries

- Bottled drinking water (one gallon per day per person, with a three- to seven-day supply recommended). Store water in sealed, unbreakable containers. Note the storage date and replace every six months.

- A supply of nonperishable canned and sealed packaged foods that do not require refrigeration or cooking (at least enough for three to seven days) and a can opener

- A change of clothing, rain gear, and sturdy shoes

- A blanket or sleeping bag for each family member

- First-aid kit, including any special prescription medications

- Toilet paper and paper towels

- Extra set of car keys

- Credit cards and cash

- Tools

- Special items for infants (e.g., disposable diapers), elderly, or disabled family members

- Extra eyeglasses, contact lenses, and supplies

- A list of physicians and their telephone numbers

- A list of important family information, important documents, and telephone numbers; copies of family immunization and health records; and the style and serial number of medical devices such as pacemakers

Careful planning and sufficient resources are critical for any response to an emergency, be it a natural disaster or a terrorist attack. Inquire about emergency plans for your children's school or daycare center. Consider becoming involved in your community emergency response team.

What more can be done nationally and globally?

National and international institutions are working together to strengthen the public health infrastructure, to more effectively monitor the threat of biological weapons, to identify actions likely to prevent the proliferation of bioweapons, and develop a coordinated plan for monitoring the worldwide emergence of infectious diseases. Investment in the public health system is the best possible defense against any outbreak of infectious disease, whether natural or deliberate. Given the ease of travel and increasing globalization, an outbreak anywhere in the world should be considered a threat to all nations.

Section 36.2

How to Recognize and Handle a Suspicious Package or Envelope

Reprinted from the Centers for Disease Control and Development, February 22, 2006.

Between September and October 2001, several letters containing *Bacillus anthracis* were sent through the mail in several areas of the United States. As a result, the Centers for Disease Control and Prevention (CDC) developed the following guidelines for recognizing and handling suspicious packages. Although there have been no recent mail-related anthrax exposures, all persons should take appropriate steps to protect themselves and others from exposure to *Bacillus anthracis* by following these guidelines for recognizing and handling suspicious packages.

Identifying Suspicious Packages and Envelopes

Some characteristics of suspicious packages and envelopes include the following:

- Inappropriate or unusual labeling:
  - Excessive postage
  - Handwritten or poorly typed addresses
  - Misspellings of common words
  - Strange return address or no return address
  - Incorrect titles or title without a name
  - Not addressed to a specific person
  - Marked with restrictions, such as "Personal," "Confidential," or "Do not x-ray"
  - Marked with any threatening language
  - Postmarked from a city or state that does not match the return address
- Appearance:
  - Powdery substance felt through or appearing on the package or envelope
  - Oily stains, discolorations, or odor
  - Lopsided or uneven envelope
  - Excessive packaging material such as masking tape, string, etc.
- Other suspicious signs:
  - Excessive weight
  - Ticking sound
  - Protruding wires or aluminum foil

If a package or envelope appears suspicious, *do not open it.*

Handling of Suspicious Packages or Envelopes

- Do not shake or empty the contents of any suspicious package or envelope.
- Do not carry the package or envelope, show it to others, or allow others to examine it.
- Put the package or envelope down on a stable surface; do not sniff, touch, taste, or look closely at it or at any contents which may have spilled.

- Alert others in the area about the suspicious package or envelope. Leave the area, close any doors, and take actions to prevent others from entering the area. If possible, shut off the ventilation system.

- Wash hands with soap and water to prevent spreading potentially infectious material to face or skin. Seek additional instructions for exposed or potentially exposed persons.

- If at work, notify a supervisor, a security officer, or a law enforcement official. If at home, contact the local law enforcement agency.

- If possible, create a list of persons who were in the room or area when this suspicious letter or package was recognized and a list of persons who also may have handled this package or letter. Give this list to both the local public health authorities and law enforcement officials.

Section 36.3

Anthrax

Reprinted from "Anthrax: What You Need to Know,"
Centers for Disease Control and Prevention, February 22, 2006.

What is anthrax?

Anthrax is a serious disease caused by *Bacillus anthracis*, a bacterium that forms spores. A bacterium is a very small organism made up of one cell. Many bacteria can cause disease. A spore is a cell that is dormant (asleep) but may come to life with the right conditions.

There are three types of anthrax:

- Skin (cutaneous)
- Lungs (inhalation)
- Digestive (gastrointestinal)

How do you get it?

Anthrax is not known to spread from one person to another.

Anthrax from animals: Humans can become infected with anthrax by handling products from infected animals or by breathing in anthrax spores from infected animal products (like wool, for example). People also can become infected with gastrointestinal anthrax by eating undercooked meat from infected animals.

Anthrax as a weapon: Anthrax also can be used as a weapon. This happened in the United States in 2001. Anthrax was deliberately spread through the postal system by sending letters with powder containing anthrax. This caused twenty-two cases of anthrax infection.

How dangerous is anthrax?

The Centers for Disease Control and Prevention classifies agents with recognized bioterrorism potential into three priority areas (A, B, and C). Anthrax is classified as a Category A agent. Category A agents are those that:

- Pose the greatest possible threat for a bad effect on public health;
- May spread across a large area or need public awareness;
- Need a great deal of planning to protect the public's health.

In most cases, early treatment with antibiotics can cure cutaneous anthrax. Even if untreated, 80 percent of people who become infected with cutaneous anthrax do not die. Gastrointestinal anthrax is more serious because between one-fourth and more than half of cases lead to death. Inhalation anthrax is much more severe. In 2001, about half of the cases of inhalation anthrax ended in death.

What are the symptoms?

The symptoms (warning signs) of anthrax are different depending on the type of the disease:

- **Cutaneous:** The first symptom is a small sore that develops into a blister. The blister then develops into a skin ulcer with a black area in the center. The sore, blister, and ulcer do not hurt.

- **Gastrointestinal:** The first symptoms are nausea, loss of appetite, bloody diarrhea, and fever, followed by bad stomach pain.

- **Inhalation:** The first symptoms of inhalation anthrax are like cold or flu symptoms and can include a sore throat, mild fever, and muscle aches. Later symptoms include cough, chest discomfort, shortness of breath, tiredness, and muscle aches. (Caution: Do not assume that just because a person has cold or flu symptoms that they have inhalation anthrax.)

How soon do infected people get sick?

Symptoms can appear within seven days of coming in contact with the bacterium for all three types of anthrax. For inhalation anthrax, symptoms can appear within a week or can take up to forty-two days to appear.

How is anthrax treated?

Antibiotics are used to treat all three types of anthrax. Early identification and treatment are important.

Prevention after exposure: Treatment is different for a person who is exposed to anthrax, but is not yet sick. Health-care providers will use antibiotics (such as ciprofloxacin, levofloxacin, doxycycline, or penicillin) combined with the anthrax vaccine to prevent anthrax infection.

Treatment after infection: Treatment is usually a sixty-day course of antibiotics. Success depends on the type of anthrax and how soon treatment begins.

Can anthrax be prevented?

There is a vaccine to prevent anthrax, but it is not yet available for the general public. Anyone who may be exposed to anthrax, including certain members of the U.S. armed forces, laboratory workers, and workers who may enter or re-enter contaminated areas, may get the vaccine. Also, in the event of an attack using anthrax as a weapon, people exposed would get the vaccine.

What should I do if I think I have anthrax?

If you are showing symptoms of anthrax infection, call your health-care provider right away.

What should I do if I think I have been exposed to anthrax?

Contact local law enforcement immediately if you think that you may have been exposed to anthrax. This includes being exposed to a suspicious package or envelope that contains powder.

What are the Centers for Disease Control and Prevention (CDC) doing to prepare for a possible anthrax attack?

CDC is working with state and local health authorities to prepare for an anthrax attack. Activities include:

- Developing plans and procedures to respond to an attack using anthrax.

- Training and equipping emergency response teams to help state and local governments control infection, gather samples, and perform tests. Educating health-care providers, media, and the general public about what to do in the event of an attack.

- Working closely with health departments, veterinarians, and laboratories to watch for suspected cases of anthrax. Developing a national electronic database to track potential cases of anthrax.

- Ensuring that there are enough safe laboratories for quick testing of suspected anthrax cases.

- Working with hospitals, laboratories, emergency response teams, and health-care providers to make sure they have the supplies they need in case of an attack.

Section 36.4

Smallpox

"What You Need to Know about Smallpox and Bioterrorism," © 2004 Texas Department of State Health Services. Reprinted with permission. For the most current information, visit http://www.dshs.state.tx.us/.

What is smallpox?

Smallpox is a serious, contagious, sometimes fatal viral disease. The name "smallpox" refers to raised bumps that appear on the face and body of an infected person. Smallpox is caused by the variola virus that has been in the human population for thousands of years. The last naturally occurring case of smallpox in the United States was in

1949, and the naturally occurring virus was eliminated from the world in 1980. Smallpox vaccinations for the general public were discontinued in the United States in 1972 because smallpox no longer occurred and because of risks associated with the vaccine.

Can smallpox be used as a bioterrorism threat?

Because smallpox was wiped out many years ago, a case of smallpox today would be the result of an intentional act. A single confirmed case of smallpox would be considered an emergency. There is no treatment for smallpox disease, and the only prevention is vaccination.

How is it spread?

People can get smallpox by being in direct, close contact (usually within six feet) with an infectious person. The virus is found in droplets of saliva released when the infectious person talks, coughs, or sneezes. Direct contact with materials such as bedding and clothing contaminated with the virus is another way people can be infected. Rarely, smallpox is spread when the virus is in the air in enclosed places such as buses and trains. Humans are the only natural hosts of variola virus. Smallpox virus is not known to be transmitted by insects or animals. People with smallpox are sometimes contagious when fever begins but are most contagious when the rash appears. At this stage, people usually are very sick and not able to move much. The infected person is contagious until the last smallpox scab falls off.

What are the symptoms?

A person does not have symptoms until seven to seventeen days after exposure. During this time, the person is not contagious.

The first symptoms include high fever, fatigue, head and body aches, and sometimes vomiting. During this phase, which may last from two to four days, the person feels too sick for normal activities.

One to four days after the first symptoms appear, the person develops a rash as small red spots on the tongue and in the mouth. These spots develop into sores that break open and spread the virus. Then a skin rash appears starting on the face and spreading to the legs and arms. Usually the rash spreads over the body within twenty-four hours. By the third day, the rash becomes raised bumps which then fill with fluid and often have a depression in the center. The bumps become pustules, which are usually round, raised and firm. These form first a crust and then a scab. These scabs fall off after about three to four weeks. Most people with smallpox recover, but death occurs in up to 30 percent of cases.

How is smallpox treated?

No medicines are available to treat smallpox once sores develop. When people have been exposed to the smallpox virus, vaccines given within four days of exposure can lessen the severity of illness or possibly prevent the illness altogether. Smallpox vaccine contains a live virus called vaccinia; it does not contain the smallpox virus. Smallpox patients can benefit from therapies such as intravenous fluids and medicine to control fever or pain. Antibiotics may be given for secondary bacterial infection. Public health officials have large supplies of drugs needed in the event of a bioterrorism attack. These supplies can be sent anywhere in the United States within twelve hours.

Can I be vaccinated for smallpox?

Smallpox vaccine is controlled by the Centers for Disease Control and Prevention (CDC) and not available to the general public. Smallpox vaccine will be made available to any community to protect people and stop the spread of the virus should a smallpox outbreak occur.

If I was vaccinated against smallpox before 1980, am I still protected?

Probably not. The vaccination has been shown to wear off in most people after ten years but may last longer if the person has been successfully vaccinated multiple times. Therefore, all people in the United States are considered susceptible to smallpox.

How will public health officials respond to a smallpox outbreak?

The Department of State Health Services and the U.S. Centers for Disease Control and Prevention have detailed plans to protect people against the use of smallpox as a biological weapon. Plans include creation and use of special teams of public health and health care workers who have been vaccinated.

If a smallpox case is found, these teams will take steps immediately to control the spread of the disease including the request of vaccine from CDC to protect people at risk of exposure. The health department also will notify the Federal Bureau of Investigation (FBI) and other appropriate authorities.

Smallpox patients will be kept away from other susceptible people and will receive the best medical care possible. Isolation prevents the virus from spreading to others.

Anyone who has had contact with a smallpox patient will be offered smallpox vaccination as soon as possible. Then the people who have had contact with those individuals also will be vaccinated. Following vaccination, these people will need to watch for any signs of smallpox. People who have been exposed to smallpox virus may be asked to take their temperatures regularly and report the results to their health department.

The smallpox vaccine also may be offered to those who have not been exposed but would like to be vaccinated. At local clinics, the risks and benefits of the vaccine will be explained and professionals will be available to answer questions.

No one will be forced to be vaccinated, even if they have been exposed to smallpox. To prevent smallpox from spreading, anyone who has been in contact with a person with smallpox but who decides not to get the vaccine may need to be isolated for at least eighteen days. During this time, they will be checked for symptoms of smallpox.

People in isolation will not be able to go to work.

How can I protect myself and my family during an outbreak?

Stay informed. Listen to the news to learn how the outbreak is affecting your community. Public health officials will share important information including areas where smallpox cases have been found and who to call and where to go if you think you have been exposed.

Follow the instructions of public health authorities.

Stay away from and keep your children away from anyone who might have smallpox.

If you think you have been exposed to smallpox virus, stay away from others and call your health department or health care provider immediately. They will tell you where to go.

Section 36.5

Plague

Reprinted from "Frequently Asked Questions (FAQ) about Plague," Centers for Disease Control and Prevention, April 5, 2005.

What is plague?

Plague is a disease caused by *Yersinia pestis* (*Y. pestis*), a bacterium found in rodents and their fleas in many areas around the world.

Why are we concerned about pneumonic plague as a bioweapon?

Yersinia pestis used in an aerosol attack could cause cases of the pneumonic form of plague. One to six days after becoming infected with the bacteria, people would develop pneumonic plague. Once people have the disease, the bacteria can spread to others who have close contact with them. Because of the delay between being exposed to the bacteria and becoming sick, people could travel over a large area before becoming contagious and possibly infecting others. Controlling the disease would then be more difficult. A bioweapon carrying *Y. pestis* is possible because the bacterium occurs in nature and could be isolated and grown in quantity in a laboratory. Even so, manufacturing an effective weapon using *Y. pestis* would require advanced knowledge and technology.

Is pneumonic plague different from bubonic plague?

Yes. Both are caused by *Yersinia pestis*, but they are transmitted differently and their symptoms differ. Pneumonic plague can be transmitted from person to person; bubonic plague cannot. Pneumonic plague affects the lungs and is transmitted when a person breathes in *Y. pestis* particles in the air. Bubonic plague is transmitted through the bite of an infected flea or exposure to infected material through a break in the skin. Symptoms include swollen, tender lymph glands called buboes. Buboes are not present in pneumonic plague. If bubonic plague is not treated, however, the bacteria can spread through the bloodstream and infect the lungs, causing a secondary case of pneumonic plague.

What are the signs and symptoms of pneumonic plague?

Patients usually have fever, weakness, and rapidly developing pneumonia with shortness of breath, chest pain, cough, and sometimes bloody or watery sputum. Nausea, vomiting, and abdominal pain may also occur. Without early treatment, pneumonic plague usually leads to respiratory failure, shock, and rapid death.

How do people become infected with pneumonic plague?

Pneumonic plague occurs when *Yersinia pestis* infects the lungs. Transmission can take place if someone breathes in *Y. pestis* particles, which could happen in an aerosol release during a bioterrorism attack. Pneumonic plague is also transmitted by breathing in *Y. pestis* suspended in respiratory droplets from a person (or animal) with pneumonic plague. Respiratory droplets are spread most readily by coughing or sneezing. Becoming infected in this way usually requires direct and close (within six feet) contact with the ill person or animal. Pneumonic plague may also occur if a person with bubonic or septicemic plague is untreated and the bacteria spread to the lungs.

Does plague occur naturally?

Yes. The World Health Organization reports one thousand to three thousand cases of plague worldwide every year. An average of five to fifteen cases occur each year in the western United States. These cases are usually scattered and occur in rural to semi-rural areas. Most cases are of the bubonic form of the disease. Naturally occurring pneumonic plague is uncommon, although small outbreaks do occur. Both types of plague are readily controlled by standard public health response measures.

Can a person exposed to pneumonic plague avoid becoming sick?

Yes. People who have had close contact with an infected person can greatly reduce the chance of becoming sick if they begin treatment within seven days of their exposure. Treatment consists of taking antibiotics for at least seven days.

How quickly would someone get sick if exposed to plague bacteria through the air?

Someone exposed to *Yersinia pestis* through the air—either from an intentional aerosol release or from close and direct exposure to someone with plague pneumonia—would become ill within one to six days.

Can pneumonic plague be treated?

Yes. To prevent a high risk of death, antibiotics should be given within twenty-four hours of the first symptoms. Several types of antibiotics are effective for curing the disease and for preventing it. Available oral medications are a tetracycline (such as doxycycline) or a fluoroquinolone (such as ciprofloxacin). For injection or intravenous use, streptomycin or gentamicin antibiotics are used. Early in the response to a bioterrorism attack, these drugs would be tested to determine which is most effective against the particular weapon that was used.

Would enough medication be available in the event of a bioterrorism attack involving pneumonic plague?

National and state public health officials have large supplies of drugs needed in the event of a bioterrorism attack. These supplies can be sent anywhere in the United States within twelve hours.

What should someone do if they suspect they or others have been exposed to plague?

Get immediate medical attention: To prevent illness, a person who has been exposed to pneumonic plague must receive antibiotic treatment without delay. If an exposed person becomes ill, antibiotics must be administered within twenty-four hours of their first symptoms to reduce the risk of death. Notify authorities: Immediately notify local or state health departments so they can begin to investigate and control the problem right away. If bioterrorism is suspected, the health departments will notify the Centers for Disease Control and Prevention (CDC), the Federal Bureau of Investigation (FBI), and other appropriate authorities.

How can the general public reduce the risk of getting pneumonic plague from another person or giving it to someone else?

If possible, avoid close contact with other people. People having direct and close contact with someone with pneumonic plague should wear tightly fitting disposable surgical masks. If surgical masks are not available, even makeshift face coverings made of layers of cloth may be helpful in an emergency. People who have been exposed to a contagious person can be protected from developing plague by receiving prompt antibiotic treatment.

How is plague diagnosed?

The first step is evaluation by a health worker. If the health worker suspects pneumonic plague, samples of the patient's blood, sputum, or lymph node aspirate are sent to a laboratory for testing. Once the laboratory receives the sample, preliminary results can be ready in less than two hours. Confirmation will take longer, usually twenty-four to forty-eight hours.

How long can plague bacteria exist in the environment?

Yersinia pestis is easily destroyed by sunlight and drying. Even so, when released into air, the bacterium will survive for up to one hour, depending on conditions.

Is a vaccine available to prevent pneumonic plague?

Currently, no plague vaccine is available in the United States. Research is in progress, but we are not likely to have vaccines for several years or more.

Section 36.6

Ricin

Reprinted from "Facts about Ricin," U.S. Centers
for Disease Control and Prevention, February 22, 2006.

What Ricin Is

Ricin is a poison that can be made from the waste left over from processing castor beans.

It can be in the form of a powder, a mist, or a pellet, or it can be dissolved in water or weak acid.

It is a stable substance. For example, it is not affected much by extreme conditions such as very hot or very cold temperatures.

Where Ricin Is Found and How It Is Used

Castor beans are processed throughout the world to make castor oil. Ricin is part of the waste "mash" produced when castor oil is made.

Ricin has some potential medical uses, such as bone marrow transplants and cancer treatment (to kill cancer cells).

How You Could Be Exposed to Ricin

It would take a deliberate act to make ricin and use it to poison people. Accidental exposure to ricin is highly unlikely.

People can breathe in ricin mist or powder and be poisoned.

Ricin can also get into water or food and then be swallowed.

Pellets of ricin, or ricin dissolved in a liquid, can be injected into people's bodies.

Depending on the route of exposure (such as injection or inhalation), as little as 500 micrograms of ricin could be enough to kill an adult. A 500-microgram dose of ricin would be about the size of the head of a pin. A greater amount would likely be needed to kill people if the ricin were swallowed.

In 1978, Georgi Markov, a Bulgarian writer and journalist who was living in London, died after he was attacked by a man with an umbrella.

The umbrella had been rigged to inject a poison ricin pellet under Markov's skin.

Some reports have indicated that ricin may have been used in the Iran-Iraq war during the 1980s and that quantities of ricin were found in Al Qaeda caves in Afghanistan.

Ricin poisoning is not contagious. It cannot be spread from person to person through casual contact.

How Ricin Works

Ricin works by getting inside the cells of a person's body and preventing the cells from making the proteins they need. Without the proteins, cells die. Eventually this is harmful to the whole body, and death may occur.

Effects of ricin poisoning depend on whether ricin was inhaled, ingested, or injected.

Signs and Symptoms of Ricin Exposure

The major symptoms of ricin poisoning depend on the route of exposure and the dose received, though many organs may be affected in severe cases.

Initial symptoms of ricin poisoning by inhalation may occur within eight hours of exposure. Following ingestion of ricin, initial symptoms typically occur in less than six hours.

Inhalation: Within a few hours of inhaling significant amounts of ricin, the likely symptoms would be respiratory distress (difficulty breathing), fever, cough, nausea, and tightness in the chest. Heavy sweating may follow as well as fluid building up in the lungs (pulmonary edema). This would make breathing even more difficult, and the skin might turn blue. Excess fluid in the lungs would be diagnosed by x-ray or by listening to the chest with a stethoscope. Finally, low blood pressure and respiratory failure may occur, leading to death. In cases of known exposure to ricin, people having respiratory symptoms that started within twelve hours of inhaling ricin should seek medical care.

Ingestion: If someone swallows a significant amount of ricin, he or she would develop vomiting and diarrhea that may become bloody. Severe dehydration may be the result, followed by low blood pressure. Other signs or symptoms may include hallucinations, seizures, and blood in the urine. Within several days, the person's liver, spleen, and kidneys might stop working, and the person could die.

Skin and eye exposure: Ricin in the powder or mist form can cause redness and pain of the skin and the eyes.

Death from ricin poisoning could take place within thirty-six to seventy-two hours of exposure, depending on the route of exposure (inhalation, ingestion, or injection) and the dose received. If death has not occurred in three to five days, the victim usually recovers.

Showing these signs and symptoms does not necessarily mean that a person has been exposed to ricin.

How Ricin Poisoning Is Treated

Because no antidote exists for ricin, the most important factor is avoiding ricin exposure in the first place. If exposure cannot be avoided, the most important factor is then getting the ricin off or out of the body as quickly as possible. Ricin poisoning is treated by giving victims supportive medical care to minimize the effects of the poisoning. The types of supportive medical care would depend on several factors, such as the route by which victims were poisoned (that is, whether poisoning was by inhalation, ingestion, or skin or eye exposure). Care could include such measures as helping victims breathe, giving them intravenous fluids (fluids given through a needle inserted into a vein), giving them medications to treat conditions such as seizure and low blood pressure, flushing their stomachs with activated charcoal (if the ricin has been very recently ingested), or washing out their eyes with water if their eyes are irritated.

How You Can Know Whether You Have Been Exposed to Ricin

If we suspect that people have inhaled ricin, a potential clue would be that a large number of people who had been close to each other suddenly developed fever, cough, and excess fluid in their lungs. These symptoms could be followed by severe breathing problems and possibly death.

No widely available, reliable test exists to confirm that a person has been exposed to ricin.

How You Can Protect Yourself, and What to Do If You Are Exposed to Ricin

First, get fresh air by leaving the area where the ricin was released. Moving to an area with fresh air is a good way to reduce the possibility of death from exposure to ricin:

- If the ricin release was outside, move away from the area where the ricin was released.

- If the ricin release was indoors, get out of the building.

If you are near a release of ricin, emergency coordinators may tell you to either evacuate the area or to "shelter in place" inside a building to avoid being exposed to the chemical.

If you think you may have been exposed to ricin, you should remove your clothing, rapidly wash your entire body with soap and water, and get medical care as quickly as possible.

Removing your clothing: Quickly take off clothing that may have ricin on it. Any clothing that has to be pulled over the head should be cut off the body instead of pulled over the head. If you are helping other people remove their clothing, try to avoid touching any contaminated areas, and remove the clothing as quickly as possible.

Washing yourself: As quickly as possible, wash any ricin from your skin with large amounts of soap and water. Washing with soap and water will help protect people from any chemicals on their bodies. If your eyes are burning or your vision is blurred, rinse your eyes with plain water for ten to fifteen minutes. If you wear contacts, remove them and put them with the contaminated clothing. Do not put the contacts back in your eyes (even if they are not disposable contacts). If you wear eyeglasses, wash them with soap and water. You can put your eyeglasses back on after you wash them.

Disposing of your clothes: After you have washed yourself, place your clothing inside a plastic bag. Avoid touching contaminated areas of the clothing. If you can't avoid touching contaminated areas, or you aren't sure where the contaminated areas are, wear rubber gloves, turn the bag inside out and use it to pick up the clothing, or put the clothing in the bag using tongs, tool handles, sticks, or similar objects. Anything that touches the contaminated clothing should also be placed in the bag. If you wear contacts, put them in the plastic bag, too.

Seal the bag, and then seal that bag inside another plastic bag. Disposing of your clothing in this way will help protect you and other people from any chemicals that might be on your clothes.

When the local or state health department or emergency personnel arrive, tell them what you did with your clothes. The health department or emergency personnel will arrange for further disposal. Do not handle the plastic bags yourself.

If someone has ingested ricin, do not induce vomiting or give fluids to drink.

Seek medical attention right away. Dial 911 and explain what has happened.

Section 36.7

Sarin

Reprinted from "Facts about Sarin," U.S. Centers
for Disease Control and Prevention, February 22, 2006.

What Sarin Is

Sarin is a human-made chemical warfare agent classified as a nerve agent. Nerve agents are the most toxic and rapidly acting of the known chemical warfare agents. They are similar to certain kinds of pesticides (insect killers) called organophosphates in terms of how they work and what kind of harmful effects they cause. However, nerve agents are much more potent than organophosphate pesticides.

Sarin originally was developed in 1938 in Germany as a pesticide.

Sarin is a clear, colorless, and tasteless liquid that has no odor in its pure form. However, sarin can evaporate into a vapor (gas) and spread into the environment.

Sarin is also known as GB.

Where Sarin Is Found and How It Is Used

Sarin and other nerve agents may have been used in chemical warfare during the Iran-Iraq War in the 1980s.

Sarin was used in two terrorist attacks in Japan in 1994 and 1995.

Sarin is not found naturally in the environment.

How People Can Be Exposed to Sarin

Following release of sarin into the air, people can be exposed through skin contact or eye contact. They can also be exposed by breathing air that contains sarin.

Sarin mixes easily with water, so it could be used to poison water. Following release of sarin into water, people can be exposed by touching or drinking water that contains sarin.

Following contamination of food with sarin, people can be exposed by eating the contaminated food.

A person's clothing can release sarin for about thirty minutes after it has come in contact with sarin vapor, which can lead to exposure of other people.

Because sarin breaks down slowly in the body, people who are repeatedly exposed to sarin may suffer more harmful health effects.

Because sarin vapor is heavier than air, it will sink to low-lying areas and create a greater exposure hazard there.

How Sarin Works

The extent of poisoning caused by sarin depends on the amount of sarin to which a person was exposed, how the person was exposed, and the length of time of the exposure.

Symptoms will appear within a few seconds after exposure to the vapor form of sarin and within a few minutes up to eighteen hours after exposure to the liquid form.

All the nerve agents cause their toxic effects by preventing the proper operation of the chemical that acts as the body's "off switch" for glands and muscles. Without an "off switch," the glands and muscles are constantly being stimulated. They may tire and no longer be able to sustain breathing function.

Sarin is the most volatile of the nerve agents, which means that it can easily and quickly evaporate from a liquid into a vapor and spread into the environment. People can be exposed to the vapor even if they do not come in contact with the liquid form of sarin.

Because it evaporates so quickly, sarin presents an immediate but short-lived threat.

Immediate Signs and Symptoms of Sarin Exposure

People may not know that they were exposed because sarin has no odor.

People exposed to a low or moderate dose of sarin by breathing contaminated air, eating contaminated food, drinking contaminated water, or touching contaminated surfaces may experience some or all of the following symptoms within seconds to hours of exposure:

• Runny nose

- Watery eyes
- Small, pinpoint pupils
- Eye pain
- Blurred vision
- Drooling and excessive sweating
- Cough
- Chest tightness
- Rapid breathing
- Diarrhea
- Increased urination
- Confusion
- Drowsiness
- Weakness
- Headache
- Nausea, vomiting, and/or abdominal pain
- Slow or fast heart rate
- Low or high blood pressure

Even a small drop of sarin on the skin can cause sweating and muscle twitching where sarin touched the skin.

Exposure to large doses of sarin by any route may result in the following harmful health effects:

- Loss of consciousness
- Convulsions
- Paralysis
- Respiratory failure possibly leading to death

Showing these signs and symptoms does not necessarily mean that a person has been exposed to sarin.

What the Long-Term Health Effects Are

Mild or moderately exposed people usually recover completely. Severely exposed people are not likely to survive. Unlike some organophosphate pesticides, nerve agents have not been associated with neurological problems lasting more than one to two weeks after the exposure.

How People Can Protect Themselves and What They Should Do If They Are Exposed to Sarin

Recovery from sarin exposure is possible with treatment, but the antidotes available must be used quickly to be effective. Therefore, the best thing to do is avoid exposure:

- Leave the area where the sarin was released and get to fresh air. Quickly moving to an area where fresh air is available is highly effective in reducing the possibility of death from exposure to sarin vapor.

  - If the sarin release was outdoors, move away from the area where the sarin was released. Go to the highest ground possible, because sarin is heavier than air and will sink to low-lying areas.

  - If the sarin release was indoors, get out of the building.

If people think they may have been exposed, they should remove their clothing, rapidly wash their entire body with soap and water, and get medical care as quickly as possible.

Removing and disposing of clothing: Quickly take off clothing that has liquid sarin on it. Any clothing that has to be pulled over the head should be cut off the body instead of pulled over the head. If possible, seal the clothing in a plastic bag. Then seal the first plastic bag in a second plastic bag. Removing and sealing the clothing in this way will help protect people from any chemicals that might be on their clothes.

If clothes were placed in plastic bags, inform either the local or state health department or emergency personnel upon their arrival. Do not handle the plastic bags.

If helping other people remove their clothing, try to avoid touching any contaminated areas, and remove the clothing as quickly as possible.

Washing the body: As quickly as possible, wash any liquid sarin from the skin with large amounts of soap and water. Washing with soap and water will help protect people from any chemicals on their bodies. Rinse the eyes with plain water for ten to fifteen minutes if they are burning or if vision is blurred.

If sarin has been swallowed, do not induce vomiting or give fluids to drink.

589

Seek medical attention immediately. Dial 911 and explain what has happened.

How Sarin Exposure Is Treated

Treatment consists of removing sarin from the body as soon as possible and providing supportive medical care in a hospital setting. Antidotes are available for sarin. They are most useful if given as soon as possible after exposure.

Section 36.8

Chlorine Gas

Reprinted from "Facts about Chlorine," U.S. Centers
for Disease Control and Prevention, February 22, 2006.

What Chlorine Is

Chlorine is an element used in industry and found in some household products.

Chlorine is sometimes in the form of a poisonous gas. Chlorine gas can be pressurized and cooled to change it into a liquid so that it can be shipped and stored. When liquid chlorine is released, it quickly turns into a gas that stays close to the ground and spreads rapidly.

Chlorine gas can be recognized by its pungent, irritating odor, which is like the odor of bleach. The strong smell may provide an adequate warning to people that they have been exposed.

Chlorine gas appears to be yellow-green in color.

Chlorine itself is not flammable, but it can react explosively or form explosive compounds with other chemicals such as turpentine and ammonia.

Where Chlorine Is Found and How It Is Used

Chlorine was used during World War I as a choking (pulmonary) agent.

Chlorine is one of the most commonly manufactured chemicals in the United States. Its most important use is as a bleach in the manufacture of paper and cloth, but it is also used to make pesticides (insect killers), rubber, and solvents.

Chlorine is used in drinking water and swimming pool water to kill harmful bacteria. It is also as used as part of the sanitation process for industrial waste and sewage.

Household chlorine bleach can release chlorine gas if it is mixed with other cleaning agents.

How People Can Be Exposed to Chlorine

People's risk for exposure depends on how close they are to the place where the chlorine was released.

If chlorine gas is released into the air, people may be exposed through skin contact or eye contact. They may also be exposed by breathing air that contains chlorine.

If chlorine liquid is released into water, people may be exposed by touching or drinking water that contains chlorine.

If chlorine liquid comes into contact with food, people may be exposed by eating the contaminated food.

Chlorine gas is heavier than air, so it would settle in low-lying areas.

How Chlorine Works

The extent of poisoning caused by chlorine depends on the amount of chlorine a person is exposed to, how the person was exposed, and the length of time of the exposure.

When chlorine gas comes into contact with moist tissues such as the eyes, throat, and lungs, an acid is produced that can damage these tissues.

Immediate Signs and Symptoms of Chlorine Exposure

During or immediately after exposure to dangerous concentrations of chlorine, the following signs and symptoms may develop:

- Coughing
- Chest tightness
- Burning sensation in the nose, throat, and eyes
- Watery eyes

- Blurred vision

- Nausea and vomiting

- Burning pain, redness, and blisters on the skin if exposed to gas, skin injury similar to frostbite if exposed to liquid chlorine

- Difficulty breathing or shortness of breath (may appear immediately if high concentrations of chlorine gas are inhaled, or may be delayed if low concentrations of chlorine gas are inhaled)

- Fluid in the lungs (pulmonary edema) within two to four hours

Showing these signs or symptoms does not necessarily mean that a person has been exposed to chlorine.

What the Long-Term Health Effects Are

Long-term complications from chlorine exposure are not found in people who survive a sudden exposure unless they suffer complications such as pneumonia during therapy. Chronic bronchitis may develop in people who develop pneumonia during therapy.

How People Can Protect Themselves, and What They Should Do If They Are Exposed to Chlorine

Leave the area where the chlorine was released and get to fresh air. Quickly moving to an area where fresh air is available is highly effective in reducing exposure to chlorine:

- If the chlorine release was outdoors, move away from the area where the chlorine was released. Go to the highest ground possible, because chlorine is heavier than air and will sink to low-lying areas.

- If the chlorine release was indoors, get out of the building.

If you think you may have been exposed, remove your clothing, rapidly wash your entire body with soap and water, and get medical care as quickly as possible.

Removing and disposing of clothing: Quickly take off clothing that has liquid chlorine on it. Any clothing that has to be pulled over the head should be cut off the body instead of pulled over the head. If possible, seal the clothing in a plastic bag. Then seal the first plastic bag in a second plastic bag. Removing and sealing the clothing in this way will help protect you and other people from any chemicals that might be on your clothes.

If you placed your clothes in plastic bags, inform either the local or state health department or emergency personnel upon their arrival. Do not handle the plastic bags.

If you are helping other people remove their clothing, try to avoid touching any contaminated areas, and remove the clothing as quickly as possible.

Washing the body: As quickly as possible, wash your entire body with large amounts of soap and water. Washing with soap and water will help protect people from any chemicals on their bodies.

If your eyes are burning or your vision is blurred, rinse your eyes with plain water for ten to fifteen minutes. If you wear contacts, remove them before rinsing your eyes, and place them in the bags with the contaminated clothing. Do not put the contacts back in your eyes. You should dispose of them even if you do not wear disposable contacts. If you wear eyeglasses, wash them with soap and water. You can put the eyeglasses back on after you wash them.

If you have ingested (swallowed) chlorine, do not induce vomiting or drink fluids.

Seek medical attention right away. Dial 911 and explain what has happened.

How Chlorine Exposure Is Treated

No antidote exists for chlorine exposure. Treatment consists of removing the chlorine from the body as soon as possible and providing supportive medical care in a hospital setting.

Part Five

Additional Help and Information

Chapter 37

Glossary of Terms Related to Respiratory Disorders

acid aerosol: Acidic liquid or solid particles that are small enough to become airborne. High concentrations of acid aerosols can be irritating to the lungs and have been associated with some respiratory diseases, such as asthma.[3]

action plan: A written set of directions or a chart that tells you what to do if asthma symptoms occur, depending on their severity. Your action plan also should tell you what to do when you do *not* feel any symptoms (i.e., preventive care).[1]

albuterol: An asthma medication.[1]

allergen: A substance that triggers an allergic reaction. Many allergens are responsible for triggering asthma, including dust mites, animal dander, mold, and cockroaches.[1]

allergic asthma: A chronic, inflammatory disorder of the airways characterized by wheezing, breathing difficulties, coughing, chest tightness, wherein these symptoms are caused by an allergic reaction to an inhaled allergen, rather than an irritant or other non-allergy factor.[1]

The terms in this glossary were reprinted from "Glossary of Asthma Terms" with permission from the Asthma and Allergy Foundation of America, © 2005, all rights reserved [marked 1]; and excerpted from *Stedman's Electronic Medical Dictionary* v.5.0, © 2000 Lippincott Williams and Wilkins [marked 2] and "The Inside Story: A Guide to Indoor Air Quality," U.S. Environmental Protection Agency, August 2007 [marked 3].

allergic rhinitis: Inflammation of the mucous membranes in the nose that is caused by an allergic reaction.[3]

allergist: A doctor that has specific training in the care of asthma and in some cases may be more familiar with current clinical guidelines than a pediatrician or general practitioner.[1]

alveoli: Tiny air sacs where oxygen is transferred into your lungs and carbon dioxide waste enters the airways in order to be exhaled out.[1]

animal dander: Tiny scales of animal skin.[3]

antioxidant: An agent that inhibits oxidation; any of numerous chemical substances, including certain natural body products and nutrients, that can neutralize the oxidant effect of free radicals and other substances.[2]

asthma: A chronic, inflammatory disorder of the airways characterized by wheezing, breathing difficulties, coughing, chest tightness, and other possible symptoms. People with asthma have very sensitive airways that are constantly on the verge of over-reacting to asthma triggers.[1]

beta-agonists: Asthma drugs that relax the muscles around the bronchial tubes ("bronchodilators"), thus opening the airways or helping keep them open. There are two main types. The long-acting type is taken every day to prevent symptoms, often in combination with a steroid. The short-acting type is used for quick relief of symptoms during an asthma episode/attack. Albuterol is the most commonly used short-acting beta-agonist.[1]

bronchial tubes: Airways in the lungs. There is one major branch going into each lung, and these then divide into many smaller branches.[1]

bronchiectasis: Chronic dilation of bronchi or bronchioles as a sequel of inflammatory disease or obstruction often associated with heavy sputum production.[2]

bronchioles: The smallest airways in the lungs.[1]

bronchitis: Inflammation of the mucous membrane of the bronchial tubes.[2]

bronchoconstriction: This is when the muscles that wrap the airways constrict tighter and tighter, pinching the airways closed.[1]

bronchodilators: Drugs that relax the muscles around the airways, thus opening the airways up. Some bronchodilators are used for quick relief of symptoms during an asthma attack. Others are taken every day to prevent symptoms.[1]

bronchopulmonary: Relating to the bronchi and the lungs.[2]

bronchopulmonary dysplasia: Chronic pulmonary insufficiency seen primarily in infants born prematurely; defined clinically as a persistent supplemental oxygen requirement at one month of age and typically seen in infants who required positive pressure ventilation.[2]

building-related illness: A discrete, identifiable disease or illness that can be traced to a specific pollutant or source within a building. (Contrast with "sick building syndrome").[3]

chemical sensitization: Evidence suggests that some people may develop health problems characterized by effects such as dizziness, eye and throat irritation, chest tightness, and nasal congestion that appear whenever they are exposed to certain chemicals. People may react to even trace amounts of chemicals to which they have become "sensitized."[3]

chronic obstructive pulmonary disease: General term used for those diseases with permanent or temporary narrowing of small bronchi, in which forced expiratory flow is slowed.[2]

control drug: A drug that some people take on a daily basis to prevent asthma symptoms and asthma attacks.[1]

corticosteroids: The most common and effective drugs used for long-term daily control of asthma (prevention of symptoms). They are most frequently inhaled using either a metered dose inhaler, dry powder inhaler, or nebulizer. Corticosteroids primarily decrease or prevent inflammation.[1]

cromolyn: An anti-inflammatory drug that may be used on a daily basis to prevent symptoms of asthma.[1]

cystic fibrosis: A congenital metabolic disorder in which secretions of exocrine glands are abnormal; excessively viscid mucus causes obstruction of passageways (including pancreatic and bile ducts, intestines, and bronchi), and the sodium and chloride content of sweat are increased throughout the patient's life.[2]

dry powder inhaler: A small device similar to a metered dose inhaler, but where the drug is in powder form. The patient exhales out a full breath, places the lips around the mouthpiece, then quickly breathes in the powder.[1]

dyspnea: Shortness of breath, a subjective difficulty or distress in breathing, usually associated with disease of the heart or lungs; occurs normally during intense physical exertion or at high altitude.[2]

edema: An accumulation of an excessive amount of watery fluid in cells or intercellular tissues.[2]

emphysema: A condition of the lung characterized by increase beyond the normal in the size of air spaces distal to the terminal bronchiole (those parts containing alveoli), with destructive changes in their walls and reduction in their number. Clinical manifestation is breathlessness on exertion, due to the combined effect (in varying degrees) of reduction of alveolar surface for gas exchange and collapse of smaller airways with trapping of alveolar gas in expiration; this causes the chest to be held in the position of inspiration ("barrel chest"), with prolonged expiration and increased residual volume.[2]

environmental tobacco smoke: Mixture of smoke from the burning end of a cigarette, pipe, or cigar and smoke exhaled by the smoker (also secondhand smoke or passive smoking).[3]

fungi: Any of a group of parasitic lower plants that lack chlorophyll, including molds and mildews.[3]

holding chamber: See spacer.

humidifier fever: A respiratory illness caused by exposure to toxins from microorganisms found in wet or moist areas in humidifiers and air conditioners. Also called air conditioner or ventilation fever.[3]

hyperoxia: An increased amount of oxygen in tissues and organs.[2]

hypersensitivity pneumonitis: A group of respiratory diseases that cause inflammation of the lung (specifically granulomatous cells). Most forms of hypersensitivity pneumonitis are caused by the inhalation of organic dusts, including molds.[3]

idiopathic pulmonary fibrosis: An acute to chronic inflammatory process or interstitial fibrosis of the lung of unknown etiology.[2]

immunotherapy: A series of shots that help build up the immune system's tolerance to an asthma trigger.[1]

inflammation: A fundamental pathologic process consisting of a dynamic complex of cytologic and chemical reactions that occur in the affected blood vessels and adjacent tissues in response to an injury or abnormal stimulation caused by a physical, chemical, or biologic agent.[2]

ipratropium bromide: A bronchodilator sometimes used for quick relief of asthma symptoms, often for people who do not tolerate beta-agonists. It is also used for people whose asthma is triggered by beta-blocker medication for the heart.[1]

leukotriene modifiers: Control drugs in the form of tablets for patients with mild to moderate persistent asthma. For mild asthma, they are sometimes considered as an alternative to inhaled steroids. For moderate asthma, they may be considered as a supplement to inhaled steroids in place of long-acting beta agonists.[1]

metered dose inhaler (MDI): The most common device people use to take asthma medication. An MDI allows you to inhale a specific amount of medicine (a "metered dose"). It consists of a metal canister, which keeps the medication under pressure, and a plastic sleeve, which helps to release the medication. When you press the canister, medicine particles are propelled toward your throat where you can inhale them.[1]

nebulizer: A device that creates a mist out of your asthma drug, which makes it easy and pleasant to breathe the drug into the lungs. The drug is placed into a small cup. Air from a small compressor converts the drug into an aerosol mist, which travels through a hose with a mouthpiece attached. By taking slow, deep breaths, the medicine is delivered into your lungs.[1]

nedocromil sodium: An inhaled medication that may be used on a daily basis to treat inflammation in the airways and prevent asthma attacks.[1]

nonallergic asthma: A chronic, inflammatory disorder of the airways characterized by wheezing, breathing difficulties, coughing, chest tightness, wherein these symptoms are caused by an inhaled irritant or other non-allergy factor; when these symptoms are not caused by allergic reactions. (See "allergic asthma" for more information.)[1]

organic compounds: Chemicals that contain carbon. Volatile organic compounds vaporize at room temperature and pressure. They are found in many indoor sources, including many common household products and building materials.[3]

peak flow: A measurement of how well you can blow air out of your lungs. If your airways become narrow and blocked due to asthma, you can't blow air out as well, and your peak flow values drop.[1]

pneumonia: Inflammation of the lung parenchyma characterized by consolidation of the affected part, the alveolar air spaces being filled with exudate, inflammatory cells, and fibrin. Most cases are due to infection by bacteria or viruses, a few to inhalation of chemicals or trauma to the chest wall, and a small minority to rickettsiae, fungi, and yeasts.[2]

pulmonary: Relating to the lungs, to the pulmonary artery, or to the aperture leading from the right ventricle into the pulmonary artery.[2]

pulmonary embolism: Embolism of pulmonary arteries, most frequently by detached fragments of thrombus from a leg or pelvic vein, commonly when thrombosis has followed an operation or confinement to bed.[2]

pulmonary hypertension: Hypertension in the pulmonary circuit; may be primary, or secondary to pulmonary or cardiac disease.[2]

radon (Rn) and radon decay products: A radioactive gas formed in the decay of uranium. The radon decay products (also called radon daughters or progeny) can be breathed into the lung where they continue to release radiation as they further decay.[3]

relief drug: A drug used as needed to relieve asthma symptoms during asthma attacks. Also called a quick-relief or rescue drug.[1]

rescue drug: Relief or quick-relief drug.[1]

respirator: An apparatus for administering artificial respiration in cases of respiratory failure.[2]

sarcoidosis: S systemic granulomatous disease of unknown cause, especially involving the lungs with resulting interstitial fibrosis, but also involving lymph nodes, skin, liver, spleen, eyes, phalangeal bones, and parotid glands.[2]

sick building syndrome: Term that refers to a set of symptoms that affect some number of building occupants during the time they spend in the building and diminish or go away during periods when they leave the building. Cannot be traced to specific pollutants or sources within the building. (Contrast with "building related illness").[3]

sinusitis: An inflammation or infection of one or more sinuses. The sinuses are hollow air spaces located around the nose and eyes.[1]

spacer: This works with your metered dose inhaler (MDI) to deliver medication more easily and effectively, and can reduce side effects.

When you use an MDI by itself, more of the medicine is left in your mouth and throat, wasting your dose and causing an unpleasant aftertaste. Spacers hold the medicine between you and the MDI, so that you can inhale it slowly and more completely. Spacers are also called holding chambers.[1]

spirometry: Test for diagnosing asthma. A spirometer is an instrument that measures the maximum volume you can exhale after breathing in as much as you can. Small spirometers are available for home use, although peak flow meters are more appropriate for most people.[1]

steroids: See corticosteroids.

theophylline: This drug is sometimes used to help control mild asthma, especially to prevent nighttime symptoms. The drug works by relaxing the muscles of your bronchial tubes.[1]

tuberculosis: A specific disease caused by infection with *Mycobacterium tuberculosis*, the tubercle bacillus, which can affect almost any tissue or organ of the body, the most common seat of the disease being the lungs.[2]

ventilation rate: The rate at which indoor air enters and leaves a building. Expressed in one of two ways: the number of changes of outdoor air per unit of time (air changes per hour, or "ach") or the rate at which a volume of outdoor air enters per unit of time (cubic feet per minute, or "cfm").[3]

ventilator: See respirator.

Chapter 38

Resource List

General

American College of Chest Physicians
3300 Dundee Road
Northbrook, IL 60062-2348
Toll-Free: 800-343-2227
Phone: 847-498-1400
Website: http://www.chestnet.org

American Lung Association
61 Broadway, 6th Floor
New York, NY 10006
Toll-Free: 800-548-8252
Phone: 212-315-8700
Website: http://www.lungusa.org

American Thoracic Society
61 Broadway
New York, NY 10006-2755
Phone: 212-315-8600
Fax: 212-315-6498
Website: http://www.thoracic.org

British Lung Foundation
73-75 Goswell Road
London, England
Great Britain
EC1V 7ER
Website: http://www.lunguk.org

Canadian Lung Association, National Office
1750 Courtwood Crescent
Suite 300
Ottawa, ON
K2C 2B5
Canada
Toll-Free: 888-566-LUNG (5864)
Phone: 613-569-6411
Fax: 613-569-8860
Website: http://www.lung.ca
E-mail: info@lung.ca

The information in this chapter was compiled from various sources deemed accurate. All contact information was verified and updated in September 2007. Inclusion does not imply endorsement. This list is intended to serve as a starting point for information gathering; it is not comprehensive.

605

National Heart, Lung, and Blood Institute

NHLBI Health Information Center
P.O. Box 30105
Bethesda, MD 20824-0105
Toll-Free: 800-575-WELL (9355)
Phone: 301-592-8573
Fax: 240-629-3246
TTY: 240-629-3255
Website: http://www.nhlbi.nih.gov
E-mail: nhlbiinfo@nhlbi.nih.gov

National Lung Health Education Program

American Association for Respiratory Care
9425 MacArthur Boulevard
Irving, TX 75063
Phone: 972-910-8555
Fax: 972-484-2720
Website: http://www.nlhep.org
E-mail: NLHEP@aarc.org

Pulmonary Education and Research Foundation (PERF)

P.O. Box 1133
Lomita, CA 90717-5133
Phone: 310-539-8390
Fax: 310-539-8390
Website: http://www.perf2ndwind.org

Acute Respiratory Distress Syndrome (ARDS)

ARDS Support Center, Inc.

7172 Regional Street, #278
Dublin, CA 94568-2324
Website: http://ards.org

Alpha-1 Antitrypsin Deficiency

Alpha-1 Association

2937 SW 27 Avenue, Suite 106
Miami, FL 33133
Toll-Free: 800-521-3025
Phone: 305-648-0088
Fax: 305-648-0089
Website: http://www.alpha1.org
E-mail: info@alpha1.org

Alpha-1 Foundation

2937 SW 27th Avenue, Suite 302
Miami, Florida 33133
Toll Free: 877-2-CURE-A1
Phone: 305-567-9888
Fax: 305-567-1317
Website: http://www.alphaone.org
E-mail: info@alphaone.org

AlphaNet, Inc.

2937 SW 27th Avenue, Suite 305
Coconut Grove, FL 33133
Toll-Free: 800-577-2638
Website: http://www.alphanet.org
E-mail: info@alphanet.org

American Liver Foundation

75 Maiden Lane, Suite 603
New York, NY 10038
Phone: 212-668-1000
Fax: 212-483-8179
Website: http://www.liverfoundation.org

Asthma

American Academy of Allergy, Asthma and Immunology
555 East Wells Street, Suite 1100
Milwaukee, WI 53202-3823
Phone: 414-272-6071
Website: http://www.aaaai.org
E-mail: info@aaaai.org

Asthma and Allergy Foundation of America
1233 20th Street, NW, Suite 402
Washington, DC 20036
Toll-Free: 800-7-ASTHMA
(727-8462)
Website: http://www.aafa.org
E-mail: Info@aafa.org

Cystic Fibrosis

Cystic Fibrosis Foundation
6931 Arlington Road
Bethesda, MD 20814
Toll-Free: 800-FIGHT CF
(344-4823)
Phone: 301-951-4422
Website: http://www.cff.org
E-mail: info@cff.org

Lung Cancer

American Cancer Society
250 Williams street NW
Atlanta, GA 30303
Toll-Free: 800-ACS-2345
TTY: 866-228-4327
Website: http://www.cancer.org

National Cancer Institute
NCI Public Inquiries Office
6116 Executive Boulevard
Room 3036A
Bethesda, MD 20892-8322
Toll-Free: 800-4-CANCER
(422-6237)
TTY: 800-332-8615
Website: http://www.cancer.gov

Lymphangioleiomyomatosis (LAM)

LAM Foundation
4015 Executive Park Drive
Suite 320
Cincinnati, OH 45241
Phone: 513-777-6889
Fax: 513-777-4109
Website: http://www.thelamfoundation.org
E-mail: info@thelamfoundation.org

Primary Ciliary Dyskinesia

PCD Foundation
29252 N. 22nd Lane
Phoenix, AZ 85085
Phone: 612-396-1179 or
623-215-2032
Fax: 623-215-6670
Website: http://www.pcdfoundation.org
E-mail: info@pcdfoundation.org

Pulmonary Fibrosis

Coalition for Pulmonary Fibrosis
1659 Branham Lane
Suite F, # 227
San Jose, CA 95118-5226
Toll-Free: 888-222-8541
Fax: 866-683-9458
Website: http://
www.coalitionforpf.org
E-mail: info@coalitionforpf.org

Pulmonary Fibrosis Foundation
1332 North Halsted Street
Suite 201
Chicago, Illinois 60622
Phone: 312-587-9272
Fax: 312-587- 9273
Website: http://
www.pulmonaryfibrosis.org

Pulmonary Hypertension

PHCentral
1309 12th Ave.
San Francisco, CA 94122
Website: http://www.phcentral.org
E-mail: info@phcentral.org

Pulmonary Hypertension Association
801 Roeder Road, Suite 400
Silver Spring, MD 20910
Toll-Free: 800-748-7274
Phone: 301-565-3004
Fax: 301-565-3994
Website: http://
www.phassociation.org

Sarcoidosis

Foundation for Sarcoidosis Research
122 South Michigan Avenue
Suite 1700
Chicago, IL 60603
Phone: 312-341-0500
Fax: 312-322-9808
Website: http://
www.stopsarcoidosis.org

National Sarcoidosis Resource Center
P.O. Box 1593
Piscataway, NJ 08854
Phone: 732-699-0733
Fax: 732-699-0882
Website: http://www.nsrc-global
.net

Sleep Apnea

American Sleep Apnea Association
1424 K Street, NW, Suite 302
Washington, DC 20005
Phone: 202-293-3650
Fax: 202-293-3656
Website: http://
www.sleepapnea.org
E-mail: asaa@sleepapnea.org

National Sleep Foundation
1522 K Street NW, Suite 500
Washington, DC 20005
Phone: 202-347-3471
Fax: 202-347-3472
Website: http://
www.sleepfoundation.org
E-mail: nsf@sleepfoundation.org

Sudden Infant Death Syndrome (SIDS)

American Academy of Pediatrics
141 Northwest Point Boulevard
Elk Grove Village, IL 60007-1098
Phone: 847-434-4000
Fax: 847-434-8000
Website: http://www.aap.org

Association of SIDS and Infant Mortality Programs (ASIP)
8280 Greensboro Drive
Suite 300
McLean, VA 22102
Toll-Free: 800-930-7437
Fax: 703-902-1320
Website: http://www.asip1.org
E-mail: asip@asip1.org

Back to Sleep
National Institute of Child
Health and Human Development
31 Center Drive, Building 31,
Room 2A32
Bethesda, MD 20892
Toll-Free: 800-505-CRIB
Fax: 301-984-1471
Website: http://
www.nichd.nih.gov
E-mail:
NICHDIRC@mail.nih.gov

C.J. Foundation for SIDS
The Don Imus-WFAN Pediatric
Center
Hackensack University Medical
Center
30 Prospect Avenue
Hackensack, NJ 07601
Toll-Free: 888-8CJ-SIDS
Phone: 201-996-5111
Fax: 201-996-5326
Website: http://www.cjsids.com
E-mail: info@cjsids.com

First Candle/SIDS Alliance
1314 Bedford Avenue, Suite 210
Baltimore, MD 21208
Toll-Free: 800-221-7437
Phone: 410-653-8226
Fax: 410-653-8709
Website: http://www.firstcandle.org
E-mail: info@firstcandle.org

National SIDS/Infant Death Resource Center
2115 Wisconsin Avenue, N.W.
Suite 601
Washington, DC 20007-2292
Toll-Free: 866-866-7437
Phone: 202-687-7466 (local)
Fax: 202-784-9777
Website: http://
www.sidscenter.org
E-mail: info@sidscenter.org

U.S. Consumer Product Safety Commission
4330 East West Highway
Bethesda, MD 20814-4408
Toll-Free: 800-638-2772
Fax: 301-504-0124
Website: http://www.cpsc.gov
E-mail: info@cpsc.gov

Tuberculosis

Francis J. Curry National Tuberculosis Center (CNTC)
3180 Eighteenth Street
Suite 101
San Francisco, CA
94110-2028
Phone: 415-502-4600
Fax: 415-502-4620
Website: http://
www.nationaltbcenter.edu
E-mail:
tbcenter@nationaltbcenter.edu

Heartland National TB Center
2303 SE Military Drive
San Antonio, TX 78223
Toll-Free: 800-TEX-LUNG
(839-5864)
Fax: 210-531-4590
Website: http://
www.heartlandntbc.org

New Jersey Medical School Global Tuberculosis Institute (GTBI)
225 Warren Street
P.O. Box 1709
Newark, NJ 07101-1709
Toll-Free: 800-4TB-DOCS
(482-3627)
Website: http://www.umdnj.edu/
globaltb

Index

Index

E

F

623

631

632

Health Reference Series
COMPLETE CATALOG

List price $87 per volume. **School and library price $78 per volume.**

Adolescent Health Sourcebook, 2nd Edition

Basic Consumer Health Information about the Physical, Mental, and Emotional Growth and Development of Adolescents, Including Medical Care, Nutritional and Physical Activity Requirements, Puberty, Sexual Activity, Acne, Tanning, Body Piercing, Common Physical Illnesses and Disorders, Eating Disorders, Attention Deficit Hyperactivity Disorder, Depression, Bullying, Hazing, and Adolescent Injuries Related to Sports, Driving, and Work

Along with Substance Abuse Information about Nicotine, Alcohol, and Drug Use, a Glossary, and Directory of Additional Resources

Edited by Joyce Brennfleck Shannon. 683 pages. 2006. 978-0-7808-0943-7.

"It is written in clear, nontechnical language aimed at general readers. . . . Recommended for public libraries, community colleges, and other agencies serving health care consumers."
— *American Reference Books Annual, 2003*

"Recommended for school and public libraries. Parents and professionals dealing with teens will appreciate the easy-to-follow format and the clearly written text. This could become a 'must have' for every high school teacher."
— *E-Streams, Jan '03*

"A good starting point for information related to common medical, mental, and emotional concerns of adolescents."
— *School Library Journal, Nov '02*

"This book provides accurate information in an easy to access format. It addresses topics that parents and caregivers might not be aware of and provides practical, useable information."
— *Doody's Health Sciences Book Review Journal, Sep-Oct '02*

"Recommended reference source."
— *Booklist, American Library Association, Sep '02*

■

AIDS Sourcebook, 3rd Edition

Basic Consumer Health Information about Acquired Immune Deficiency Syndrome (AIDS) and Human Immunodeficiency Virus (HIV) Infection, Including Facts about Transmission, Prevention, Diagnosis, Treatment, Opportunistic Infections, and Other Complications, with a Section for Women and Children, Including Details about Associated Gynecological Concerns, Pregnancy, and Pediatric Care

Along with Updated Statistical Information, Reports on Current Research Initiatives, a Glossary, and Directories of Internet, Hotline, and Other Resources

Edited by Dawn D. Matthews. 664 pages. 2003. 978-0-7808-0631-3.

"The 3rd edition of the *AIDS Sourcebook*, part of Omnigraphics' *Health Reference Series*, is a welcome update. . . . This resource is highly recommended for academic and public libraries."
— *American Reference Books Annual, 2004*

"Excellent sourcebook. This continues to be a highly recommended book. There is no other book that provides as much information as this book provides."
— *AIDS Book Review Journal, Dec-Jan '00*

"Recommended reference source."
— *Booklist, American Library Association, Dec '99*

■

Alcoholism Sourcebook, 2nd Edition

Basic Consumer Health Information about Alcohol Use, Abuse, and Dependence, Featuring Facts about the Physical, Mental, and Social Health Effects of Alcohol Addiction, Including Alcoholic Liver Disease, Pancreatic Disease, Cardiovascular Disease, Neurological Disorders, and the Effects of Drinking during Pregnancy

Along with Information about Alcohol Treatment, Medications, and Recovery Programs, in Addition to Tips for Reducing the Prevalence of Underage Drinking, Statistics about Alcohol Use, a Glossary of Related Terms, and Directories of Resources for More Help and Information

Edited by Amy L. Sutton. 653 pages. 2006. 978-0-7808-0942-0.

"This title is one of the few reference works on alcoholism for general readers. For some readers this will be a welcome complement to the many self-help books on the market. Recommended for collections serving general readers and consumer health collections."
— *E-Streams, Mar '01*

"This book is an excellent choice for public and academic libraries."
— *American Reference Books Annual, 2001*

"Recommended reference source."
— *Booklist, American Library Association, Dec '00*

"Presents a wealth of information on alcohol use and abuse and its effects on the body and mind, treatment, and prevention."
— *SciTech Book News, Dec '00*

"Important new health guide which packs in the latest consumer information about the problems of alcoholism."
— *Reviewer's Bookwatch, Nov '00*

SEE ALSO Drug Abuse Sourcebook

Allergies Sourcebook, 3rd Edition

Basic Consumer Health Information about Allergic Disorders, Such as Anaphylaxis, Hives, Eczema, Rhinitis, Sinusitis, and Conjunctivitis, and Their Triggers, Including Pollen, Mold, Dust Mites, Animal Dander, Insects, Chemicals, Food, Food Additives, and Medications;

Along with Advice about the Diagnosis and Treatment of Allergy Symptoms, a Glossary of Related Terms, a Directory of Resources for Help and Information, and Suggestions for Additional Reading

Edited by Amy L. Sutton. 598 pages. 2007. 978-0-7808-0950-5.

"This book brings a great deal of useful material together. . . . This is an excellent addition to public and consumer health library collections."
— *American Reference Books Annual, 2003*

"This second edition would be useful to laypersons with little or advanced knowledge of the subject matter. This book would also serve as a resource for nursing and other health care professions students. It would be useful in public, academic, and hospital libraries with consumer health collections." — *E-Streams, Jul '02*

∎

Alternative Medicine Sourcebook

SEE Complementary & Alternative Medicine Sourcebook

∎

Alzheimer's Disease Sourcebook, 3rd Edition

Basic Consumer Health Information about Alzheimer's Disease, Other Dementias, and Related Disorders, Including Multi-Infarct Dementia, AIDS Dementia Complex, Dementia with Lewy Bodies, Huntington's Disease, Wernicke-Korsakoff Syndrome (Alcohol-Related Dementia), Delirium, and Confusional States

Along with Information for People Newly Diagnosed with Alzheimer's Disease and Caregivers, Reports Detailing Current Research Efforts in Prevention, Diagnosis, and Treatment, Facts about Long-Term Care Issues, and Listings of Sources for Additional Information

Edited by Karen Bellenir. 645 pages. 2003. 978-0-7808-0666-5.

"This very informative and valuable tool will be a great addition to any library serving consumers, students and health care workers."
— *American Reference Books Annual, 2004*

"This is a valuable resource for people affected by dementias such as Alzheimer's. It is easy to navigate and includes important information and resources."
— *Doody's Review Service, Feb '04*

"Recommended reference source."
— *Booklist, American Library Association, Oct '99*

SEE ALSO *Brain Disorders Sourcebook*

Arthritis Sourcebook, 2nd Edition

Basic Consumer Health Information about Osteoarthritis, Rheumatoid Arthritis, Other Rheumatic Disorders, Infectious Forms of Arthritis, and Diseases with Symptoms Linked to Arthritis, Featuring Facts about Diagnosis, Pain Management, and Surgical Therapies

Along with Coping Strategies, Research Updates, a Glossary, and Resources for Additional Help and Information

Edited by Amy L. Sutton. 593 pages. 2004. 978-0-7808-0667-2.

"This easy-to-read volume is recommended for consumer health collections within public or academic libraries." — *E-Streams, May '05*

"As expected, this updated edition continues the excellent reputation of this series in providing sound, usable health information. . . . Highly recommended."
— *American Reference Books Annual, 2005*

"Excellent reference." — *The Bookwatch, Jan '05*

∎

Asthma Sourcebook, 2nd Edition

Basic Consumer Health Information about the Causes, Symptoms, Diagnosis, and Treatment of Asthma in Infants, Children, Teenagers, and Adults, Including Facts about Different Types of Asthma, Common Co-Occurring Conditions, Asthma Management Plans, Triggers, Medications, and Medication Delivery Devices

Along with Asthma Statistics, Research Updates, a Glossary, a Directory of Asthma-Related Resources, and More

Edited by Karen Bellenir. 609 pages. 2006. 978-0-7808-0866-9.

"A worthwhile reference acquisition for public libraries and academic medical libraries whose readers desire a quick introduction to the wide range of asthma information."
— *Choice, Association of College & Research Libraries, Jun '01*

"Recommended reference source."
— *Booklist, American Library Association, Feb '01*

"Highly recommended." — *The Bookwatch, Jan '01*

"There is much good information for patients and their families who deal with asthma daily."
— *American Medical Writers Association Journal, Winter '01*

"This informative text is recommended for consumer health collections in public, secondary school, and community college libraries and the libraries of universities with a large undergraduate population."
— *American Reference Books Annual, 2001*

∎

Attention Deficit Disorder Sourcebook

Basic Consumer Health Information about Attention Deficit/Hyperactivity Disorder in Children and Adults,

Including Facts about Causes, Symptoms, Diagnostic Criteria, and Treatment Options Such as Medications, Behavior Therapy, Coaching, and Homeopathy

Along with Reports on Current Research Initiatives, Legal Issues, and Government Regulations, and Featuring a Glossary of Related Terms, Internet Resources, and a List of Additional Reading Material

Edited by Dawn D. Matthews. 470 pages. 2002. 978-0-7808-0624-5.

"Recommended reference source."
— Booklist, American Library Association, Jan '03

"This book is recommended for all school libraries and the reference or consumer health sections of public libraries." — American Reference Books Annual, 2003

Back & Neck Sourcebook, 2nd Edition

Basic Consumer Health Information about Spinal Pain, Spinal Cord Injuries, and Related Disorders, Such as Degenerative Disk Disease, Osteoarthritis, Scoliosis, Sciatica, Spina Bifida, and Spinal Stenosis, and Featuring Facts about Maintaining Spinal Health, Self-Care, Pain Management, Rehabilitative Care, Chiropractic Care, Spinal Surgeries, and Complementary Therapies

Along with Suggestions for Preventing Back and Neck Pain, a Glossary of Related Terms, and a Directory of Resources

Edited by Amy L. Sutton. 633 pages. 2004. 978-0-7808-0738-9.

"Recommended . . . an easy to use, comprehensive medical reference book." — E-Streams, Sep '05

"The strength of this work is its basic, easy-to-read format. Recommended." — Reference and User Services Quarterly, American Library Association, Winter '97

Blood & Circulatory Disorders Sourcebook, 2nd Edition

Basic Consumer Health Information about the Blood and Circulatory System and Related Disorders, Such as Anemia and Other Hemoglobin Diseases, Cancer of the Blood and Associated Bone Marrow Disorders, Clotting and Bleeding Problems, and Conditions That Affect the Veins, Blood Vessels, and Arteries, Including Facts about the Donation and Transplantation of Bone Marrow, Stem Cells, and Blood and Tips for Keeping the Blood and Circulatory System Healthy

Along with a Glossary of Related Terms and Resources for Additional Help and Information

Edited by Amy L. Sutton. 659 pages. 2005. 978-0-7808-0746-4.

"Highly recommended pick for basic consumer health reference holdings at all levels."
— The Bookwatch, Aug '05

"Recommended reference source."
— Booklist, American Library Association, Feb '99

"An important reference sourcebook written in simple language for everyday, non-technical users. "
— Reviewer's Bookwatch, Jan '99

Brain Disorders Sourcebook, 2nd Edition

Basic Consumer Health Information about Acquired and Traumatic Brain Injuries, Infections of the Brain, Epilepsy and Seizure Disorders, Cerebral Palsy, and Degenerative Neurological Disorders, Including Amyotrophic Lateral Sclerosis (ALS), Dementias, Multiple Sclerosis, and More

Along with Information on the Brain's Structure and Function, Treatment and Rehabilitation Options, Reports on Current Research Initiatives, a Glossary of Terms Related to Brain Disorders and Injuries, and a Directory of Sources for Further Help and Information

Edited by Sandra J. Judd. 625 pages. 2005. 978-0-7808-0744-0.

"Highly recommended pick for basic consumer health reference holdings at all levels."
— The Bookwatch, Aug '05

"Belongs on the shelves of any library with a consumer health collection." — E-Streams, Mar '00

"Recommended reference source."
— Booklist, American Library Association, Oct '99

SEE ALSO Alzheimer's Disease Sourcebook

Breast Cancer Sourcebook, 2nd Edition

Basic Consumer Health Information about Breast Cancer, Including Facts about Risk Factors, Prevention, Screening and Diagnostic Methods, Treatment Options, Complementary and Alternative Therapies, Post-Treatment Concerns, Clinical Trials, Special Risk Populations, and New Developments in Breast Cancer Research

Along with Breast Cancer Statistics, a Glossary of Related Terms, and a Directory of Resources for Additional Help and Information

Edited by Sandra J. Judd. 595 pages. 2004. 978-0-7808-0668-9.

"This book will be an excellent addition to public, community college, medical, and academic libraries."
— American Reference Books Annual, 2006

"It would be a useful reference book in a library or on loan to women in a support group."
— Cancer Forum, Mar '03

"Recommended reference source."
— Booklist, American Library Association, Jan '02

"This reference source is highly recommended. It is quite informative, comprehensive and detailed in nature, and yet it offers practical advice in easy-to-read language. It could be thought of as the 'bible' of breast cancer for the consumer." — *E-Streams, Jan '02*

"From the pros and cons of different screening methods and results to treatment options, *Breast Cancer Sourcebook* provides the latest information on the subject." — *Library Bookwatch, Dec '01*

"This thoroughgoing, very readable reference covers all aspects of breast health and cancer.... Readers will find much to consider here. Recommended for all public and patient health collections." — *Library Journal, Sep '01*

SEE ALSO *Cancer Sourcebook for Women, Women's Health Concerns Sourcebook*

■

Breastfeeding Sourcebook

Basic Consumer Health Information about the Benefits of Breastmilk, Preparing to Breastfeed, Breastfeeding as a Baby Grows, Nutrition, and More, Including Information on Special Situations and Concerns Such as Mastitis, Illness, Medications, Allergies, Multiple Births, Prematurity, Special Needs, and Adoption

Along with a Glossary and Resources for Additional Help and Information

Edited by Jenni Lynn Colson. 388 pages. 2002. 978-0-7808-0332-9.

"Particularly useful is the information about professional lactation services and chapters on breastfeeding when returning to work.... *Breastfeeding Sourcebook* will be useful for public libraries, consumer health libraries, and technical schools offering nurse assistant training, especially in areas where Internet access is problematic." — *American Reference Books Annual, 2003*

SEE ALSO *Pregnancy & Birth Sourcebook*

■

Burns Sourcebook

Basic Consumer Health Information about Various Types of Burns and Scalds, Including Flame, Heat, Cold, Electrical, Chemical, and Sun Burns

Along with Information on Short-Term and Long-Term Treatments, Tissue Reconstruction, Plastic Surgery, Prevention Suggestions, and First Aid

Edited by Allan R. Cook. 604 pages. 1999. 978-0-7808-0204-9.

"This is an exceptional addition to the series and is highly recommended for all consumer health collections, hospital libraries, and academic medical centers." — *E-Streams, Mar '00*

"This key reference guide is an invaluable addition to all health care and public libraries in confronting this ongoing health issue." — *American Reference Books Annual, 2000*

"Recommended reference source." — *Booklist, American Library Association, Dec '99*

SEE ALSO *Dermatological Disorders Sourcebook*

Cancer Sourcebook, 5th Edition

Basic Consumer Health Information about Major Forms and Stages of Cancer, Featuring Facts about Head and Neck Cancers, Lung Cancers, Gastrointestinal Cancers, Genitourinary Cancers, Lymphomas, Blood Cell Cancers, Endocrine Cancers, Skin Cancers, Bone Cancers, Metastatic Cancers, and More

Along with Facts about Cancer Treatments, Cancer Risks and Prevention, a Glossary of Related Terms, Statistical Data, and a Directory of Resources for Additional Information

Edited by Karen Bellenir. 1,133 pages. 2007. 978-0-7808-0947-5.

"With cancer being the second leading cause of death for Americans, a prodigious work such as this one, which locates centrally so much cancer-related information, is clearly an asset to this nation's citizens and others." — *Journal of the National Medical Association, 2004*

"This title is recommended for health sciences and public libraries with consumer health collections." — *E-Streams, Feb '01*

"... can be effectively used by cancer patients and their families who are looking for answers in a language they can understand. Public and hospital libraries should have it on their shelves." — *American Reference Books Annual, 2001*

"Recommended reference source." — *Booklist, American Library Association, Dec '00*

SEE ALSO *Breast Cancer Sourcebook, Cancer Sourcebook for Women, Pediatric Cancer Sourcebook, Prostate Cancer Sourcebook*

■

Cancer Sourcebook for Women, 3rd Edition

Basic Consumer Health Information about Leading Causes of Cancer in Women, Featuring Facts about Gynecologic Cancers and Related Concerns, Such as Breast Cancer, Cervical Cancer, Endometrial Cancer, Uterine Sarcoma, Vaginal Cancer, Vulvar Cancer, and Common Non-Cancerous Gynecologic Conditions, in Addition to Facts about Lung Cancer, Colorectal Cancer, and Thyroid Cancer in Women

Along with Information about Cancer Risk Factors, Screening and Prevention, Treatment Options, and Tips on Coping with Life after Cancer Treatment, a Glossary of Cancer Terms, and a Directory of Resources for Additional Help and Information

Edited by Amy L. Sutton. 715 pages. 2006. 978-0-7808-0867-6.

"An excellent addition to collections in public, consumer health, and women's health libraries." — *American Reference Books Annual, 2003*

"Overall, the information is excellent, and complex topics are clearly explained. As a reference book for the consumer it is a valuable resource to assist them to make informed decisions about cancer and its treatments." — *Cancer Forum, Nov '02*

"Highly recommended for academic and medical reference collections." — *Library Bookwatch, Sep '02*

"This is a highly recommended book for any public or consumer library, being reader friendly and containing accurate and helpful information." — *E-Streams, Aug '02*

"Recommended reference source." — *Booklist, American Library Association, Jul '02*

SEE ALSO *Breast Cancer Sourcebook, Women's Health Concerns Sourcebook*

■

Cancer Survivorship Sourcebook

Basic Consumer Health Information about the Physical, Educational, Emotional, Social, and Financial Needs of Cancer Patients from Diagnosis, through Cancer Treatment, and Beyond, Including Facts about Researching Specific Types of Cancer and Learning about Clinical Trials and Treatment Options, and Featuring Tips for Coping with the Side Effects of Cancer Treatments and Adjusting to Life after Cancer Treatment Concludes

Along with Suggestions for Caregivers, Friends, and Family Members of Cancer Patients, a Glossary of Cancer Care Terms, and Directories of Related Resources

Edited by Karen Bellenir. 6561 pages. 2007. 978-0-7808-0985-7.

■

Cardiovascular Diseases & Disorders Sourcebook, 3rd Edition

Basic Consumer Health Information about Heart and Vascular Diseases and Disorders, Such as Angina, Heart Attacks, Arrhythmias, Cardiomyopathy, Valve Disease, Atherosclerosis, and Aneurysms, with Information about Managing Cardiovascular Risk Factors and Maintaining Heart Health, Medications and Procedures Used to Treat Cardiovascular Disorders, and Concerns of Special Significance to Women

Along with Reports on Current Research Initiatives, a Glossary of Related Medical Terms, and a Directory of Sources for Further Help and Information

Edited by Sandra J. Judd. 713 pages. 2005. 978-0-7808-0739-6.

"This updated sourcebook is still the best first stop for comprehensive introductory information on cardiovascular diseases." — *American Reference Books Annual, 2006*

"Recommended for public libraries and libraries supporting health care professionals." — *E-Streams, Sep '05*

"This should be a standard health library reference." — *The Bookwatch, Jun '05*

"Recommended reference source." — *Booklist, American Library Association, Dec '00*

"... comprehensive format provides an extensive overview on this subject." — *Choice, Association of College & Research Libraries*

■

Caregiving Sourcebook

Basic Consumer Health Information for Caregivers, Including a Profile of Caregivers, Caregiving Responsibilities and Concerns, Tips for Specific Conditions, Care Environments, and the Effects of Caregiving

Along with Facts about Legal Issues, Financial Information, and Future Planning, a Glossary, and a Listing of Additional Resources

Edited by Joyce Brennfleck Shannon. 600 pages. 2001. 978-0-7808-0331-2.

"Essential for most collections." — *Library Journal, Apr 1, 2002*

"An ideal addition to the reference collection of any public library. Health sciences information professionals may also want to acquire the *Caregiving Sourcebook* for their hospital or academic library for use as a ready reference tool by health care workers interested in aging and caregiving." — *E-Streams, Jan '02*

"Recommended reference source." — *Booklist, American Library Association, Oct '01*

■

Child Abuse Sourcebook

Basic Consumer Health Information about the Physical, Sexual, and Emotional Abuse of Children, with Additional Facts about Neglect, Munchausen Syndrome by Proxy (MSBP), Shaken Baby Syndrome, and Controversial Issues Related to Child Abuse, Such as Withholding Medical Care, Corporal Punishment, and Child Maltreatment in Youth Sports, and Featuring Facts about Child Protective Services, Foster Care, Adoption, Parenting Challenges, and Other Abuse Prevention Efforts

Along with a Glossary of Related Terms and Resources for Additional Help and Information

Edited by Dawn D. Matthews. 620 pages. 2004. 978-0-7808-0705-1.

"A valuable and highly recommended resource for school, academic and public libraries whether used on its own or as a starting point for more in-depth research." — *E-Streams, Apr '05*

"Every week the news brings cases of child abuse or neglect, so it is useful to have a source that supplies so much helpful information. . . . Recommended. Public and academic libraries, and child welfare offices." — *Choice, Association of College & Research Libraries, Mar '05*

"Packed with insights on all kinds of issues, from foster care and adoption to parenting and abuse prevention." — *The Bookwatch, Nov '04*

SEE ALSO: *Domestic Violence Sourcebook*

Childhood Diseases & Disorders Sourcebook

Basic Consumer Health Information about Medical Problems Often Encountered in Pre-Adolescent Children, Including Respiratory Tract Ailments, Ear Infections, Sore Throats, Disorders of the Skin and Scalp, Digestive and Genitourinary Diseases, Infectious Diseases, Inflammatory Disorders, Chronic Physical and Developmental Disorders, Allergies, and More

Along with Information about Diagnostic Tests, Common Childhood Surgeries, and Frequently Used Medications, with a Glossary of Important Terms and Resource Directory

Edited by Chad T. Kimball. 662 pages. 2003. 978-0-7808-0458-6.

"This is an excellent book for new parents and should be included in all health care and public libraries."
—American Reference Books Annual, 2004

SEE ALSO: Healthy Children Sourcebook

■

Colds, Flu & Other Common Ailments Sourcebook

Basic Consumer Health Information about Common Ailments and Injuries, Including Colds, Coughs, the Flu, Sinus Problems, Headaches, Fever, Nausea and Vomiting, Menstrual Cramps, Diarrhea, Constipation, Hemorrhoids, Back Pain, Dandruff, Dry and Itchy Skin, Cuts, Scrapes, Sprains, Bruises, and More

Along with Information about Prevention, Self-Care, Choosing a Doctor, Over-the-Counter Medications, Folk Remedies, and Alternative Therapies, and Including a Glossary of Important Terms and a Directory of Resources for Further Help and Information

Edited by Chad T. Kimball. 638 pages. 2001. 978-0-7808-0435-7.

"A good starting point for research on common illnesses. It will be a useful addition to public and consumer health library collections."
—American Reference Books Annual, 2002

"Will prove valuable to any library seeking to maintain a current, comprehensive reference collection of health resources. . . . Excellent reference."
—The Bookwatch, Aug '01

"Recommended reference source."
—Booklist, American Library Association, Jul '01

■

Communication Disorders Sourcebook

Basic Information about Deafness and Hearing Loss, Speech and Language Disorders, Voice Disorders, Balance and Vestibular Disorders, and Disorders of Smell, Taste, and Touch

Edited by Linda M. Ross. 533 pages. 1996. 978-0-7808-0077-9.

"This is skillfully edited and is a welcome resource for the layperson. It should be found in every public and medical library."
—Booklist Health Sciences Supplement, American Library Association, Oct '97

■

Complementary & Alternative Medicine Sourcebook, 3rd Edition

Basic Consumer Health Information about Complementary and Alternative Medical Therapies, Including Acupuncture, Ayurveda, Traditional Chinese Medicine, Herbal Medicine, Homeopathy, Naturopathy, Biofeedback, Hypnotherapy, Yoga, Art Therapy, Aromatherapy, Clinical Nutrition, Vitamin and Mineral Supplements, Chiropractic, Massage, Reflexology, Crystal Therapy, Therapeutic Touch, and More

Along with Facts about Alternative and Complementary Treatments for Specific Conditions Such as Cancer, Diabetes, Osteoarthritis, Chronic Pain, Menopause, Gastrointestinal Disorders, Headaches, and Mental Illness, a Glossary, and a Resource List for Additional Help and Information

Edited by Sandra J. Judd. 657 pages. 2006. 978-0-7808-0864-5.

"Recommended for public, high school, and academic libraries that have consumer health collections. Hospital libraries that also serve the public will find this to be a useful resource." —E-Streams, Feb '03

"Recommended reference source."
—Booklist, American Library Association, Jan '03

"An important alternate health reference."
—MBR Bookwatch, Oct '02

"A great addition to the reference collection of every type of library." —American Reference Books Annual, 2000

■

Congenital Disorders Sourcebook, 2nd Edition

Basic Consumer Health Information about Nonhereditary Birth Defects and Disorders Related to Prematurity, Gestational Injuries, Congenital Infections, and Birth Complications, Including Heart Defects, Hydrocephalus, Spina Bifida, Cleft Lip and Palate, Cerebral Palsy, and More

Along with Facts about the Prevention of Birth Defects, Fetal Surgery and Other Treatment Options, Research Initiatives, a Glossary of Related Terms, and Resources for Additional Information and Support

Edited by Sandra J. Judd. 647 pages. 2006. 978-0-7808-0945-1.

"Recommended reference source."
—Booklist, American Library Association, Oct '97

SEE ALSO Pregnancy & Birth Sourcebook

■

Contagious Diseases Sourcebook

Basic Consumer Health Information about Infectious Diseases Spread by Person-to-Person Contact through

Direct Touch, Airborne Transmission, Sexual Contact, or Contact with Blood or Other Body Fluids, Including Hepatitis, Herpes, Influenza, Lice, Measles, Mumps, Pinworm, Ringworm, Severe Acute Respiratory Syndrome (SARS), Streptococcal Infections, Tuberculosis, and Others

Along with Facts about Disease Transmission, Antimicrobial Resistance, and Vaccines, with a Glossary and Directories of Resources for More Information

Edited by Karen Bellenir. 643 pages. 2004. 978-0-7808-0736-5.

"This easy-to-read volume is recommended for consumer health collections within public or academic libraries." — *E-Streams, May '05*

"This informative book is highly recommended for public libraries, consumer health collections, and secondary schools and undergraduate libraries." — *American Reference Books Annual, 2005*

"Excellent reference." — *The Bookwatch, Jan '05*

■

Death & Dying Sourcebook, 2nd Edition

Basic Consumer Health Information about End-of-Life Care and Related Perspectives and Ethical Issues, Including End-of-Life Symptoms and Treatments, Pain Management, Quality-of-Life Concerns, the Use of Life Support, Patients' Rights and Privacy Issues, Advance Directives, Physician-Assisted Suicide, Caregiving, Organ and Tissue Donation, Autopsies, Funeral Arrangements, and Grief

Along with Statistical Data, Information about the Leading Causes of Death, a Glossary, and Directories of Support Groups and Other Resources

Edited by Joyce Brennfleck Shannon. 653 pages. 2006. 978-0-7808-0871-3.

"Public libraries, medical libraries, and academic libraries will all find this sourcebook a useful addition to their collections." — *American Reference Books Annual, 2001*

"An extremely useful resource for those concerned with death and dying in the United States." — *Respiratory Care, Nov '00*

"Recommended reference source." — *Booklist, American Library Association, Aug '00*

"This book is a definite must for all those involved in end-of-life care." — *Doody's Review Service, 2000*

■

Dental Care & Oral Health Sourcebook, 2nd Edition

Basic Consumer Health Information about Dental Care, Including Oral Hygiene, Dental Visits, Pain Management, Cavities, Crowns, Bridges, Dental Implants, and Fillings, and Other Oral Health Concerns, Such as Gum Disease, Bad Breath, Dry Mouth, Genetic and Developmental Abnormalities, Oral Cancers, Orthodontics, and Temporomandibular Disorders

Along with Updates on Current Research in Oral Health, a Glossary, a Directory of Dental and Oral Health Organizations, and Resources for People with Dental and Oral Health Disorders

Edited by Amy L. Sutton. 609 pages. 2003. 978-0-7808-0634-4.

"This book could serve as a turning point in the battle to educate consumers in issues concerning oral health." — *American Reference Books Annual, 2004*

"Unique source which will fill a gap in dental sources for patients and the lay public. A valuable reference tool even in a library with thousands of books on dentistry. Comprehensive, clear, inexpensive, and easy to read and use. It fills an enormous gap in the health care literature." — *Reference & User Services Quarterly, American Library Association, Summer '98*

"Recommended reference source." — *Booklist, American Library Association, Dec '97*

■

Depression Sourcebook

Basic Consumer Health Information about Unipolar Depression, Bipolar Disorder, Postpartum Depression, Seasonal Affective Disorder, and Other Types of Depression in Children, Adolescents, Women, Men, the Elderly, and Other Selected Populations

Along with Facts about Causes, Risk Factors, Diagnostic Criteria, Treatment Options, Coping Strategies, Suicide Prevention, a Glossary, and a Directory of Sources for Additional Help and Information

Edited by Karen Bellenir. 602 pages. 2002. 978-0-7808-0611-5.

"*Depression Sourcebook* is of a very high standard. Its purpose, which is to serve as a reference source to the lay reader, is very well served." — *Journal of the National Medical Association, 2004*

"Invaluable reference for public and school library collections alike." — *Library Bookwatch, Apr '03*

"Recommended for purchase." — *American Reference Books Annual, 2003*

■

Dermatological Disorders Sourcebook, 2nd Edition

Basic Consumer Health Information about Conditions and Disorders Affecting the Skin, Hair, and Nails, Such as Acne, Rosacea, Rashes, Dermatitis, Pigmentation Disorders, Birthmarks, Skin Cancer, Skin Injuries, Psoriasis, Scleroderma, and Hair Loss, Including Facts about Medications and Treatments for Dermatological Disorders and Tips for Maintaining Healthy Skin, Hair, and Nails

Along with Information about How Aging Affects the Skin, a Glossary of Related Terms, and a Directory of Resources for Additional Help and Information

Edited by Amy L. Sutton. 645 pages. 2005. 978-0-7808-0795-2.

"... comprehensive, easily read reference book."
—*Doody's Health Sciences Book Reviews, Oct '97*

SEE ALSO *Burns Sourcebook*

Diabetes Sourcebook, 3rd Edition

Basic Consumer Health Information about Type 1 Diabetes (Insulin-Dependent or Juvenile-Onset Diabetes), Type 2 Diabetes (Noninsulin-Dependent or Adult-Onset Diabetes), Gestational Diabetes, Impaired Glucose Tolerance (IGT), and Related Complications, Such as Amputation, Eye Disease, Gum Disease, Nerve Damage, and End-Stage Renal Disease, Including Facts about Insulin, Oral Diabetes Medications, Blood Sugar Testing, and the Role of Exercise and Nutrition in the Control of Diabetes

Along with a Glossary and Resources for Further Help and Information

Edited by Dawn D. Matthews. 622 pages. 2003. 978-0-7808-0629-0.

"This edition is even more helpful than earlier versions. . . . It is a truly valuable tool for anyone seeking readable and authoritative information on diabetes."
—*American Reference Books Annual, 2004*

"An invaluable reference." —*Library Journal, May '00*

Selected as one of the 250 "Best Health Sciences Books of 1999." —*Doody's Rating Service, Mar-Apr '00*

"Provides useful information for the general public."
—*Healthlines, University of Michigan Health Management Research Center, Sep/Oct '99*

". . . provides reliable mainstream medical information . . . belongs on the shelves of any library with a consumer health collection." —*E-Streams, Sep '99*

"Recommended reference source."
—*Booklist, American Library Association, Feb '99*

Diet & Nutrition Sourcebook, 3rd Edition

Basic Consumer Health Information about Dietary Guidelines and the Food Guidance System, Recommended Daily Nutrient Intakes, Serving Proportions, Weight Control, Vitamins and Supplements, Nutrition Issues for Different Life Stages and Lifestyles, and the Needs of People with Specific Medical Concerns, Including Cancer, Celiac Disease, Diabetes, Eating Disorders, Food Allergies, and Cardiovascular Disease

Along with Facts about Federal Nutrition Support Programs, a Glossary of Nutrition and Dietary Terms, and Directories of Additional Resources for More Information about Nutrition

Edited by Joyce Brennfleck Shannon. 633 pages. 2006. 978-0-7808-0800-3.

"This book is an excellent source of basic diet and nutrition information." —*Booklist Health Sciences Supplement, American Library Association, Dec '00*

"This reference document should be in any public library, but it would be a very good guide for beginning students in the health sciences. If the other books in this publisher's series are as good as this, they should all be in the health sciences collections."
—*American Reference Books Annual, 2000*

"This book is an excellent general nutrition reference for consumers who desire to take an active role in their health care for prevention. Consumers of all ages who select this book can feel confident they are receiving current and accurate information." —*Journal of Nutrition for the Elderly, Vol. 19, No. 4, 2000*

SEE ALSO *Digestive Diseases & Disorders Sourcebook, Eating Disorders Sourcebook, Gastrointestinal Diseases & Disorders Sourcebook, Vegetarian Sourcebook*

Digestive Diseases & Disorders Sourcebook

Basic Consumer Health Information about Diseases and Disorders that Impact the Upper and Lower Digestive System, Including Celiac Disease, Constipation, Crohn's Disease, Cyclic Vomiting Syndrome, Diarrhea, Diverticulosis and Diverticulitis, Gallstones, Heartburn, Hemorrhoids, Hernias, Indigestion (Dyspepsia), Irritable Bowel Syndrome, Lactose Intolerance, Ulcers, and More

Along with Information about Medications and Other Treatments, Tips for Maintaining a Healthy Digestive Tract, a Glossary, and Directory of Digestive Diseases Organizations

Edited by Karen Bellenir. 335 pages. 2000. 978-0-7808-0327-5.

"This title would be an excellent addition to all public or patient-research libraries."
—*American Reference Books Annual, 2001*

"This title is recommended for public, hospital, and health sciences libraries with consumer health collections." —*E-Streams, Jul-Aug '00*

"Recommended reference source."
—*Booklist, American Library Association, May '00*

SEE ALSO *Eating Disorders Sourcebook, Gastrointestinal Diseases & Disorders Sourcebook*

Disabilities Sourcebook

Basic Consumer Health Information about Physical and Psychiatric Disabilities, Including Descriptions of Major Causes of Disability, Assistive and Adaptive Aids, Workplace Issues, and Accessibility Concerns

Along with Information about the Americans with Disabilities Act, a Glossary, and Resources for Additional Help and Information

Edited by Dawn D. Matthews. 616 pages. 2000. 978-0-7808-0389-3.

"It is a must for libraries with a consumer health section." —*American Reference Books Annual, 2002*

"A much needed addition to the Omnigraphics *Health Reference Series*. A current reference work to provide people with disabilities, their families, caregivers or those who work with them, a broad range of information in one volume, has not been available until now. . . . It is recommended for all public and academic library reference collections." — *E-Streams, May '01*

"An excellent source book in easy-to-read format covering many current topics; highly recommended for all libraries." — *Choice, Association of College & Research Libraries, Jan '01*

"Recommended reference source."
— *Booklist, American Library Association, Jul '00*

Domestic Violence Sourcebook, 2nd Edition

Basic Consumer Health Information about the Causes and Consequences of Abusive Relationships, Including Physical Violence, Sexual Assault, Battery, Stalking, and Emotional Abuse, and Facts about the Effects of Violence on Women, Men, Young Adults, and the Elderly, with Reports about Domestic Violence in Selected Populations, and Featuring Facts about Medical Care, Victim Assistance and Protection, Prevention Strategies, Mental Health Services, and Legal Issues

Along with a Glossary of Related Terms and Resources for Additional Help and Information

Edited by Dawn D. Matthews. 628 pages. 2004. 978-0-7808-0669-6.

"Educators, clergy, medical professionals, police, and victims and their families will benefit from this realistic and easy-to-understand resource."
— *American Reference Books Annual, 2005*

"Recommended for all collections supporting consumer health information. It should also be considered for any collection needing general, readable information on domestic violence." — *E-Streams, Jan '05*

"This sourcebook complements other books in its field, providing a one-stop resource . . . Recommended."
— *Choice, Association of College & Research Libraries, Jan '05*

"Interested lay persons should find the book extremely beneficial. . . . A copy of *Domestic Violence and Child Abuse Sourcebook* should be in every public library in the United States."
— *Social Science & Medicine, No. 56, 2003*

"This is important information. The Web has many resources but this sourcebook fills an important societal need. I am not aware of any other resources of this type." — *Doody's Review Service, Sep '01*

"Recommended reference source."
— *Booklist, American Library Association, Apr '01*

"Important pick for college-level health reference libraries." — *The Bookwatch, Mar '01*

"Because this problem is so widespread and because this book includes a lot of issues within one volume, this work is recommended for all public libraries."
— *American Reference Books Annual, 2001*

SEE ALSO Child Abuse Sourcebook

Drug Abuse Sourcebook, 2nd Edition

Basic Consumer Health Information about Illicit Substances of Abuse and the Misuse of Prescription and Over-the-Counter Medications, Including Depressants, Hallucinogens, Inhalants, Marijuana, Stimulants, and Anabolic Steroids

Along with Facts about Related Health Risks, Treatment Programs, Prevention Programs, a Glossary of Abuse and Addiction Terms, a Glossary of Drug-Related Street Terms, and a Directory of Resources for More Information

Edited by Catherine Ginther. 607 pages. 2004. 978-0-7808-0740-2.

"Commendable for organizing useful, normally scattered government and association-produced data into a logical sequence."
— *American Reference Books Annual, 2006*

"This easy-to-read volume is recommended for consumer health collections within public or academic libraries." — *E-Streams, Sep '05*

"An excellent library reference."
— *The Bookwatch, May '05*

"Containing a wealth of information, this book will be useful to the college student just beginning to explore the topic of substance abuse. This resource belongs in libraries that serve a lower-division undergraduate or community college clientele as well as the general public." — *Choice, Association of College & Research Libraries, Jun '01*

"Recommended reference source."
— *Booklist, American Library Association, Feb '01*

SEE ALSO Alcoholism Sourcebook

Ear, Nose & Throat Disorders Sourcebook, 2nd Edition

Basic Consumer Health Information about Disorders of the Ears, Hearing Loss, Vestibular Disorders, Nasal and Sinus Problems, Throat and Vocal Cord Disorders, and Otolaryngologic Cancers, Including Facts about Ear Infections and Injuries, Genetic and Congenital Deafness, Sensorineural Hearing Disorders, Tinnitus, Vertigo, Ménière Disease, Rhinitis, Sinusitis, Snoring, Sore Throats, Hoarseness, and More

Along with Reports on Current Research Initiatives, a Glossary of Related Medical Terms, and a Directory of Sources for Further Help and Information

Edited by Sandra J. Judd. 659 pages. 2006. 978-0-7808-0872-0.

"Overall, this sourcebook is helpful for the consumer seeking information on ENT issues. It is recommended for public libraries."
—*American Reference Books Annual, 1999*

"Recommended reference source."
—*Booklist, American Library Association, Dec '98*

■

Eating Disorders Sourcebook, 2nd Edition

Basic Consumer Health Information about Anorexia Nervosa, Bulimia Nervosa, Binge Eating, Compulsive Exercise, Female Athlete Triad, and Other Eating Disorders, Including Facts about Body Image and Other Cultural and Age-Related Risk Factors, Prevention Efforts, Adverse Health Effects, Treatment Options, and the Recovery Process

Along with Guidelines for Healthy Weight Control, a Glossary, and Directories of Additional Resources

Edited by Joyce Brennfleck Shannon. 585 pages. 2007. 978-0-7808-0948-2.

"Recommended for health science libraries that are open to the public, as well as hospital libraries. This book is a good resource for the consumer who is concerned about eating disorders." — *E-Streams, Mar '02*

"This volume is another convenient collection of excerpted articles. Recommended for school and public library patrons; lower-division undergraduates; and two-year technical program students."
—*Choice, Association of College & Research Libraries, Jan '02*

"Recommended reference source."
— *Booklist, American Library Association, Oct '01*

SEE ALSO *Diet & Nutrition Sourcebook, Digestive Diseases & Disorders Sourcebook, Gastrointestinal Diseases & Disorders Sourcebook*

■

Emergency Medical Services Sourcebook

Basic Consumer Health Information about Preventing, Preparing for, and Managing Emergency Situations, When and Who to Call for Help, What to Expect in the Emergency Room, the Emergency Medical Team, Patient Issues, and Current Topics in Emergency Medicine

Along with Statistical Data, a Glossary, and Sources of Additional Help and Information

Edited by Jenni Lynn Colson. 494 pages. 2002. 978-0-7808-0420-3.

"Handy and convenient for home, public, school, and college libraries. Recommended."
— *Choice, Association of College & Research Libraries, Apr '03*

"This reference can provide the consumer with answers to most questions about emergency care in the United States, or it will direct them to a resource where the answer can be found."
—*American Reference Books Annual, 2003*

"Recommended reference source."
— *Booklist, American Library Association, Feb '03*

■

Endocrine & Metabolic Disorders Sourcebook

Basic Information for the Layperson about Pancreatic and Insulin-Related Disorders Such as Pancreatitis, Diabetes, and Hypoglycemia; Adrenal Gland Disorders Such as Cushing's Syndrome, Addison's Disease, and Congenital Adrenal Hyperplasia; Pituitary Gland Disorders Such as Growth Hormone Deficiency, Acromegaly, and Pituitary Tumors; Thyroid Disorders Such as Hypothyroidism, Graves' Disease, Hashimoto's Disease, and Goiter; Hyperparathyroidism; and Other Diseases and Syndromes of Hormone Imbalance or Metabolic Dysfunction

Along with Reports on Current Research Initiatives

Edited by Linda M. Shin. 574 pages. 1998. 978-0-7808-0207-0.

"Omnigraphics has produced another needed resource for health information consumers."
—*American Reference Books Annual, 2000*

"Recommended reference source."
— *Booklist, American Library Association, Dec '98*

■

Environmental Health Sourcebook, 2nd Edition

Basic Consumer Health Information about the Environment and Its Effect on Human Health, Including the Effects of Air Pollution, Water Pollution, Hazardous Chemicals, Food Hazards, Radiation Hazards, Biological Agents, Household Hazards, Such as Radon, Asbestos, Carbon Monoxide, and Mold, and Information about Associated Diseases and Disorders, Including Cancer, Allergies, Respiratory Problems, and Skin Disorders

Along with Information about Environmental Concerns for Specific Populations, a Glossary of Related Terms, and Resources for Further Help and Information

Edited by Dawn D. Matthews. 673 pages. 2003. 978-0-7808-0632-0.

"This recently updated edition continues the level of quality and the reputation of the numerous other volumes in Omnigraphics' *Health Reference Series*."
— *American Reference Books Annual, 2004*

"An excellent updated edition."
—*The Bookwatch, Oct '03*

"Recommended reference source."
— *Booklist, American Library Association, Sep '98*

"This book will be a useful addition to anyone's library." — *Choice Health Sciences Supplement, Association of College & Research Libraries, May '98*

". . . a good survey of numerous environmentally induced physical disorders . . . a useful addition to anyone's library."
—*Doody's Health Sciences Book Reviews, Jan '98*

Ethnic Diseases Sourcebook

Basic Consumer Health Information for Ethnic and Racial Minority Groups in the United States, Including General Health Indicators and Behaviors, Ethnic Diseases, Genetic Testing, the Impact of Chronic Diseases, Women's Health, Mental Health Issues, and Preventive Health Care Services

Along with a Glossary and a Listing of Additional Resources

Edited by Joyce Brennfleck Shannon. 664 pages. 2001. 978-0-7808-0336-7.

"Recommended for health sciences libraries where public health programs are a priority."
— E-Streams, Jan '02

"Not many books have been written on this topic to date, and the *Ethnic Diseases Sourcebook* is a strong addition to the list. It will be an important introductory resource for health consumers, students, health care personnel, and social scientists. It is recommended for public, academic, and large hospital libraries."
— American Reference Books Annual, 2002

"Recommended reference source."
— Booklist, American Library Association, Oct '01

"Will prove valuable to any library seeking to maintain a current, comprehensive reference collection of health resources.... An excellent source of health information about genetic disorders which affect particular ethnic and racial minorities in the U.S."
— The Bookwatch, Aug '01

Eye Care Sourcebook, 2nd Edition

Basic Consumer Health Information about Eye Care and Eye Disorders, Including Facts about the Diagnosis, Prevention, and Treatment of Common Refractive Problems Such as Myopia, Hyperopia, Astigmatism, and Presbyopia, and Eye Diseases, Including Glaucoma, Cataract, Age-Related Macular Degeneration, and Diabetic Retinopathy

Along with a Section on Vision Correction and Refractive Surgeries, Including LASIK and LASEK, a Glossary, and Directories of Resources for Additional Help and Information

Edited by Amy L. Sutton. 543 pages. 2003. 978-0-7808-0635-1.

"... a solid reference tool for eye care and a valuable addition to a collection."
— American Reference Books Annual, 2004

Family Planning Sourcebook

Basic Consumer Health Information about Planning for Pregnancy and Contraception, Including Traditional Methods, Barrier Methods, Hormonal Methods, Permanent Methods, Future Methods, Emergency Contraception, and Birth Control Choices for Women at Each Stage of Life

Along with Statistics, a Glossary, and Sources of Additional Information

Edited by Amy Marcaccio Keyzer. 520 pages. 2001. 978-0-7808-0379-4.

"Recommended for public, health, and undergraduate libraries as part of the circulating collection."
— E-Streams, Mar '02

"Information is presented in an unbiased, readable manner, and the sourcebook will certainly be a necessary addition to those public and high school libraries where Internet access is restricted or otherwise problematic." — American Reference Books Annual, 2002

"Recommended reference source."
— Booklist, American Library Association, Oct '01

"Will prove valuable to any library seeking to maintain a current, comprehensive reference collection of health resources.... Excellent reference."
— The Bookwatch, Aug '01

SEE ALSO Pregnancy & Birth Sourcebook

Fitness & Exercise Sourcebook, 3rd Edition

Basic Consumer Health Information about the Physical and Mental Benefits of Fitness, Including Cardiorespiratory Endurance, Muscular Strength, Muscular Endurance, and Flexibility, with Facts about Sports Nutrition and Exercise-Related Injuries and Tips about Physical Activity and Exercises for People of All Ages and for People with Health Concerns

Along with Advice on Selecting and Using Exercise Equipment, Maintaining Exercise Motivation, a Glossary of Related Terms, and a Directory of Resources for More Help and Information

Edited by Amy L. Sutton. 663 pages. 2007. 978-0-7808-0946-8.

"This work is recommended for all general reference collections."
— American Reference Books Annual, 2002

"Highly recommended for public, consumer, and school grades fourth through college." — E-Streams, Nov '01

"Recommended reference source."
— Booklist, American Library Association, Oct '01

"The information appears quite comprehensive and is considered reliable.... This second edition is a welcomed addition to the series."
— Doody's Review Service, Sep '01

Food Safety Sourcebook

Basic Consumer Health Information about the Safe Handling of Meat, Poultry, Seafood, Eggs, Fruit Juices, and Other Food Items, and Facts about Pesticides, Drinking Water, Food Safety Overseas, and the Onset, Duration, and Symptoms of Foodborne Illnesses, Including Types of Pathogenic Bacteria, Parasitic Protozoa, Worms, Viruses, and Natural Toxins

Along with the Role of the Consumer, the Food Handler, and the Government in Food Safety; a Glossary, and Resources for Additional Help and Information

Edited by Dawn D. Matthews. 339 pages. 1999. 978-0-7808-0326-8.

"This book is recommended for public libraries and universities with home economic and food science programs." — *E-Streams, Nov '00*

"Recommended reference source." — *Booklist, American Library Association, May '00*

"This book takes the complex issues of food safety and foodborne pathogens and presents them in an easily understood manner. [It does] an excellent job of covering a large and often confusing topic." — *American Reference Books Annual, 2000*

■

Forensic Medicine Sourcebook

Basic Consumer Information for the Layperson about Forensic Medicine, Including Crime Scene Investigation, Evidence Collection and Analysis, Expert Testimony, Computer-Aided Criminal Identification, Digital Imaging in the Courtroom, DNA Profiling, Accident Reconstruction, Autopsies, Ballistics, Drugs and Explosives Detection, Latent Fingerprints, Product Tampering, and Questioned Document Examination

Along with Statistical Data, a Glossary of Forensics Terminology, and Listings of Sources for Further Help and Information

Edited by Annemarie S. Muth. 574 pages. 1999. 978-0-7808-0232-2.

"Given the expected widespread interest in its content and its easy to read style, this book is recommended for most public and all college and university libraries." — *E-Streams, Feb '01*

"Recommended for public libraries." — *Reference & User Services Quarterly, American Library Association, Spring 2000*

"Recommended reference source." — *Booklist, American Library Association, Feb '00*

"A wealth of information, useful statistics, references are up-to-date and extremely complete. This wonderful collection of data will help students who are interested in a career in any type of forensic field. It is a great resource for attorneys who need information about types of expert witnesses needed in a particular case. It also offers useful information for fiction and nonfiction writers whose work involves a crime. A fascinating compilation. All levels." — *Choice, Association of College & Research Libraries, Jan '00*

"There are several items that make this book attractive to consumers who are seeking certain forensic data. . . . This is a useful current source for those seeking general forensic medical answers." — *American Reference Books Annual, 2000*

Gastrointestinal Diseases & Disorders Sourcebook, 2nd Edition

Basic Consumer Health Information about the Upper and Lower Gastrointestinal (GI) Tract, Including the Esophagus, Stomach, Intestines, Rectum, Liver, and Pancreas, with Facts about Gastroesophageal Reflux Disease, Gastritis, Hernias, Ulcers, Celiac Disease, Diverticulitis, Irritable Bowel Syndrome, Hemorrhoids, Gastrointestinal Cancers, and Other Diseases and Disorders Related to the Digestive Process

Along with Information about Commonly Used Diagnostic and Surgical Procedures, Statistics, Reports on Current Research Initiatives and Clinical Trials, a Glossary, and Resources for Additional Help and Information

Edited by Sandra J. Judd. 681 pages. 2006. 978-0-7808-0798-3.

". . . very readable form. The successful editorial work that brought this material together into a useful and understandable reference makes accessible to all readers information that can help them more effectively understand and obtain help for digestive tract problems." — *Choice, Association of College & Research Libraries, Feb '97*

SEE ALSO *Diet & Nutrition Sourcebook, Digestive Diseases & Disorders Sourcebook, Eating Disorders Sourcebook*

■

Genetic Disorders Sourcebook, 3rd Edition

Basic Consumer Health Information about Hereditary Diseases and Disorders, Including Facts about the Human Genome, Genetic Inheritance Patterns, Disorders Associated with Specific Genes, Such as Sickle Cell Disease, Hemophilia, and Cystic Fibrosis, Chromosome Disorders, Such as Down Syndrome, Fragile X Syndrome, and Turner Syndrome, and Complex Diseases and Disorders Resulting from the Interaction of Environmental and Genetic Factors, Such as Allergies, Cancer, and Obesity

Along with Facts about Genetic Testing, Suggestions for Parents of Children with Special Needs, Reports on Current Research Initiatives, a Glossary of Genetic Terminology, and Resources for Additional Help and Information

Edited by Karen Bellenir. 777 pages. 2004. 978-0-7808-0742-6.

"This text is recommended for any library with an interest in providing consumer health resources." — *E-Streams, Aug '05*

"This is a valuable resource for anyone wishing to have an understandable description of any of the topics or disorders included. The editor succeeds in making complex genetic issues understandable." — *Doody's Book Review Service, May '05*

"A good acquisition for public libraries." — *American Reference Books Annual, 2005*

◼

Head Trauma Sourcebook

Basic Information for the Layperson about Open-Head and Closed-Head Injuries, Treatment Advances, Recovery, and Rehabilitation

Along with Reports on Current Research Initiatives

Edited by Karen Bellenir. 414 pages. 1997. 978-0-7808-0208-7.

Headache Sourcebook

Basic Consumer Health Information about Migraine, Tension, Cluster, Rebound and Other Types of Headaches, with Facts about the Cause and Prevention of Headaches, the Effects of Stress and the Environment, Headaches during Pregnancy and Menopause, and Childhood Headaches

Along with a Glossary and Other Resources for Additional Help and Information

Edited by Dawn D. Matthews. 362 pages. 2002. 978-0-7808-0337-4.

◼

Healthy Aging Sourcebook

Basic Consumer Health Information about Maintaining Health through the Aging Process, Including Advice on Nutrition, Exercise, and Sleep, Help in Making Decisions about Midlife Issues and Retirement, and Guidance Concerning Practical and Informed Choices in Health Consumerism

Along with Data Concerning the Theories of Aging, Different Experiences in Aging by Minority Groups, and Facts about Aging Now and Aging in the Future; and Featuring a Glossary, a Guide to Consumer Help, Additional Suggested Reading, and Practical Resource Directory

Edited by Jenifer Swanson. 536 pages. 1999. 978-0-7808-0390-9.

SEE ALSO *Physical & Mental Issues in Aging Sourcebook*

◼

Healthy Children Sourcebook

Basic Consumer Health Information about the Physical and Mental Development of Children between the Ages of 3 and 12, Including Routine Health Care, Preventative Health Services, Safety and First Aid,

Healthy Sleep, Dental Care, Nutrition, and Fitness, and Featuring Parenting Tips on Such Topics as Bedwetting, Choosing Day Care, Monitoring TV and Other Media, and Establishing a Foundation for Substance Abuse Prevention

Along with a Glossary of Commonly Used Pediatric Terms and Resources for Additional Help and Information.

Edited by Chad T. Kimball. 647 pages. 2003. 978-0-7808-0247-6.

SEE ALSO *Childhood Diseases & Disorders Sourcebook*

◼

Healthy Heart Sourcebook for Women

Basic Consumer Health Information about Cardiac Issues Specific to Women, Including Facts about Major Risk Factors and Prevention, Treatment and Control Strategies, and Important Dietary Issues

Along with a Special Section Regarding the Pros and Cons of Hormone Replacement Therapy and Its Impact on Heart Health, and Additional Help, Including Recipes, a Glossary, and a Directory of Resources

Edited by Dawn D. Matthews. 336 pages. 2000. 978-0-7808-0329-9.

SEE ALSO *Cardiovascular Diseases & Disorders Sourcebook, Women's Health Concerns Sourcebook*

◼

Hepatitis Sourcebook

Basic Consumer Health Information about Hepatitis A, Hepatitis B, Hepatitis C, and Other Forms of Hepatitis, Including Autoimmune Hepatitis, Alcoholic Hepatitis, Nonalcoholic Steatohepatitis, and Toxic Hepatitis, with

Facts about Risk Factors, Screening Methods, Diagnostic Tests, and Treatment Options

Along with Information on Liver Health, Tips for People Living with Chronic Hepatitis, Reports on Current Research Initiatives, a Glossary of Terms Related to Hepatitis, and a Directory of Sources for Further Help and Information

Edited by Sandra J. Judd. 597 pages. 2005. 978-0-7808-0749-5.

"Highly recommended."
— American Reference Books Annual, 2006

Household Safety Sourcebook

Basic Consumer Health Information about Household Safety, Including Information about Poisons, Chemicals, Fire, and Water Hazards in the Home

Along with Advice about the Safe Use of Home Maintenance Equipment, Choosing Toys and Nursery Furniture, Holiday and Recreation Safety, a Glossary, and Resources for Further Help and Information

Edited by Dawn D. Matthews. 606 pages. 2002. 978-0-7808-0338-1.

"This work will be useful in public libraries with large consumer health and wellness departments."
— American Reference Books Annual, 2003

"As a sourcebook on household safety this book meets its mark. It is encyclopedic in scope and covers a wide range of safety issues that are commonly seen in the home."   — E-Streams, Jul '02

Hypertension Sourcebook

Basic Consumer Health Information about the Causes, Diagnosis, and Treatment of High Blood Pressure, with Facts about Consequences, Complications, and Co-Occurring Disorders, Such as Coronary Heart Disease, Diabetes, Stroke, Kidney Disease, and Hypertensive Retinopathy, and Issues in Blood Pressure Control, Including Dietary Choices, Stress Management, and Medications

Along with Reports on Current Research Initiatives and Clinical Trials, a Glossary, and Resources for Additional Help and Information

Edited by Dawn D. Matthews and Karen Bellenir. 613 pages. 2004. 978-0-7808-0674-0.

"Academic, public, and medical libraries will want to add the Hypertension Sourcebook to their collections."
— E-Streams, Aug '05

"The strength of this source is the wide range of information given about hypertension."
— American Reference Books Annual, 2005

Immune System Disorders Sourcebook, 2nd Edition

Basic Consumer Health Information about Disorders of the Immune System, Including Immune System Function and Response, Diagnosis of Immune Disorders, Information about Inherited Immune Disease, Acquired Immune Disease, and Autoimmune Diseases, Including Primary Immune Deficiency, Acquired Immunodeficiency Syndrome (AIDS), Lupus, Multiple Sclerosis, Type 1 Diabetes, Rheumatoid Arthritis, and Graves' Disease

Along with Treatments, Tips for Coping with Immune Disorders, a Glossary, and a Directory of Additional Resources.

Edited by Joyce Brennfleck Shannon. 671 pages. 2005. 978-0-7808-0748-8.

"Highly recommended for academic and public libraries." — American Reference Books Annual, 2006

"The updated second edition is a 'must' for any consumer health library seeking a solid resource covering the treatments, symptoms, and options for immune disorder sufferers. . . . An excellent guide."
— MBR Bookwatch, Jan '06

Infant & Toddler Health Sourcebook

Basic Consumer Health Information about the Physical and Mental Development of Newborns, Infants, and Toddlers, Including Neonatal Concerns, Nutrition Recommendations, Immunization Schedules, Common Pediatric Disorders, Assessments and Milestones, Safety Tips, and Advice for Parents and Other Caregivers

Along with a Glossary of Terms and Resource Listings for Additional Help

Edited by Jenifer Swanson. 585 pages. 2000. 978-0-7808-0246-9.

"As a reference for the general public, this would be useful in any library."   — E-Streams, May '01

"Recommended reference source."
— Booklist, American Library Association, Feb '01

"This is a good source for general use."
— American Reference Books Annual, 2001

Infectious Diseases Sourcebook

Basic Consumer Health Information about Non-Contagious Bacterial, Viral, Prion, Fungal, and Parasitic Diseases Spread by Food and Water, Insects and Animals, or Environmental Contact, Including Botulism, E. Coli, Encephalitis, Legionnaires' Disease, Lyme Disease, Malaria, Plague, Rabies, Salmonella, Tetanus, and Others, and Facts about Newly Emerging Diseases, Such as Hantavirus, Mad Cow Disease, Monkeypox, and West Nile Virus

Along with Information about Preventing Disease Transmission, the Threat of Bioterrorism, and Current Research Initiatives, with a Glossary and Directory of Resources for More Information

Edited by Karen Bellenir. 634 pages. 2004. 978-0-7808-0675-7.

"This reference continues the excellent tradition of the *Health Reference Series* in consolidating a wealth of information on a selected topic into a format that is easy to use and accessible to the general public."
— *American Reference Books Annual, 2005*

"Recommended for public and academic libraries."
— *E-Streams, Jan '05*

Injury & Trauma Sourcebook

Basic Consumer Health Information about the Impact of Injury, the Diagnosis and Treatment of Common and Traumatic Injuries, Emergency Care, and Specific Injuries Related to Home, Community, Workplace, Transportation, and Recreation

Along with Guidelines for Injury Prevention, a Glossary, and a Directory of Additional Resources

Edited by Joyce Brennfleck Shannon. 696 pages. 2002. 978-0-7808-0421-0.

"This publication is the most comprehensive work of its kind about injury and trauma."
— *American Reference Books Annual, 2003*

"This sourcebook provides concise, easily readable, basic health information about injuries. . . . This book is well organized and an easy to use reference resource suitable for hospital, health sciences and public libraries with consumer health collections."
— *E-Streams, Nov '02*

"Practitioners should be aware of guides such as this in order to facilitate their use by patients and their families."
— *Doody's Health Sciences Book Review Journal, Sep-Oct '02*

"Recommended reference source."
— *Booklist, American Library Association, Sep '02*

"Highly recommended for academic and medical reference collections."
— *Library Bookwatch, Sep '02*

Kidney & Urinary Tract Diseases & Disorders Sourcebook

SEE *Urinary Tract & Kidney Diseases & Disorders Sourcebook*

Learning Disabilities Sourcebook, 2nd Edition

Basic Consumer Health Information about Learning Disabilities, Including Dyslexia, Developmental Speech and Language Disabilities, Non-Verbal Learning Disorders, Developmental Arithmetic Disorder, Developmental Writing Disorder, and Other Conditions That Impede Learning Such as Attention Deficit/Hyperactivity Disorder, Brain Injury, Hearing Impairment, Klinefelter Syndrome, Dyspraxia, and Tourette's Syndrome

Along with Facts about Educational Issues and Assistive Technology, Coping Strategies, a Glossary of Related Terms, and Resources for Further Help and Information

Edited by Dawn D. Matthews. 621 pages. 2003. 978-0-7808-0626-9.

"The second edition of Learning Disabilities Sourcebook far surpasses the earlier edition in that it is more focused on information that will be useful as a consumer health resource."
— *American Reference Books Annual, 2004*

"Teachers as well as consumers will find this an essential guide to understanding various syndromes and their latest treatments. [An] invaluable reference for public and school library collections alike."
— *Library Bookwatch, Apr '03*

Named "Outstanding Reference Book of 1999."
— *New York Public Library, Feb '00*

"An excellent candidate for inclusion in a public library reference section. It's a great source of information. Teachers will also find the book useful. Definitely worth reading."
— *Journal of Adolescent & Adult Literacy, Feb 2000*

"Readable . . . provides a solid base of information regarding successful techniques used with individuals who have learning disabilities, as well as practical suggestions for educators and family members. Clear language, concise descriptions, and pertinent information for contacting multiple resources add to the strength of this book as a useful tool." — *Choice, Association of College & Research Libraries, Feb '99*

"Recommended reference source."
— *Booklist, American Library Association, Sep '98*

"A useful resource for libraries and for those who don't have the time to identify and locate the individual publications." — *Disability Resources Monthly, Sep '98*

Leukemia Sourcebook

Basic Consumer Health Information about Adult and Childhood Leukemias, Including Acute Lymphocytic Leukemia (ALL), Chronic Lymphocytic Leukemia (CLL), Acute Myelogenous Leukemia (AML), Chronic Myelogenous Leukemia (CML), and Hairy Cell Leukemia, and Treatments Such as Chemotherapy, Radiation Therapy, Peripheral Blood Stem Cell and Marrow Transplantation, and Immunotherapy

Along with Tips for Life During and After Treatment, a Glossary, and Directories of Additional Resources

Edited by Joyce Brennfleck Shannon. 587 pages. 2003. 978-0-7808-0627-6.

"Unlike other medical books for the layperson, . . . the language does not talk down to the reader. . . . This volume is highly recommended for all libraries."
— *American Reference Books Annual, 2004*

". . . a fine title which ranges from diagnosis to alternative treatments, staging, and tips for life during and after diagnosis." — *The Bookwatch, Dec '03*

Liver Disorders Sourcebook

Basic Consumer Health Information about the Liver and How It Works; Liver Diseases, Including Cancer, Cirrhosis, Hepatitis, and Toxic and Drug Related Diseases; Tips for Maintaining a Healthy Liver; Laboratory Tests, Radiology Tests, and Facts about Liver Transplantation

Along with a Section on Support Groups, a Glossary, and Resource Listings

Edited by Joyce Brennfleck Shannon. 591 pages. 2000. 978-0-7808-0383-1.

"A valuable resource."
—American Reference Books Annual, 2001

"This title is recommended for health sciences and public libraries with consumer health collections."
—E-Streams, Oct '00

"Recommended reference source."
—Booklist, American Library Association, Jun '00

■

Lung Disorders Sourcebook

Basic Consumer Health Information about Emphysema, Pneumonia, Tuberculosis, Asthma, Cystic Fibrosis, and Other Lung Disorders, Including Facts about Diagnostic Procedures, Treatment Strategies, Disease Prevention Efforts, and Such Risk Factors as Smoking, Air Pollution, and Exposure to Asbestos, Radon, and Other Agents

Along with a Glossary and Resources for Additional Help and Information

Edited by Dawn D. Matthews. 678 pages. 2002. 978-0-7808-0339-8.

"This title is a great addition for public and school libraries because it provides concise health information on the lungs."
—American Reference Books Annual, 2003

"Highly recommended for academic and medical reference collections." *—Library Bookwatch, Sep '02*

SEE ALSO Respiratory Diseases & Disorders Sourcebook

■

Medical Tests Sourcebook, 2nd Edition

Basic Consumer Health Information about Medical Tests, Including Age-Specific Health Tests, Important Health Screenings and Exams, Home-Use Tests, Blood and Specimen Tests, Electrical Tests, Scope Tests, Genetic Testing, and Imaging Tests, Such as X-Rays, Ultrasound, Computed Tomography, Magnetic Resonance Imaging, Angiography, and Nuclear Medicine

Along with a Glossary and Directory of Additional Resources

Edited by Joyce Brennfleck Shannon. 654 pages. 2004. 978-0-7808-0670-2.

"Recommended for hospital and health sciences

libraries with consumer health collections."
—E-Streams, Mar '00

"This is an overall excellent reference with a wealth of general knowledge that may aid those who are reluctant to get vital tests performed."
—Today's Librarian, Jan '00

"A valuable reference guide."
—American Reference Books Annual, 2000

■

Men's Health Concerns Sourcebook, 2nd Edition

Basic Consumer Health Information about the Medical and Mental Concerns of Men, Including Theories about the Shorter Male Lifespan, the Leading Causes of Death and Disability, Physical Concerns of Special Significance to Men, Reproductive and Sexual Concerns, Sexually Transmitted Diseases, Men's Mental and Emotional Health, and Lifestyle Choices That Affect Wellness, Such as Nutrition, Fitness, and Substance Use

Along with a Glossary of Related Terms and a Directory of Organizational Resources in Men's Health

Edited by Robert Aquinas McNally. 644 pages. 2004. 978-0-7808-0671-9.

"A very accessible reference for non-specialist general readers and consumers." *—The Bookwatch, Jun '04*

"This comprehensive resource and the series are highly recommended."
—American Reference Books Annual, 2000

"Recommended reference source."
—Booklist, American Library Association, Dec '98

■

Mental Health Disorders Sourcebook, 3rd Edition

Basic Consumer Health Information about Mental and Emotional Health and Mental Illness, Including Facts about Depression, Bipolar Disorder, and Other Mood Disorders, Phobias, Post-Traumatic Stress Disorder (PTSD), Obsessive-Compulsive Disorder, and Other Anxiety Disorders, Impulse Control Disorders, Eating Disorders, Personality Disorders, and Psychotic Disorders, Including Schizophrenia and Dissociative Disorders

Along with Statistical Information, a Special Section Concerning Mental Health Issues in Children and Adolescents, a Glossary, and Directories of Resources for Additional Help and Information

Edited by Karen Bellenir. 661 pages. 2005. 978-0-7808-0747-1.

"Recommended for public libraries and academic libraries with an undergraduate program in psychology."
—American Reference Books Annual, 2006

"Recommended reference source."
—Booklist, American Library Association, Jun '00

Mental Retardation Sourcebook

Basic Consumer Health Information about Mental Retardation and Its Causes, Including Down Syndrome, Fetal Alcohol Syndrome, Fragile X Syndrome, Genetic Conditions, Injury, and Environmental Sources

Along with Preventive Strategies, Parenting Issues, Educational Implications, Health Care Needs, Employment and Economic Matters, Legal Issues, a Glossary, and a Resource Listing for Additional Help and Information

Edited by Joyce Brennfleck Shannon. 642 pages. 2000. 978-0-7808-0377-0.

"Public libraries will find the book useful for reference and as a beginning research point for students, parents, and caregivers."
— *American Reference Books Annual, 2001*

"The strength of this work is that it compiles many basic fact sheets and addresses for further information in one volume. It is intended and suitable for the general public. This sourcebook is relevant to any collection providing health information to the general public."
— *E-Streams, Nov '00*

"From preventing retardation to parenting and family challenges, this covers health, social and legal issues and will prove an invaluable overview."
— *Reviewer's Bookwatch, Jul '00*

Movement Disorders Sourcebook

Basic Consumer Health Information about Neurological Movement Disorders, Including Essential Tremor, Parkinson's Disease, Dystonia, Cerebral Palsy, Huntington's Disease, Myasthenia Gravis, Multiple Sclerosis, and Other Early-Onset and Adult-Onset Movement Disorders, Their Symptoms and Causes, Diagnostic Tests, and Treatments

Along with Mobility and Assistive Technology Information, a Glossary, and a Directory of Additional Resources

Edited by Joyce Brennfleck Shannon. 655 pages. 2003. 978-0-7808-0628-3.

". . . a good resource for consumers and recommended for public, community college and undergraduate libraries." — *American Reference Books Annual, 2004*

Muscular Dystrophy Sourcebook

Basic Consumer Health Information about Congenital, Childhood-Onset, and Adult-Onset Forms of Muscular Dystrophy, Such as Duchenne, Becker, Emery-Dreifuss, Distal, Limb-Girdle, Facioscapulohumeral (FSHD), Myotonic, and Ophthalmoplegic Muscular Dystrophies, Including Facts about Diagnostic Tests, Medical and Physical Therapies, Management of Co-Occurring Conditions, and Parenting Guidelines

Along with Practical Tips for Home Care, a Glossary, and Directories of Additional Resources

Edited by Joyce Brennfleck Shannon. 577 pages. 2004. 978-0-7808-0676-4.

"This book is highly recommended for public and academic libraries as well as health care offices that support the information needs of patients and their families."
— *E-Streams, Apr '05*

"Excellent reference." — *The Bookwatch, Jan '05*

Obesity Sourcebook

Basic Consumer Health Information about Diseases and Other Problems Associated with Obesity, and Including Facts about Risk Factors, Prevention Issues, and Management Approaches

Along with Statistical and Demographic Data, Information about Special Populations, Research Updates, a Glossary, and Source Listings for Further Help and Information

Edited by Wilma Caldwell and Chad T. Kimball. 376 pages. 2001. 978-0-7808-0333-6.

"The book synthesizes the reliable medical literature on obesity into one easy-to-read and useful resource for the general public."
— *American Reference Books Annual, 2002*

"This is a very useful resource book for the lay public."
— *Doody's Review Service, Nov '01*

"Well suited for the health reference collection of a public library or an academic health science library that serves the general population." — *E-Streams, Sep '01*

"Recommended reference source."
— *Booklist, American Library Association, Apr '01*

"Recommended pick both for specialty health library collections and any general consumer health reference collection." — *The Bookwatch, Apr '01*

Oral Health Sourcebook

SEE Dental Care & Oral Health Sourcebook

Osteoporosis Sourcebook

Basic Consumer Health Information about Primary and Secondary Osteoporosis and Juvenile Osteoporosis and Related Conditions, Including Fibrous Dysplasia, Gaucher Disease, Hyperthyroidism, Hypophosphatasia, Myeloma, Osteopetrosis, Osteogenesis Imperfecta, and Paget's Disease

Along with Information about Risk Factors, Treatments, Traditional and Non-Traditional Pain Management, a Glossary of Related Terms, and a Directory of Resources

Edited by Allan R. Cook. 584 pages. 2001. 978-0-7808-0239-1.

"This would be a book to be kept in a staff or patient library. The targeted audience is the layperson, but the therapist who needs a quick bit of information on a particular topic will also find the book useful."
— *Physical Therapy, Jan '02*

"This resource is recommended as a great reference source for public, health, and academic libraries, and is another triumph for the editors of Omnigraphics."
— *American Reference Books Annual, 2002*

"Recommended for all public libraries and general health collections, especially those supporting patient education or consumer health programs."
— *E-Streams, Nov '01*

"Will prove valuable to any library seeking to maintain a current, comprehensive reference collection of health resources. . . . From prevention to treatment and associated conditions, this provides an excellent survey."
— *The Bookwatch, Aug '01*

"Recommended reference source."
— *Booklist, American Library Association, Jul '01*

SEE ALSO *Healthy Aging Sourcebook, Physical & Mental Issues in Aging Sourcebook, Women's Health Concerns Sourcebook*

■

Pain Sourcebook, 2nd Edition

Basic Consumer Health Information about Specific Forms of Acute and Chronic Pain, Including Muscle and Skeletal Pain, Nerve Pain, Cancer Pain, and Disorders Characterized by Pain, Such as Fibromyalgia, Shingles, Angina, Arthritis, and Headaches

Along with Information about Pain Medications and Management Techniques, Complementary and Alternative Pain Relief Options, Tips for People Living with Chronic Pain, a Glossary, and a Directory of Sources for Further Information

Edited by Karen Bellenir. 670 pages. 2002. 978-0-7808-0612-2.

"A source of valuable information. . . . This book offers help to nonmedical people who need information about pain and pain management. It is also an excellent reference for those who participate in patient education."
— *Doody's Review Service, Sep '02*

"Highly recommended for academic and medical reference collections."
— *Library Bookwatch, Sep '02*

"The text is readable, easily understood, and well indexed. This excellent volume belongs in all patient education libraries, consumer health sections of public libraries, and many personal collections."
— *American Reference Books Annual, 1999*

"The information is basic in terms of scholarship and is appropriate for general readers. Written in journalistic style . . . intended for non-professionals. Quite thorough in its coverage of different pain conditions and summarizes the latest clinical information regarding pain treatment."
— *Choice, Association of College and Research Libraries, Jun '98*

"Recommended reference source."
— *Booklist, American Library Association, Mar '98*

■

Pediatric Cancer Sourcebook

Basic Consumer Health Information about Leukemias, Brain Tumors, Sarcomas, Lymphomas, and Other Cancers in Infants, Children, and Adolescents, Including Descriptions of Cancers, Treatments, and Coping Strategies

Along with Suggestions for Parents, Caregivers, and Concerned Relatives, a Glossary of Cancer Terms, and Resource Listings

Edited by Edward J. Prucha. 587 pages. 1999. 978-0-7808-0245-2.

"An excellent source of information. Recommended for public, hospital, and health science libraries with consumer health collections."
— *E-Streams, Jun '00*

"Recommended reference source."
— *Booklist, American Library Association, Feb '00*

"A valuable addition to all libraries specializing in health services and many public libraries."
— *American Reference Books Annual, 2000*

SEE ALSO *Childhood Diseases & Disorders Sourcebook, Healthy Children Sourcebook*

■

Physical & Mental Issues in Aging Sourcebook

Basic Consumer Health Information on Physical and Mental Disorders Associated with the Aging Process, Including Concerns about Cardiovascular Disease, Pulmonary Disease, Oral Health, Digestive Disorders, Musculoskeletal and Skin Disorders, Metabolic Changes, Sexual and Reproductive Issues, and Changes in Vision, Hearing, and Other Senses

Along with Data about Longevity and Causes of Death, Information on Acute and Chronic Pain, Descriptions of Mental Concerns, a Glossary of Terms, and Resource Listings for Additional Help

Edited by Jenifer Swanson. 660 pages. 1999. 978-0-7808-0233-9.

"This is a treasure of health information for the layperson."
— *Choice Health Sciences Supplement, Association of College & Research Libraries, May '00*

"Recommended for public libraries."
— *American Reference Books Annual, 2000*

"Recommended reference source."
— *Booklist, American Library Association, Oct '99*

SEE ALSO *Healthy Aging Sourcebook*

■

Podiatry Sourcebook, 2nd Edition

Basic Consumer Health Information about Disorders, Diseases, Deformities, and Injuries that Affect the Foot and Ankle, Including Sprains, Corns, Calluses, Bunions, Plantar Warts, Plantar Fasciitis, Neuromas, Clubfoot, Flat Feet, Achilles Tendonitis, and Much More

Along with Information about Selecting a Foot Care Specialist, Foot Fitness, Shoes and Socks, Diagnostic Tests and Corrective Procedures, Financial Assistance for Corrective Devices, a Glossary of Related Terms, and a Directory of Resources for Additional Help and Information

Edited by Ivy L. Alexander. 543 pages. 2007. 978-0-7808-0944-4.

"Recommended reference source."
— *Booklist, American Library Association, Feb '02*

"There is a lot of information presented here on a topic that is usually only covered sparingly in most larger comprehensive medical encyclopedias."
— *American Reference Books Annual, 2002*

■

Pregnancy & Birth Sourcebook, 2nd Edition

Basic Consumer Health Information about Conception and Pregnancy, Including Facts about Fertility, Infertility, Pregnancy Symptoms and Complications, Fetal Growth and Development, Labor, Delivery, and the Postpartum Period, as Well as Information about Maintaining Health and Wellness during Pregnancy and Caring for a Newborn

Along with Information about Public Health Assistance for Low-Income Pregnant Women, a Glossary, and Directories of Agencies and Organizations Providing Help and Support

Edited by Amy L. Sutton. 626 pages. 2004. 978-0-7808-0672-6.

"Will appeal to public and school reference collections strong in medicine and women's health. . . . Deserves a spot on any medical reference shelf."
— *The Bookwatch, Jul '04*

"A well-organized handbook. Recommended."
— *Choice, Association of College & Research Libraries, Apr '98*

"Recommended reference source."
— *Booklist, American Library Association, Mar '98*

"Recommended for public libraries."
— *American Reference Books Annual, 1998*

SEE ALSO Breastfeeding Sourcebook, Congenital Disorders Sourcebook, Family Planning Sourcebook

■

Prostate & Urological Disorders Sourcebook

Basic Consumer Health Information about Urogenital and Sexual Disorders in Men, Including Prostate and Other Andrological Cancers, Prostatitis, Benign Prostatic Hyperplasia, Testicular and Penile Trauma, Cryptorchidism, Peyronie Disease, Erectile Dysfunction, and Male Factor Infertility, and Facts about Commonly Used Tests and Procedures, Such as Prostatectomy, Vasectomy, Vasectomy Reversal, Penile Implants, and Semen Analysis

Along with a Glossary of Andrological Terms and a Directory of Resources for Additional Information

Edited by Karen Bellenir. 631 pages. 2005. 978-0-7808-0797-6.

Prostate Cancer Sourcebook

Basic Consumer Health Information about Prostate Cancer, Including Information about the Associated Risk Factors, Detection, Diagnosis, and Treatment of Prostate Cancer

Along with Information on Non-Malignant Prostate Conditions, and Featuring a Section Listing Support and Treatment Centers and a Glossary of Related Terms

Edited by Dawn D. Matthews. 358 pages. 2001. 978-0-7808-0324-4.

"Recommended reference source."
— *Booklist, American Library Association, Jan '02*

"A valuable resource for health care consumers seeking information on the subject. . . . All text is written in a clear, easy-to-understand language that avoids technical jargon. Any library that collects consumer health resources would strengthen their collection with the addition of the *Prostate Cancer Sourcebook.*"
— *American Reference Books Annual, 2002*

SEE ALSO Men's Health Concerns Sourcebook

■

Reconstructive & Cosmetic Surgery Sourcebook

Basic Consumer Health Information on Cosmetic and Reconstructive Plastic Surgery, Including Statistical Information about Different Surgical Procedures, Things to Consider Prior to Surgery, Plastic Surgery Techniques and Tools, Emotional and Psychological Considerations, and Procedure-Specific Information

Along with a Glossary of Terms and a Listing of Resources for Additional Help and Information

Edited by M. Lisa Weatherford. 374 pages. 2001. 978-0-7808-0214-8.

"An excellent reference that addresses cosmetic and medically necessary reconstructive surgeries. . . . The style of the prose is calm and reassuring, discussing the many positive outcomes now available due to advances in surgical techniques."
— *American Reference Books Annual, 2002*

"Recommended for health science libraries that are open to the public, as well as hospital libraries that are open to the patients. This book is a good resource for the consumer interested in plastic surgery."
— *E-Streams, Dec '01*

"Recommended reference source."
— *Booklist, American Library Association, Jul '01*

■

Rehabilitation Sourcebook

Basic Consumer Health Information about Rehabilitation for People Recovering from Heart Surgery, Spinal Cord Injury, Stroke, Orthopedic Impairments, Amputation, Pulmonary Impairments, Traumatic Injury, and More, Including Physical Therapy, Occupational Therapy, Speech/Language Therapy, Massage Therapy, Dance Therapy, Art Therapy, and Recreational Therapy

Along with Information on Assistive and Adaptive Devices, a Glossary, and Resources for Additional Help and Information

Edited by Dawn D. Matthews. 531 pages. 1999. 978-0-7808-0236-0.

"This is an excellent resource for public library reference and health collections."
— *American Reference Books Annual, 2001*

"Recommended reference source."
— *Booklist, American Library Association, May '00*

■

Respiratory Diseases & Disorders Sourcebook

Basic Information about Respiratory Diseases and Disorders, Including Asthma, Cystic Fibrosis, Pneumonia, the Common Cold, Influenza, and Others, Featuring Facts about the Respiratory System, Statistical and Demographic Data, Treatments, Self-Help Management Suggestions, and Current Research Initiatives

Edited by Allan R. Cook and Peter D. Dresser. 771 pages. 1995. 978-0-7808-0037-3.

"Designed for the layperson and for patients and their families coping with respiratory illness. . . . an extensive array of information on diagnosis, treatment, management, and prevention of respiratory illnesses for the general reader." — *Choice, Association of College & Research Libraries, Jun '96*

"A highly recommended text for all collections. It is a comforting reminder of the power of knowledge that good books carry between their covers."
— *Academic Library Book Review, Spring '96*

"A comprehensive collection of authoritative information presented in a nontechnical, humanitarian style for patients, families, and caregivers."
— *Association of Operating Room Nurses, Sep/Oct '95*

SEE ALSO *Lung Disorders Sourcebook*

■

Sexually Transmitted Diseases Sourcebook, 3rd Edition

Basic Consumer Health Information about Chlamydial Infections, Gonorrhea, Hepatitis, Herpes, HIV/AIDS, Human Papillomavirus, Pubic Lice, Scabies, Syphilis, Trichomoniasis, Vaginal Infections, and Other Sexually Transmitted Diseases, Including Facts about Risk Factors, Symptoms, Diagnosis, Treatment, and the Prevention of Sexually Transmitted Infections

Along with Updates on Current Research Initiatives, a Glossary of Related Terms, and Resources for Additional Help and Information

Edited by Amy L. Sutton. 629 pages. 2006. 978-0-7808-0824-9.

"Recommended for consumer health collections in public libraries, and secondary school and community college libraries."
— *American Reference Books Annual, 2002*

"Every school and public library should have a copy of this comprehensive and user-friendly reference book."
— *Choice, Association of College & Research Libraries, Sep '01*

"This is a highly recommended book. This is an especially important book for all school and public libraries."
— *AIDS Book Review Journal, Jul-Aug '01*

"Recommended reference source."
— *Booklist, American Library Association, Apr '01*

■

Sleep Disorders Sourcebook, 2nd Edition

Basic Consumer Health Information about Sleep and Sleep Disorders, Including Insomnia, Sleep Apnea, Restless Legs Syndrome, Narcolepsy, Parasomnias, and Other Health Problems That Affect Sleep, Plus Facts about Diagnostic Procedures, Treatment Strategies, Sleep Medications, and Tips for Improving Sleep Quality

Along with a Glossary of Related Terms and Resources for Additional Help and Information

Edited by Amy L. Sutton. 567 pages. 2005. 978-0-7808-0743-3.

"This book will be useful for just about everybody, especially the 40 million Americans with sleep disorders."
— *American Reference Books Annual, 2006*

"Recommended for public libraries and libraries supporting health care professionals." — *E-Streams, Sep '05*

". . . key medical library acquisition."
— *The Bookwatch, Jun '05*

■

Smoking Concerns Sourcebook

Basic Consumer Health Information about Nicotine Addiction and Smoking Cessation, Featuring Facts about the Health Effects of Tobacco Use, Including Lung and Other Cancers, Heart Disease, Stroke, and Respiratory Disorders, Such as Emphysema and Chronic Bronchitis

Along with Information about Smoking Prevention Programs, Suggestions for Achieving and Maintaining a Smoke-Free Lifestyle, Statistics about Tobacco Use, Reports on Current Research Initiatives, a Glossary of Related Terms, and Directories of Resources for Additional Help and Information

Edited by Karen Bellenir. 621 pages. 2004. 978-0-7808-0323-7.

"Provides everything needed for the student or general reader seeking practical details on the effects of tobacco use." — *The Bookwatch, Mar '05*

"Public libraries and consumer health care libraries will find this work useful."
— *American Reference Books Annual, 2005*

Sports Injuries Sourcebook, 3rd Edition

Basic Consumer Health Information about Sprains and Strains, Fractures, Growth Plate Injuries, Overtraining Injuries, and Injuries to the Head, Face, Shoulders, Elbows, Hands, Spinal Column, Knees, Ankles, and Feet, and with Facts about Heat-Related Illness, Steroids and Sport Supplements, Protective Equipment, Diagnostic Procedures, Treatment Options, and Rehabilitation

Along with a Glossary of Related Terms and a Directory of Resources for Additional Help and Information

Edited by Sandra J. Judd. 651 pages. 2007. 978-0-7808-0949-9.

"This is an excellent reference for consumers and it is recommended for public, community college, and undergraduate libraries."
— *American Reference Books Annual, 2003*

"Recommended reference source."
— *Booklist, American Library Association, Feb '03*

■

Stress-Related Disorders Sourcebook

Basic Consumer Health Information about Stress and Stress-Related Disorders, Including Stress Origins and Signals, Environmental Stress at Work and Home, Mental and Emotional Stress Associated with Depression, Post-Traumatic Stress Disorder, Panic Disorder, Suicide, and the Physical Effects of Stress on the Cardiovascular, Immune, and Nervous Systems

Along with Stress Management Techniques, a Glossary, and a Listing of Additional Resources

Edited by Joyce Brennfleck Shannon. 610 pages. 2002. 978-0-7808-0560-6.

"Well written for a general readership, the *Stress-Related Disorders Sourcebook* is a useful addition to the health reference literature."
— *American Reference Books Annual, 2003*

"I am impressed by the amount of information. It offers a thorough overview of the causes and consequences of stress for the layperson. . . . A well-done and thorough reference guide for professionals and nonprofessionals alike." — *Doody's Review Service, Dec '02*

■

Stroke Sourcebook

Basic Consumer Health Information about Stroke, Including Ischemic, Hemorrhagic, Transient Ischemic Attack (TIA), and Pediatric Stroke, Stroke Triggers and Risks, Diagnostic Tests, Treatments, and Rehabilitation Information

Along with Stroke Prevention Guidelines, Legal and Financial Information, a Glossary, and a Directory of Additional Resources

Edited by Joyce Brennfleck Shannon. 606 pages. 2003. 978-0-7808-0630-6.

"This volume is highly recommended and should be in every medical, hospital, and public library."
— *American Reference Books Annual, 2004*

"Highly recommended for the amount and variety of topics and information covered." — *Choice, Nov '03*

■

Surgery Sourcebook

Basic Consumer Health Information about Inpatient and Outpatient Surgeries, Including Cardiac, Vascular, Orthopedic, Ocular, Reconstructive, Cosmetic, Gynecologic, and Ear, Nose, and Throat Procedures and More

Along with Information about Operating Room Policies and Instruments, Laser Surgery Techniques, Hospital Errors, Statistical Data, a Glossary, and Listings of Sources for Further Help and Information

Edited by Annemarie S. Muth and Karen Bellenir. 596 pages. 2002. 978-0-7808-0380-0.

"Large public libraries and medical libraries would benefit from this material in their reference collections."
— *American Reference Books Annual, 2004*

"Invaluable reference for public and school library collections alike." — *Library Bookwatch, Apr '03*

■

Thyroid Disorders Sourcebook

Basic Consumer Health Information about Disorders of the Thyroid and Parathyroid Glands, Including Hypothyroidism, Hyperthyroidism, Graves Disease, Hashimoto Thyroiditis, Thyroid Cancer, and Parathyroid Disorders, Featuring Facts about Symptoms, Risk Factors, Tests, and Treatments

Along with Information about the Effects of Thyroid Imbalance on Other Body Systems, Environmental Factors That Affect the Thyroid Gland, a Glossary, and a Directory of Additional Resources

Edited by Joyce Brennfleck Shannon. 599 pages. 2005. 978-0-7808-0745-7.

"Recommended for consumer health collections."
— *American Reference Books Annual, 2006*

"Highly recommended pick for basic consumer health reference holdings at all levels."
— *The Bookwatch, Aug '05*

■

Transplantation Sourcebook

Basic Consumer Health Information about Organ and Tissue Transplantation, Including Physical and Financial Preparations, Procedures and Issues Relating to Specific Solid Organ and Tissue Transplants, Rehabilitation, Pediatric Transplant Information, the Future of Transplantation, and Organ and Tissue Donation

Along with a Glossary and Listings of Additional Resources

Edited by Joyce Brennfleck Shannon. 628 pages. 2002. 978-0-7808-0322-0.

"Along with these advances [in transplantation technology] have come a number of daunting questions for potential transplant patients, their families, and their health care providers. This reference text is the best single tool to address many of these questions. . . . It will be a much-needed addition to the reference collections in health care, academic, and large public libraries."
— *American Reference Books Annual, 2003*

"Recommended for libraries with an interest in offering consumer health information." — *E-Streams, Jul '02*

"This is a unique and valuable resource for patients facing transplantation and their families."
— *Doody's Review Service, Jun '02*

Traveler's Health Sourcebook

Basic Consumer Health Information for Travelers, Including Physical and Medical Preparations, Transportation Health and Safety, Essential Information about Food and Water, Sun Exposure, Insect and Snake Bites, Camping and Wilderness Medicine, and Travel with Physical or Medical Disabilities

Along with International Travel Tips, Vaccination Recommendations, Geographical Health Issues, Disease Risks, a Glossary, and a Listing of Additional Resources

Edited by Joyce Brennfleck Shannon. 613 pages. 2000. 978-0-7808-0384-8.

"Recommended reference source."
— *Booklist, American Library Association, Feb '01*

"This book is recommended for any public library, any travel collection, and especially any collection for the physically disabled."
— *American Reference Books Annual, 2001*

SEE ALSO *Worldwide Health Sourcebook*

Urinary Tract & Kidney Diseases & Disorders Sourcebook, 2nd Edition

Basic Consumer Health Information about the Urinary System, Including the Bladder, Urethra, Ureters, and Kidneys, with Facts about Urinary Tract Infections, Incontinence, Congenital Disorders, Kidney Stones, Cancers of the Urinary Tract and Kidneys, Kidney Failure, Dialysis, and Kidney Transplantation

Along with Statistical and Demographic Information, Reports on Current Research in Kidney and Urologic Health, a Summary of Commonly Used Diagnostic Tests, a Glossary of Related Terms, and a Directory of Resources for Additional Help and Information

Edited by Ivy L. Alexander. 649 pages. 2005. 978-0-7808-0750-1.

"A good choice for a consumer health information library or for a medical library needing information to refer to their patients."
— *American Reference Books Annual, 2006*

Vegetarian Sourcebook

Basic Consumer Health Information about Vegetarian Diets, Lifestyle, and Philosophy, Including Definitions of Vegetarianism and Veganism, Tips about Adopting Vegetarianism, Creating a Vegetarian Pantry, and Meeting Nutritional Needs of Vegetarians, with Facts Regarding Vegetarianism's Effect on Pregnant and Lactating Women, Children, Athletes, and Senior Citizens

Along with a Glossary of Commonly Used Vegetarian Terms and Resources for Additional Help and Information

Edited by Chad T. Kimball. 360 pages. 2002. 978-0-7808-0439-5.

"Organizes into one concise volume the answers to the most common questions concerning vegetarian diets and lifestyles. This title is recommended for public and secondary school libraries." — *E-Streams, Apr '03*

"Invaluable reference for public and school library collections alike." — *Library Bookwatch, Apr '03*

"The articles in this volume are easy to read and come from authoritative sources. The book does not necessarily support the vegetarian diet but instead provides the pros and cons of this important decision. The Vegetarian Sourcebook is recommended for public libraries and consumer health libraries."
— *American Reference Books Annual, 2003*

SEE ALSO *Diet & Nutrition Sourcebook*

Women's Health Concerns Sourcebook, 2nd Edition

Basic Consumer Health Information about the Medical and Mental Concerns of Women, Including Maintaining Health and Wellness, Gynecological Concerns, Breast Health, Sexuality and Reproductive Issues, Menopause, Cancer in Women, Leading Causes of Death and Disability among Women, Physical Concerns of Special Significance to Women, and Women's Mental and Emotional Health

Along with a Glossary of Related Terms and Directories of Resources for Additional Help and Information

Edited by Amy L. Sutton. 746 pages. 2004. 978-0-7808-0673-3.

"This is a useful reference book, which makes the reader knowledgeable about several issues that concern women's health. It is recommended for public libraries and home library collections." — *E-Streams, May '05*

"A useful addition to public and consumer health library collections."
— *American Reference Books Annual, 2005*

"A highly recommended title."
— *The Bookwatch, May '04*

"Handy compilation. There is an impressive range of diseases, devices, disorders, procedures, and other physical and emotional issues covered . . . well organized, illustrated, and indexed." — *Choice, Association of College & Research Libraries, Jan '98*

SEE ALSO *Breast Cancer Sourcebook, Cancer Sourcebook for Women, Healthy Heart Sourcebook for Women, Osteoporosis Sourcebook*

Workplace Health & Safety Sourcebook

Basic Consumer Health Information about Workplace Health and Safety, Including the Effect of Workplace Hazards on the Lungs, Skin, Heart, Ears, Eyes, Brain, Reproductive Organs, Musculoskeletal System, and Other Organs and Body Parts

Along with Information about Occupational Cancer, Personal Protective Equipment, Toxic and Hazardous Chemicals, Child Labor, Stress, and Workplace Violence

Edited by Chad T. Kimball. 626 pages. 2000. 978-0-7808-0231-5.

"As a reference for the general public, this would be useful in any library." *—E-Streams, Jun '01*

"Provides helpful information for primary care physicians and other caregivers interested in occupational medicine. . . . General readers; professionals."
— Choice, Association of College & Research Libraries, May '01

"Recommended reference source."
— Booklist, American Library Association, Feb '01

"Highly recommended." *— The Bookwatch, Jan '01*

Worldwide Health Sourcebook

Basic Information about Global Health Issues, Including Malnutrition, Reproductive Health, Disease Dispersion and Prevention, Emerging Diseases, Risky Health Behaviors, and the Leading Causes of Death

Along with Global Health Concerns for Children, Women, and the Elderly, Mental Health Issues, Research and Technology Advancements, and Economic, Environmental, and Political Health Implications, a Glossary, and a Resource Listing for Additional Help and Information

Edited by Joyce Brennfleck Shannon. 614 pages. 2001. 978-0-7808-0330-5.

"Named an Outstanding Academic Title."
— Choice, Association of College & Research Libraries, Jan '02

"Yet another handy but also unique compilation in the extensive *Health Reference Series*, this is a useful work because many of the international publications reprinted or excerpted are not readily available. Highly recommended." *— Choice, Association of College & Research Libraries, Nov '01*

"Recommended reference source."
— Booklist, American Library Association, Oct '01

SEE ALSO *Traveler's Health Sourcebook*

661

Teen Health Series
Helping Young Adults Understand, Manage, and Avoid Serious Illness

List price $65 per volume. **School and library price $58 per volume.**

Alcohol Information for Teens
Health Tips about Alcohol and Alcoholism

Including Facts about Underage Drinking, Preventing Teen Alcohol Use, Alcohol's Effects on the Brain and the Body, Alcohol Abuse Treatment, Help for Children of Alcoholics, and More

Edited by Joyce Brennfleck Shannon. 370 pages. 2005. 978-0-7808-0741-9.

"Boxed facts and tips add visual interest to the well-researched and clearly written text."
— Curriculum Connection, Apr '06

Allergy Information for Teens
Health Tips about Allergic Reactions Such as Anaphylaxis, Respiratory Problems, and Rashes

Including Facts about Identifying and Managing Allergies to Food, Pollen, Mold, Animals, Chemicals, Drugs, and Other Substances

Edited by Karen Bellenir. 410 pages. 2006. 978-0-7808-0799-0.

Asthma Information for Teens
Health Tips about Managing Asthma and Related Concerns

Including Facts about Asthma Causes, Triggers, Symptoms, Diagnosis, and Treatment

Edited by Karen Bellenir. 386 pages. 2005. 978-0-7808-0770-9.

"Highly recommended for medical libraries, public school libraries, and public libraries."
— American Reference Books Annual, 2006

"It is so clearly written and well organized that even hesitant readers will be able to find the facts they need, whether for reports or personal information. . . . A succinct but complete resource."
— School Library Journal, Sep '05

Body Information for Teens
Health Tips about Maintaining Well-Being for a Lifetime

Including Facts about the Development and Functioning of the Body's Systems, Organs, and Structures and the Health Impact of Lifestyle Choices

Edited by Sandra Augustyn Lawton. 458 pages. 2007. 978-0-7808-0443-2.

Cancer Information for Teens
Health Tips about Cancer Awareness, Prevention, Diagnosis, and Treatment

Including Facts about Frequently Occurring Cancers, Cancer Risk Factors, and Coping Strategies for Teens Fighting Cancer or Dealing with Cancer in Friends or Family Members

Edited by Wilma R. Caldwell. 428 pages. 2004. 978-0-7808-0678-8.

"Recommended for school libraries, or consumer libraries that see a lot of use by teens."
— E-Streams, May '05

"A valuable educational tool."
— American Reference Books Annual, 2005

"Young adults and their parents alike will find this new addition to the *Teen Health Series* an important reference to cancer in teens."
— Children's Bookwatch, Feb '05

Complementary and Alternative Medicine Information for Teens
Health Tips about Non-Traditional and Non-Western Medical Practices

Including Information about Acupuncture, Chiropractic Medicine, Dietary and Herbal Supplements, Hypnosis, Massage Therapy, Prayer and Spirituality, Reflexology, Yoga, and More

Edited by Sandra Augustyn Lawton. 405 pages. 2006. 978-0-7808-0966-6.

Diabetes Information for Teens
Health Tips about Managing Diabetes and Preventing Related Complications

Including Information about Insulin, Glucose Control, Healthy Eating, Physical Activity, and Learning to Live with Diabetes

Edited by Sandra Augustyn Lawton. 410 pages. 2006. 978-0-7808-0811-9.

663

Diet Information for Teens, 2nd Edition

Health Tips about Diet and Nutrition

Including Facts about Dietary Guidelines, Food Groups, Nutrients, Healthy Meals, Snacks, Weight Control, Medical Concerns Related to Diet, and More

Edited by Karen Bellenir. 432 pages. 2006. 978-0-7808-0820-1.

"Full of helpful insights and facts throughout the book. . . . An excellent resource to be placed in public libraries or even in personal collections."
— *American Reference Books Annual, 2002*

"Recommended for middle and high school libraries and media centers as well as academic libraries that educate future teachers of teenagers. It is also a suitable addition to health science libraries that serve patrons who are interested in teen health promotion and education."
— *E-Streams, Oct '01*

"This comprehensive book would be beneficial to collections that need information about nutrition, dietary guidelines, meal planning, and weight control. . . . This reference is so easy to use that its purchase is recommended."
— *The Book Report, Sep-Oct '01*

"This book is written in an easy to understand format describing issues that many teens face every day, and then provides thoughtful explanations so that teens can make informed decisions. This is an interesting book that provides important facts and information for today's teens."
— *Doody's Health Sciences Book Review Journal, Jul-Aug '01*

"A comprehensive compendium of diet and nutrition. The information is presented in a straightforward, plain-spoken manner. This title will be useful to those working on reports on a variety of topics, as well as to general readers concerned about their dietary health."
— *School Library Journal, Jun '01*

Drug Information for Teens, 2nd Edition

Health Tips about the Physical and Mental Effects of Substance Abuse

Including Information about Marijuana, Inhalants, Club Drugs, Stimulants, Hallucinogens, Opiates, Prescription and Over-the-Counter Drugs, Herbal Products, Tobacco, Alcohol, and More

Edited by Sandra Augustyn Lawton. 468 pages. 2006. 978-0-7808-0862-1.

"A clearly written resource for general readers and researchers alike."
— *School Library Journal*

"This book is well-balanced. . . . a must for public and school libraries."
— *VOYA: Voice of Youth Advocates, Dec '03*

"The chapters are quick to make a connection to their teenage reading audience. The prose is straightforward and the book lends itself to spot reading. It should be useful both for practical information and for research, and it is suitable for public and school libraries."
— *American Reference Books Annual, 2003*

"Recommended reference source."
— *Booklist, American Library Association, Feb '03*

"This is an excellent resource for teens and their parents. Education about drugs and substances is key to discouraging teen drug abuse and this book provides this much needed information in a way that is interesting and factual." — *Doody's Review Service, Dec '02*

Eating Disorders Information for Teens

Health Tips about Anorexia, Bulimia, Binge Eating, and Other Eating Disorders

Including Information on the Causes, Prevention, and Treatment of Eating Disorders, and Such Other Issues as Maintaining Healthy Eating and Exercise Habits

Edited by Sandra Augustyn Lawton. 337 pages. 2005. 978-0-7808-0783-9.

"An excellent resource for teens and those who work with them."
— *VOYA: Voice of Youth Advocates, Apr '06*

"A welcome addition to high school and undergraduate libraries." — *American Reference Books Annual, 2006*

"This book covers the topic in a lucid manner but delves deeper into every aspect of an eating disorder. A solid addition for any nonfiction or reference collection."
— *School Library Journal, Dec '05*

Fitness Information for Teens

Health Tips about Exercise, Physical Well-Being, and Health Maintenance

Including Facts about Aerobic and Anaerobic Conditioning, Stretching, Body Shape and Body Image, Sports Training, Nutrition, and Activities for Non-Athletes

Edited by Karen Bellenir. 425 pages. 2004. 978-0-7808-0679-5.

"Another excellent offering from Omnigraphics in their *Teen Health Series*. . . . This book will be a great addition to any public, junior high, senior high, or secondary school library."
— *American Reference Books Annual, 2005*

Learning Disabilities Information for Teens

Health Tips about Academic Skills Disorders and Other Disabilities That Affect Learning

Including Information about Common Signs of Learning Disabilities, School Issues, Learning to Live with a Learning Disability, and Other Related Issues

Edited by Sandra Augustyn Lawton. 337 pages. 2005. 978-0-7808-0796-9.

"This book provides a wealth of information for any reader interested in the signs, causes, and consequences

of learning disabilities, as well as related legal rights and educational interventions. . . . Public and academic libraries should want this title for both students and general readers."
— *American Reference Books Annual, 2006*

Mental Health Information for Teens, 2nd Edition

Health Tips about Mental Wellness and Mental Illness

Including Facts about Mental and Emotional Health, Depression and Other Mood Disorders, Anxiety Disorders, Behavior Disorders, Self-Injury, Psychosis, Schizophrenia, and More

Edited by Karen Bellenir. 400 pages. 2006. 978-0-7808-0863-8.

"In both language and approach, this user-friendly entry in the *Teen Health Series* is on target for teens needing information on mental health concerns."
— *Booklist, American Library Association, Jan '02*

"Readers will find the material accessible and informative, with the shaded notes, facts, and embedded glossary insets adding appropriately to the already interesting and succinct presentation."
— *School Library Journal, Jan '02*

"This title is highly recommended for any library that serves adolescents and parents/caregivers of adolescents."
— *E-Streams, Jan '02*

"Recommended for high school libraries and young adult collections in public libraries. Both health professionals and teenagers will find this book useful."
— *American Reference Books Annual, 2002*

"This is a nice book written to enlighten the society, primarily teenagers, about common teen mental health issues. It is highly recommended to teachers and parents as well as adolescents."
— *Doody's Review Service, Dec '01*

Sexual Health Information for Teens

Health Tips about Sexual Development, Human Reproduction, and Sexually Transmitted Diseases

Including Facts about Puberty, Reproductive Health, Chlamydia, Human Papillomavirus, Pelvic Inflammatory Disease, Herpes, AIDS, Contraception, Pregnancy, and More

Edited by Deborah A. Stanley. 391 pages. 2003. 978-0-7808-0445-6.

"This work should be included in all high school libraries and many larger public libraries. . . . highly recommended."
— *American Reference Books Annual, 2004*

"*Sexual Health* approaches its subject with appropriate seriousness and offers easily accessible advice and information."
— *School Library Journal, Feb '04*

Skin Health Information for Teens

Health Tips about Dermatological Concerns and Skin Cancer Risks

Including Facts about Acne, Warts, Hives, and Other Conditions and Lifestyle Choices, Such as Tanning, Tattooing, and Piercing, That Affect the Skin, Nails, Scalp, and Hair

Edited by Robert Aquinas McNally. 429 pages. 2003. 978-0-7808-0446-3.

"This volume, as with others in the series, will be a useful addition to school and public library collections."
— *American Reference Books Annual, 2004*

"There is no doubt that this reference tool is valuable."
— *VOYA: Voice of Youth Advocates, Feb '04*

"This volume serves as a one-stop source and should be a necessity for any health collection."
— *Library Media Connection*

Sports Injuries Information for Teens

Health Tips about Sports Injuries and Injury Protection

Including Facts about Specific Injuries, Emergency Treatment, Rehabilitation, Sports Safety, Competition Stress, Fitness, Sports Nutrition, Steroid Risks, and More

Edited by Joyce Brennfleck Shannon. 405 pages. 2003. 978-0-7808-0447-0.

"This work will be useful in the young adult collections of public libraries as well as high school libraries."
— *American Reference Books Annual, 2004*

Suicide Information for Teens

Health Tips about Suicide Causes and Prevention

Including Facts about Depression, Risk Factors, Getting Help, Survivor Support, and More

Edited by Joyce Brennfleck Shannon. 368 pages. 2005. 978-0-7808-0737-2.

Tobacco Information for Teens

Health Tips about the Hazards of Using Cigarettes, Smokeless Tobacco, and Other Nicotine Products

Including Facts about Nicotine Addiction, Immediate and Long-Term Health Effects of Tobacco Use, Related Cancers, Smoking Cessation, Tobacco Use Prevention, and Tobacco Use Statistics

Edited by Karen Bellenir. 440 pages. 2007. 978-0-7808-0976-5.

Health Reference Series

Injury & Trauma Sourcebook

Learning Disabili...

Leukemia Sourc...

Liver Disorders...

Lung Disorders...

Medical Tests S...

Men's Health C...

   Edition

Mental Health Disorders Sourcebook, 3rd
   Edition

Mental Retardation Sourcebook

Movement Disorders Sourcebook

Multiple Sclerosis Sourcebook

Muscular Dystrophy Sourcebook

Obesity Sourcebook

Osteoporosis Sourcebook

Pain Sourcebook, 3rd Edition

Pediatric Cancer Sourcebook

Physical & Mental Issues in Aging
   Sourcebook

Podiatry Sourcebook, 2nd Edition

Pregnancy & Birth Sourcebook, 2nd
   Edition

Prostate Cancer Sourcebook

Prostate & Urological Disorders Sourcebook

Reconstructive & Cosmetic Surgery
   Sourcebook

Rehabilitation Sourcebook

Respiratory Disorders Sourcebook, 2nd
   Edition

Sexually Transmitted Diseases Sourcebook,
   3rd Edition

Sleep Disorders Sourcebook, 2nd Edition

Smoking Concerns Sourcebook

Sports Injuries Sourcebook, 3rd Edition

Stress-Related Disorders Sourcebook, 2nd
   Edition

Stroke Sourcebook, 2nd Edition

Surgery Sourcebook, 2nd Edition

Thyroid Disorders Sourcebook

Transplantation Sourcebook

...rcebook

...iseases &

...2nd Edition

...Sourcebook, 2nd

...Sourcebook

...ook

Teen Health Series

Abuse and Violence Information for
   Teens

Alcohol Information for Teens

Allergy Information for Teens

Asthma Information for Teens

Body Information for Teens

Cancer Information for Teens

Complementary & Alternative
   Medicine Information for Teens

Diabetes Information for Teens

Diet Information for Teens, 2nd Edition

Drug Information for Teens, 2nd Edition

Eating Disorders Information for Teens

Fitness Information for Teens, 2nd
   Edition

Learning Disabilities Information for
   Teens

Mental Health Information for Teens,
   2nd Edition

Pregnancy Information for Teens

Sexual Health Information for Teens,
   2nd Edition

Skin Health Information for Teens

Sleep Information for Teens

Sports Injuries Information for Teens,
   2nd Edition

Stress Information for Teens

Suicide Information for Teens

Tobacco Information for Teens